Changing witl

A casebook of neuro-linguistic programming in medical practice

Radcliffe Medical Press
Oxford • San Francisco

Radcliffe Medical Press Ltd
18 Marcham Road
Abingdon
Oxon OX14 1AA
United Kingdom

www.radcliffe-oxford.com
The Radcliffe Medical Press electronic catalogue and online ordering facility.
Direct sales to anywhere in the world.

British Library Cataloguing in Publication Data

A catalogue record for this book is available from the British Library.

ISBN 1 85775 810 2

Typeset by Advance Typesetting Ltd, Oxfordshire
Printed and bound by TJ International Ltd, Padstow, Cornwall

Contents

Foreword

'I just want things to be like they were before I got ill.' As a psychotherapist and an NLP trainer I have heard this many times over the years. If things really were just the same as they were before this person became ill, we might reasonably expect a repeat of what happened before. Other things being equal, they would become ill again.

When I first heard this I understood the wish of patients to return to normality, but I also felt that I needed a way to provoke a reassessment and some new thinking. I wanted to explore with them what would need to be different so that a better life might be possible.

> 'I just want things to be like they were before I got ill.'
> 'So you want to be ill again?!'

Of course that is the last thing either of us wanted. What they wanted was for things to be *different*. However, whenever we want things to be different this means that some things are going to have to change.

This book is called *Changing with NLP*. Change is one of those interesting words that has an extraordinary variety of uses – you need to change this dressing, Prozac changed him, the profession's views on complementary medicine have changed somewhat. Change may involve replacing or substituting (change this dressing), making something different (Prozac changed him), or altering, varying or modifying something (the profession's views on complementary medicine have changed somewhat). However, when I first opened Lewis Walker's manuscript I know that my interest and enthusiasm would have been greatly tempered had the book merely been entitled *Altering, Varying* or *Modifying With NLP*. For often these are no more than subsets of change. Although change can include these, the kind of change that patients frequently require involves a lot more. Often the change that is needed is not just symptomatic but systemic.

In my experience, the most profound change occurs when things become distinctively different either through *radical internal transformation* or the *replacement of critical elements* by other and different ones. This is change that impacts on the functioning of the whole system. Physicians who know how to achieve this have great leverage. Their interventions are profound and generative. *Changing with NLP* offers you the tools to achieve this systemic change.

For this reason, the pages which follow can make almost any physician more effective. They offer protocols which can be immediately applied. These derive from a way of thinking that is known as neuro-linguistic programming (NLP).

NLP has been around for almost 30 years. Its forte lies in looking for what works and figuring out how it works – not why, but how – so that successful strategies can be replicated and made available to others. When you start looking at what works, it becomes clear that some things work better than others – be they procedures, protocols or thinking patterns. We might even say that the same is true of people, because certain ways of living are just more effective than others. If we take this approach to the limit we move beyond what works to what is outstanding – we enter the realm of excellence. This is where NLP mostly lives. It is why NLP is often described as the study of excellence.

Suppose we want to know how some people – be they patients or physicians – seem to live longer with more vitality or rarely become ill. Suppose we want to ascertain how some people – be they patients or physicians – recover from illness or deal with grief, loss and trauma so much better than others. If we are to answer these questions, we will need to know at a fine level of detail just what it is they do internally that makes this possible.

NLP seeks to answer these questions, to isolate the key elements and make these available to others in universally available templates. These can then be individually tailored to particular needs. These templates are the techniques of NLP. After so many years of exploring and working with people, we now have a very considerable number of them. You will find some of the most powerful ones in this book.

I first became aware of just how valuable these interventions could be for doctors in 1988 when I was asked by physicians at the University of Padova to create a full-scale NLP practitioner training scheme exclusively for doctors. Spread over two years, it amounted to 24 days in total. It was as much an education for me as it was for them. While they were learning how to apply NLP, I was learning how to adjust to the unique mixture of micro- and macro-concerns that informed their learning. In the course of this time I came to appreciate that their first concern was highly practical, almost technical and decidedly 'micro'. They wanted particular techniques to address specific problems. Only later, when these had proved effective, did they reveal their higher-level aspirations. Then they wanted to focus on the macro-issue of healing *per se*, and why these techniques worked. I was moved by how desperately they wanted to help their patients and how frequently they felt unable to really deliver.

In the years since then, I have encountered this blend of micro-pragmatism and macro-altruism in many of the doctors whom I have trained. They have told me how demoralising it can be when they feel as if they are just writing prescriptions when so much more is needed. Possessing the NLP tools and technology seems to allow them to intervene in a more profound and complete way. This of course produces much greater job satisfaction. It also has one other extraordinarily important by-product. Many times I have seen physicians recover the passion that first drew them to their calling.

That is why I am so delighted that Lewis Walker has gathered together this NLP material and is making it available in such a comprehensive and original format. As you move on through these different techniques you may well want to explore further. If this is indeed the case, I would encourage you to do some 'hands-on' work and take an NLP training course – as every clinician knows, there is no substitute for direct experience.

Right now, however, you have in your hands an invaluable resource. The chapters which follow contain a wealth of clinical experience. They offer numerous case histories and coherent explanations as to why particular interventions actually work. In addition, they contain helpful hints and practical step-by-step guides.

Whether you want to learn this way of thinking so that you can generate new systemic interventions, or you just want rapid access to what has been developed for the benefit of your patients, I believe that you will find *Changing with NLP* a real sourcebook for healing – for both patient and physician.

Ian McDermott
International Teaching Seminars
January 2004

Foreword

I have been deeply involved in the field of neuro-linguistic programming (NLP) for the past 25 years, first as student and editor, and later as trainer, author and developer of new patterns of intervention. I am as fascinated by NLP now as I was in those early days of exciting initial explorations into the structure of internal experience – how to effectively turn problems into solutions. In part, NLP arose in reaction to the various therapies of the 1970s which focused on content rather than on process, and which assumed that change, if it occurred at all, was likely to be a long, slow and laborious process, with pain and catharsis as its currency. Today I am still in awe of how quickly NLP interventions can help people to change lifelong limitations in as little as one brief session. When you know which part of the structure to alter, rapid and painless change can be disarmingly easy.

In the early days of NLP we were very pragmatic in searching for what worked, finding out *how* it worked, and then applying this with wanton experimentation to a variety of different problems. The results were what counted, with research and academic considerations being left somewhat on the sidelines. Running in parallel with NLP's rise in the public eye over this period has been the ascent of cognitive–behavioural therapy (CBT) in the academic domain. Both fields share similar epistemologies and methodologies and seek to change troublesome problems by changing sequences of thoughts, emotions and behaviours. It is clear to me that these fields have mutually influenced each other over the years, but NLP is a much more detailed and specific elaboration of the principles of the CBT model. It is equally clear that any medical professional who is armed with the practical tools of NLP will have a significantly beneficial effect on his or her patients, enabling them to eliminate much mental suffering, as well as the physical disease and suffering that often follow this.

I first met Lewis Walker when he attended one of my seminars on transforming self-concept. His insightful observations and questions certainly kept me on my toes. He has wide experience and a deep grasp of the underlying concepts, together with a capacity for thinking 'out of the box', successfully using and applying NLP processes in ways that few others even consider. He also has the ability to tailor NLP techniques to the challenges of daily medical practice. One of his important professional aims is to encourage his colleagues to incorporate the fruits of the NLP approach within mainstream medicine, in order to help clients to make the emotional and behavioural changes that are needed to support medical treatment. I know that for those physicians who take this message to heart, *Changing with NLP* will act as a powerful stepping stone in the fulfilment of these aims.

Steve Andreas
NLP trainer, developer and author
Boulder, CO
January 2004

About the author

Dr Lewis Walker FRCP (Glas) graduated from Aberdeen University in 1981, and spent the next five years training in hospital general medicine, initially at Glasgow Royal Infirmary, where he obtained the MRCP (UK) in 1984, and subsequently at Raigmore Hospital, Inverness. In 1986 he began vocational training for general practice, and in 1989 he joined what is now a seven-doctor training practice at Ardach Health Centre, Buckie, on the Moray Firth Coast. He was elected Fellow of the Royal College of Physicians of Glasgow in 1998.

In the early 1990s, fascinated by what made people 'tick', he developed a keen interest in behavioural change mechanisms, which led him to study both classical and Ericksonian hypnosis, together with neuro-linguistic programming (NLP). To date he has undertaken certified courses at the level of Practitioner, Master Practitioner, Health Practitioner and Trainer of NLP. With numerous other short courses in addition attesting to his wide experience, he has also trained with many of the leaders and developers in the NLP field. He holds the Certificate of Accreditation of the British Society of Medical and Dental Hypnosis (Scotland), and is also a Trainer of Hypnosis. He is the author of *Consulting with NLP: neuro-linguistic programming in the medical consultation*, published by Radcliffe Medical Press. He can be contacted at lewis.walker@ardach.grampian.scot.nhs.uk

Acknowledgements

As the co-developers of NLP, John Grinder and Richard Bandler deserve much credit for their original codification of the early patterns of intervention upon which the field has developed since the early 1970s. In particular, I have found John Grinder to be most approachable 'online', and have personally benefited greatly from our numerous discussions – an eye-opening experience. Seminal contributor Robert Dilts has been an innovator of numerous new models and patterns, many of which you will read about in due course.

My thanks go to Ian McDermott, a well-respected UK-based trainer and multiple author who once again read the manuscript and provided some useful fine-tuning feedback. I appreciate his thoughtful foreword and continuing support in our mutual aim of extending the fruits of the NLP approach to as many as possible in professional and public domains.

NLP trainer, author, publisher and developer, Steve Andreas, cast his 'editorial eye' over the original manuscript and asked some thought-provoking questions! I very much value the contributions in his foreword. He and his wife Connirae were instrumental in developing the grief resolution pattern which has wide practical application in medicine.

I finally got round to training with John Overdurf and Julie Silverthorn, supplementing my gains from their highly popular tape-assisted learning material with some hands-on tuition. As they say, living is indeed learning.

In the last decade or so I have explored the training of many of the different schools of NLP, learning much about the strengths of each approach together with examples of what not to do. The following growing list of world-renowned trainers attests to this experience (from first to most recent): Willie Monteiro, Ian McDermott, Tad James, Robert Dilts, David Shephard, Tim Hallbom, Suzi Smith, Richard Bandler, Paul McKenna, Michael Breen, Tom Vizzini, Kim McFarland, Steve Andreas, John Overdurf and Julie Silverthorn. The synthesis of this experience has in large part resulted in *Changing with NLP*.

Once again my general practice partner Bill Jaffrey has provided much background support and encouragement over the long haul that a venture such as this involves. My other partners – Gordon Pringle, Colin Menzies, Angus Gallacher, Berny Welsh and retainers Kathryn Arnould and Claire Hood – have all referred patients to me for interventions, some of which you will read about in due course.

I have had the privilege of belonging to two practice groups over the years. James Beattie, John Duncan, Gavin Stark, Pat Mulcahy, Hilary Johnstone and Colin Harris were all part of the original Inverurie group which met regularly over the winter months for eight years. The core Ardach group – Bill Jaffrey, Gordon Pringle, Janice Simpson, Liz Daniel and Rita Easton – has met consistently for three years. The disciplined practice and discussion that such groups encourage are fundamental to continuing skills development – and are great fun to boot!

My editorial team of Gillian Nineham, Jamie Etherington and Paula Moran have performed all the behind-the-scenes work which make a venture like this both possible and successfully come to fruition – my thanks to you all.

Once again my wife Pam and my children Lindsay and Kerry were very tolerant of the many evenings and weekends taken up when I was in writing mode. This time, though, I fulfilled my earlier promise of a second computer, and the laptop prevented much argument about online access. My pledge for the next book – yes, there is more to come – is to do most of the writing in daylight hours.

Sadly, my father died last year when I was in the early stages of planning this project. Of his many characteristics, one that stood out – and which I have obviously inadvertently modelled to some degree – was his tremendous capacity for work. He was never happier than when he was busy working with his hands on some practical assignment. His delight in dealing with the patterns and structure of the external world mirrored my own fascination with those of the subjective inner world. Therefore I think it is quite fitting that I dedicate *Changing with NLP* to his memory.

There is a wealth of clinical material and NLP applications in the following pages. All the case scenarios have arisen from day-to-day patient encounters in general practice. I have changed various details in order to protect identities and preserve anonymity while remaining entirely congruent with the process of each intervention. My patients have taught me a great deal about what is possible with the NLP approach, and have helped in so many ways to further refine my skills.

Finally, I have attempted to give full credit to those NLP trainers and innovators who have developed particular patterns of intervention. I am entirely responsible for any errors of omission or misattribution, and I shall be only too happy to set the record straight in future editions if you provide me with more accurate, verifiable information.

Preparation

CHAPTER 1

Starting the journey ...

Introduction

Having picked this book up and begun reading through it, I am assuming that you are interested in the process that lies behind all effective change. From the outset, though, I want to ask you a question: 'Just how easy is it for people to change?' And by 'change' I mean the ability to develop new thinking patterns, new behaviours and new responses to old situations so that they really can *do something different* – both subjectively and objectively – different in a way that enhances their life, increases their personal choices and allows them to be healthier as a result. How easy is that?

And what about *you?* How easy it for *you* to change? As you think back through your own personal history, how many times have you successfully changed a chronic habit or behaviour that was unhealthy? Have you ever stopped smoking, planned to lose and then lost a significant amount of weight, cured yourself of a phobia, overcome depression, started and maintained an exercise programme, or any of myriad other things? I wonder if you found it easy – or, like most people, a bit of a struggle. A struggle that you sometimes won and sometimes lost.

For the most part, most people find change less than easy. They know what they should do, ought to do, have to do, must do and really should not do. Yet despite the weight of will-power that is brought to bear on the situation, things remain much the same. 'Old habits die hard', as the saying goes. After an initial 'supreme' effort in which a little headway is made, the increasingly stiff resistance that is encountered often puts paid to seemingly well-laid plans. We see this every day with the patients who consult with us – and if we are honest, we can see it in our own reflection in the mirror.

So what kinds of things am I talking about? Well, if you are a general practitioner or in any way involved in family medicine you can probably review a day's consultations and several examples will jump into your mind. How many people come for nicotine replacement patches yet are unlikely to see the month out before smoking just as much as before? Think of the women who 'don't eat enough to keep a sparrow alive' yet who are grossly overweight and blame it all on a non-existent under-active thyroid gland. Others may have spent years secretly binge eating and then vomiting. And of course there are the 'worried well' who are addicted to fortnightly appointments for your reassuring words. Perhaps, too, the chronically depressed and anxious. You may find that several other categories come to mind as well. Never fear – help is at hand in the second part of this book – *Practice*.

Are things any different for hospital physicians and surgeons? Think of your difficult diabetic patients who just do not seem interested in controlling their blood sugar or cannot seem to manage their weight no matter how hard they try. Think of the revolving door of admission and discharge for those with chronic lung disease induced by smoking – yet they either fail to heed advice about stopping or simply cannot put it into action. And there is the grossly obese gallstone sufferer who needs an operation yet is a major anaesthetic risk – she may diet for months yet remain the same weight. As an oncologist you may know that up to 80% of cancers may be preventable by behavioural change – yet instead you have an ever increasing workload. Later we shall explore the kinds of change mechanisms that can help to deal not only with these issues, but also with those of chronic pain and other cancer symptoms.

If you are a psychiatrist, are you immune from this? Well, the short answer is 'no'. Although it may be challenging to deal with patients who have severe and recurring psychosis, you are also likely to have a significant number of patients who are depressed. You probably know that following medication there is a 50% chance of relapse after two years in this group – and an even higher risk after each subsequent relapse. Yet with cognitive therapy the long-term relapse rate may be as low as 25%. The approaches you will learn about here may encourage you to change your current practice. And what about conditions such as post-traumatic stress disorder? Newer treatments have changed the outlook for sufferers, and we shall explore one such method in particular in due course.

Perhaps you are a counsellor or a nurse, or you are working in a profession allied to medicine. You probably deal with a multitude of different issues in your efforts to help people to change. For counsellors in particular, your caseload may well consist of patients with chronic unresolved grief reactions or dysfunctional codependent-type relationships. These types of longstanding issues can often challenge your abilities to facilitate useful change to the limit. You will be most interested to know that there are approaches for both of these issues which can result in major change in one session. Yet you might find that difficult to believe at first!

No matter which branch of medicine and its allied professions you belong to, you may have found collectively, over the years, that change is less than easy for both you and your patients. You can probably bring to mind myriad examples from your personal experience of patients who seemed stuck in their ways, unable to move forwards. No matter how you have approached it so far, and despite your best efforts, the result has been the same.

Yet what if you were able to understand the whole process of change in a new way? What if you were able to discern from first principles the pivotal points that unlocked the door to acquiring new behaviours more easily and rapidly? What if you were able to assess each uniquely presenting patient and match them with a technique to obtain the kinds of results you both want? Is that something you would like to add to your therapeutic armamentarium?

We shall cover a lot of ground in the successive chapters of *Changing with NLP*. And I would ask you to consider the following question as you digest the various elements I have to offer throughout this book: 'If the process of change really is as easy as this ... which patients can I apply this material to first?'

First steps ...

It is now a decade since I first started exploring the field of neuro-linguistic programming (NLP) and began applying it to the daily trials and tribulations of the many patients who sit in my consulting-room chair. The fruits of those many encounters have resulted in this book. From my perspective – and of course I may be a little biased here – NLP is a behavioural technology which not only can really help patients to change quickly, it also is easy to learn and apply in any medical consultation.

In the rest of this book I shall explain exactly what NLP is and how you personally can incorporate it into your daily clinical practice.

As a brief synopsis, NLP is mainly an attitude of mind which has given birth to many techniques which obtain results in the real world. It is an attitude of intense curiosity about people. It involves getting curious about the structure of their internal world and how it manifests in behaviours – some of which may lead to problems, while others lead to solutions. By modelling people who obtain exceptional results with patients – whether those people are doctors, nurses, psychologists, therapists, counsellors, etc. – and finding out *how* they do what they do, NLP has opened the door for all those interested in gaining these skills to acquire them rapidly.

NLP is composed of three parts:

* *neuro* – how we use our neurology to think and feel
* *linguistic* – how we use language to influence others *and* ourselves
* *programming* – how we act to achieve the goals that we set.

The first book about NLP I ever read was *Frogs into Princes* (Bandler and Grinder, 1979). It was so riveting that I couldn't put it down – I even read it at the breakfast table. It unveiled a whole new world which on the one hand had a healthy scepticism about the current psychotherapeutic paradigms of the day and on the other instilled an attitude of playful experimentation. The kind of experimentation that was firmly based on carefully calibrating to the moment-by-moment responses of the patient, and adjusting the next steps of the inter-vention to the in-time feedback received. From that day on – prior to embarking on further training – I excitedly began to try out the approach with a variety of patients.

One of the very first patients was Marilyn, a lady in her early fifties. Tragically, 18 months previously, she had lost her son who was in his mid-twenties – in a horrific accident. Six months later her father died of disseminated prostatic cancer. This double-onset bereavement had left her with a prolonged grief reaction. She had been on antidepressants and received some counselling but there was little improvement. That particular day she was the last patient in my pre-lunchtime surgery.

She spoke about her double loss again and tears welled up in her eyes. I reached over and anchored (*see* later) the feeling of grief to her left knee. I decided to see whether I could change her state by asking her if she had memories of a favourite holiday they had all been on together. I struck lucky! She looked up to her left as the tears stopped, then showed the beginnings of a smile which then increased as she told me about their trip to Jamaica several years previously. She broke into laughter as she related a tale about a clown who had performed an amusing sketch in a stage show with a parrot. As she laughed I reached over and anchored that response to her right knee. I waited until she was in a more neutral state once again and then, with an air of positive expectation, I reached across and fired off both anchors on her knees simultaneously.

A semi-glazed look came across her eyes. Her breathing rate increased, and her face then developed a bright vascular flush. Her eyelids fluttered and closed. Then she swooned and looked as if she was going to slide off the chair on to the floor. Thinking to myself 'Oh shit!', I reached over to stabilise her on the chair. I wondered how I might explain this one to the Medical Defence Union! I could just hear them saying 'You did what? You touched both her knees and she swooned? What exactly were you trying to do?!'

The patient was in a trance-like state for about three minutes, although at the time it seemed more like 30. When she came round she said she felt fine, and she went home. I spent the rest of that day wondering what might transpire. I had asked her to phone the next day to report further on her experi-ences. She said that she had slept very deeply and peacefully that night, with dreams of happier times with her son and father. Now, for the first time in months, she felt as if a weight had been lifted. I was secretly delighted and vowed to experiment some more – although with knuckles rather than knees! And also with an improved grief resolution process (*see* Chapter 12).

My second patient was Janine, a woman in her early thirties. She had come requesting antibiotics for a dental abscess. As I surveyed her case records I could see that this was the fourth such episode this year. I asked her why she had not been to see the dentist to get the problem sorted out once and for all. She looked at me sheepishly and told me that she couldn't – she had a dental phobia. She had not been to the dentist since she was eight years old. On that occasion she had required several extractions which had been performed in the dentist's office under a general anaesthetic. Kicking and screaming, she had been strapped down and held down in the chair by several people while the dreaded gas mask had been positioned over her face. Since that day she had not returned! I could feel myself identifying with a similar episode in my own personal history.

I asked her if she was interested in getting rid of the phobia once and for all. When I explained the procedure (straight from the book) she agreed to give it a go on the basis that if it did not work she would be no worse off – such confidence! I asked her to imagine that she was watching herself standing over there. That 'other her' was going to watch a video rerun of the eight-year-old Janine from before the incident happened, through the event until she was completely safe again. This rerun was to be seen in black-and-white – like an old-time movie – way over there in the distance. Dissociated from the memory in this way, she had no emotion as she watched it again from this safe distance. I told her to ask the 'other her' to comfort young Janine after the event, and then re-integrated all three of them together.

Janine's first response was: 'Is that it? You must be joking'. However, try as she might, she was unable to recapture any of her old fearful feelings. She left rather bemused. About a month later I saw her in the high street. She pulled a huge smile to show me the gap left from her recent extraction. She had decided to make a dental appointment and see what happened. She reasoned that if she could not get through the dentist's front door she would just cancel the appointment. However, she was amazed at how calm she remained throughout. Once again, I was impressed by how this straightforward technique could deal with a fear that had lasted 25 years. You can read further about this process (the *phobia cure*) and how it has been updated in Chapter 10.

Many aspects of NLP have been built on the models of Milton Erickson, a psychiatrist who was adept at conversational change. He was very skilful in the use of stories and metaphors which, although they had no superficial resemblance to the presenting problem, struck a deeper chord so that patients changed in their own way. He was one of the first therapeutic wizards to be modelled by

Bandler and Grinder, and stories about him abound. One that I particularly liked was when Erickson was the visiting specialist at a psychiatric hospital. The other psychiatrists presented their patients to him one by one and he worked his therapeutic magic. There was a whole line of patients sitting outside the office awaiting their turn.

One such patient was an adolescent who had what would today be described as 'extreme oppositional behaviour'. He watched the other patients go in, spend quite some time with Erickson, and then come out again with a glazed far-away look in their eyes. This had happened several times before his turn, and you could imagine the trepidation he might have felt when he was called next. He entered the room and Erickson gestured to the seat in front of him. Just as he was sitting down, Erickson said to him 'Just how surprised will you be when your behaviour completely changes next week?' With a bemused look, he replied 'I'll be very surprised!' Then Erickson dismissed him with no more ado.

The other psychiatrists present thought that Erickson had decided not to work with the lad. Yet the very next week the adolescent's behaviour changed completely! He was no longer oppositional. Personally I thought this was a bit far-fetched, and decided to experiment. I had been visiting the elderly mother of one of my patients who was in a terminal decline. Her daughter, a smoker, who had previously asked for help in stopping the habit, escorted me to the door. We were talking about how she was coping with her mother when, entirely out of the blue, as a non sequitur, I posed the same question, gazing at her expectantly: 'Just how surprised will you be when you stop smoking next week?' She gave her head a quick shake and, with a very puzzled and mystified look, replied 'I *will* be surprised'. I then carried on the conversation as if no interruption had occurred.

The matter was not mentioned at all until, at a visit to her mother several weeks later, the daughter spontaneously said that she had stopped smoking. She was not entirely clear how this had come about but, with a cheeky grin, said she thought that I had had something to do with it. Now I would not want you to run away with the idea that this is all you need to do to get someone to stop smoking – if that were the case it would be very easy indeed. This particular patient had already expressed a desire to stop, and my intervention fortuitously came at the right time for her. And it was aided by a pattern interrupt that gave her a momentary deep trance experience.

These three early successful experiences with NLP interventions, after having simply read about it in a book and applied it with wanton experimentation (as I did in those early days), laid a very firm foundation of curiosity about behavioural change patterns which persists to this day. I wonder just which of you readers will find this happening for you ... now or in a short while.

Stepping stones

NLP was developed at a time when there was a reaction to the more dominant analytical therapies of the day which saw change as a long drawn-out process. The co-founders, Richard Bandler and John Grinder, were more interested in practical results than in abstract theories *about* what worked. They and their fellow practitioners viewed each person as a unique individual who had a systematic way of organising their subjective experience to produce a problem or a solution. Given that the particular solution for one person might be quite different to that for another, even within the same class of problems, they followed the dictum '*do whatever it takes to get the result you want*'. Therefore partly as a reaction to the therapy of the day, and partly because they did not appear to do exactly the same thing twice, they eschewed the kind of evidence base that modern medicine now demands. Thus there is little if any meaningful research to support the efficacy of NLP interventions.

The huge growth in popularity of NLP within the general population over the last 25 years has been paralleled by the rising success of cognitive–behavioural therapy (CBT) within academia over the same time frame. CBT has become the most researched therapy of modern times. Its outcome and efficacy studies leave the analytical therapies well behind – CBT works and has sackloads of proof to back it up. As I began to research CBT methodologies, I found that NLP and CBT had not only paralleled each other's rise over the years, but also shared similar basic assumptions about information processing in individuals in health and disease. Indeed, it became clear to me that there had also been a major cross-fertilisation of ideas and techniques between the two therapies.

Assumptions of CBT

Here are the basic assumptions of the CBT model as set out by Clark and Steer in *Frontiers of Cognitive Therapy* (Salkovskis, 1996: 76–7).

1   *Individuals actively construct their reality.* This core tenet suggests that individuals play an active part in using the incoming sensory data from the world to construct an interpretation of the world which is based on that information. This is a synthetic process that involves all perception, learning and knowing. As such, each individual develops his or her own personalised meanings about events which, if maladaptive, may give rise to clinical symptoms.

2   *Cognition mediates affect and behaviour.* Our thoughts, emotions and behaviours interact reciprocally with one another. How we think, feel and behave

forms a feedback loop which can maintain chronic symptoms such as depression and anxiety.

3   *Cognition is knowable and accessible.* It is entirely possible to access the thoughts associated with psychological disorder (including visual and auditory imagery) – even those on the fringe of consciousness, which allow access to faulty information processing. This is the typical *negative automatic thought* which it is central to both uncover and re-mediate in anxiety and depression.

4   *Cognitive change is central to the human change process.* This is a cornerstone of CBT. It asserts that for meaningful emotional and behavioural change to occur, cognitive processes (thoughts and imagery) must change first. This can be achieved either directly by working on the various cognitions themselves (cognitive restructuring) or indirectly by engaging in a behaviour that ultimately changes thoughts (*in vivo* exposure therapies).

For comparison we shall look next at the presuppositions of NLP.

Presuppositions of NLP

The presuppositions of NLP are the underlying assumptions of the NLP model which have accrued over the years with field testing. They can be viewed as a set of beliefs which, when acted upon, ensure that communication and change flow in an active, dynamic, recursive loop. NLP practitioners do not regard them as the literal 'truth', but merely as a set of filters which can enhance any therapeutic intervention. Here are some of the basic presuppositions, which you can compare and contrast with the assumptions of CBT.

1   *Everyone has their own unique model of the world.* We all have different filters, life experiences, beliefs and values which frame our interpretation of the world 'out there'. No two individuals will have exactly the same internal representation of an external event, yet these representations can be altered to expand our 'map' of the world.

2   *Present behaviour is the best choice available at this moment in time.* We respond in the present moment on the basis of the patterns of behaviour that we have learned in the past. These patterns are the result of interactions between thoughts, emotions and behaviours which attempted to gain something of importance for us back then. They remain our current best choice for good or ill until we have an opportunity to change and update them.

3   *Mind and body are one unified system.* Changing our thoughts can change our physiological responses. Changing our physiology (movement, posture, etc.) can change our thoughts. Our communication is both verbal and non-verbal, and as such we need to pay attention to the whole message – mind and body.

4   *There is only feedback.* In any communication or therapeutic intervention (which is a series of communications) you can move either towards or away from your outcome. Honing your calibration skills so that you can 'read' people more effectively will give you the feedback necessary to know where you are in the process and what to do next.

5   *Behind every behaviour is a positive intention for that individual.* NLP assumes that every behaviour, whether labelled good or bad, is trying to do something of positive value for that person. By separating out the positive intention from the behaviour itself we can find other more acceptable ways to fulfil the same outcome. This is a prime assumption underlying many NLP techniques.

6   *Change occurs by reordering and resequencing representational systems.* Every problem can be broken down into a strategy – the sequence of thoughts, images, sounds and feelings that drive the behaviours. These are called representational systems. Changing their order and sequence can markedly modify the behaviours.

There are other NLP presuppositions which, by and large, say the same thing in a slightly different way. Yet if you contrast these with the assumptions underlying CBT, you will see that they overlap to a major degree – in fact they are virtually synonymous. Outcome- and process-based research on CBT has shown *what* works and *why* it works. CBT has similar epistemologies and methodologies to NLP, and as we shall see as *Changing with NLP* unfolds, they also share a similar set of 'how to's'. The skills-based processes of effective change are very alike, even though individual techniques may initially appear to differ substantially.

Although some of this may be anathema to those who are steeped in the NLP model (I extend my apologies to anyone who is offended), it is my view that both NLP and CBT are simply the names of overlapping categories of effective models of change. Their many similarities at the process level not only outweigh their various operational differences with regard to techniques, but also more readily open up the door to NLP approaches for more formalised research procedures. Although this does not necessarily validate NLP through the 'back door', it may allow those who are already well versed in CBT to incorporate more from this fascinating field. For those who are new to both therapies, many insights will be gained into pragmatic and practical change patterns for the everyday world.

And what is the advantage for those in the medical field? Well, it seems to me that the NLP approach in particular simplifies the processes of change and enables the techniques to be much more easily learned and assimilated within a shorter period of time. You will also find as you continue reading on into the next part of the book, on practice, that they can all be incorporated into your everyday consulting in a fairly straightforward way.

How to get the most out of this book

Changing with NLP is arranged in three parts. The first part – *Preparation* – explores validated processes of learning and changing, building them into one cohesive model. We then map across the various NLP principles of change to give us our working model upon which the rest of the book is based. There is also a chapter on the anatomy of change, which grounds the various cognitive processes in the neuro-anatomical pathways of the brain. Fear not, though – you do not need to know any complicated neurology! If you are the kind of learner who is interested in assimilating the concepts and related background theory first, then this first part is definitely the place to start.

The second part – *Practice* – is the 'meat' of the book. Starting with simple NLP techniques, each of the 12 chapters builds on the one before it, nesting the skills together so that you can learn more effortlessly. The chapter format consists of a mixture of case histories, elucidation of the particular change process so that you can use it easily, and a section connecting theory to practice. You might want to consider reading them in order for maximum skills integration. If you are the kind of learner who is interested in practical applications that you can immediately use with patients, you may want to bypass the early chapters and dive straight into the second part of the book.

The third part – *Possibility* – is a pot-pourri of various topics. I shall give an outline of how to apply the various techniques in conditions such as anxiety, depression, addictions, chronic pain and cancer. I shall also explore Freud from an NLP perspective with an analysis of transference and projective identification. In the chapter on 'The dark side of the force', I shall share my thoughts on the potential abuses of any powerful technology such as NLP – this is important from a medico-legal perspective. The book ends with a look at what the future may hold.

Whenever you are learning new material, it pays dividends to ask a series of questions of each section. If you consider your mind to be like an unformatted floppy disk – a big stretch of the imagination, I know – then questions can help to format new information in a way that not only helps you recall it more easily, but also aids the integration of your developing skills. Use the following questions liberally as you read along.

* *Why* is he using that particular case study to highlight specific points?
* *Why* does he think this particular topic is important? What is in it for me?
* *What* is the key information I need to know in this section?
* *What* other areas outwith NLP does this material connect to?
* Am I sure I know *how* this process actually works now?
* Am I sure I know *how* I am going to implement this in my daily practice?

- *Which* of my current patients can I use this particular process with?
- *What* will happen if I continue to use this material in the future?

How to learn more easily

The fields of accelerated learning have a whole variety of strategies that can help you to get the most out of your reading and study time. The following guidelines have all been shown to improve your learning and retention of salient information.

- Ensure that you are in a good learning state before starting each section (*see* Exercise 2 at the end of this chapter).
- The effects of primacy and recency mean that short periods of study (45 minutes) and rest breaks (10 minutes) help you to retain more information.
- Associations with other disciplines and fields of enquiry will surface spontaneously as you read. Take the time to jot these down in the margins.
- Using all your senses, vividly imagine being in each experience as it is described. See it from the viewpoint of the health professional, the patient and an objective observer.
- Think about where, when and with whom you would use each skill as you go along. Note down which patients come to mind.
- Briefly review the previous section before starting the next one.
- Find an interested colleague and make a firm commitment to working through each of the techniques together.
- Find every opportunity you can to use this material both in your consulting *and* in everyday life.

What should I do if I get confused?

The feeling of confusion can be quite uncomfortable – you probably know what that is like for you. It is usually a feeling that we do our best to avoid at all costs. When you are learning new material and new applications, it is quite possible that you may become confused from time to time. Why does this happen? Well, no one comes to new learning as a completely clean slate, ready to fully absorb everything. Each of us has all the material we already know categorised and stored in various neural networks in our brain. Most of this is out of our conscious awareness, yet at the same time the material has been deeply grooved and patterned for our automatic use – almost without thinking. We can think of this as our current 'map' of existing knowledge.

New knowledge and new learning may come from an entirely different map – a completely new way of seeing things. When we take this new information into our neurology, several things can happen. Initially we may experience a feeling of cognitive dissonance – we struggle to fit it together with what we already know. The main danger here, of course, is that we will simply reject it out of hand and fail to update our maps! If the material is similar in some way to what we already know, we will then file it away in the appropriate category, but little real learning will have taken place.

Confusion is often a sign that real learning is actually taking place right now. When two dissimilar maps – the known and the as yet unknown – begin the process of integrating together, our previously fairly neat categories may initially get thrown into disarray. It may take a little time for this to sort itself out, so that the end result is a new category with the best of the old and the new incorporated together. Neurobiologists have confirmed that a huge amount of protein synthesis goes on in a nerve cell at this point. Often it requires a circadian rhythm – a good night's sleep – for this to resolve spontaneously and be fully incorporated.

So if you get that feeling of confusion, recognise it for what it is – a signal that you are definitely learning something new. If you don't get it – beware!

What should I do if I feel uncomfortable when using the techniques?

This is a very common response when attempting to utilise new techniques for the first time. Some people find that they cannot remember all of the steps and need a 'crib sheet'. Perhaps they feel self-conscious when using the technique 'live' with a patient. This may even be the time when an increasing level of discomfort makes you abandon ship! So what is really going on here? To answer this question we need a short discourse on the stages of learning. Learning theorists have shown that whenever you learn a new skill you are likely to pass through the following four stages:

1   *unconscious incompetence* – when you don't yet know what you don't know. This is the state of ignorance *before* attempting something new
2   *conscious incompetence* – when you know *what* you want to do, but your current abilities do not yet match your vision of flowing flawlessness. You are likely to make many mistakes in this phase
3   *conscious competence* – when you know *how* to do it and – if there are no distractions – you perform reasonably well. You still need more practice, though
4   *unconscious competence* – when everything in the process flows together easily without any need for conscious attention to the steps.

Stages 2 and 3 are the cause of much of the discomfort you may be feeling. Yet these very stages are the ones during which the vast majority of the real learning is taking place. You are literally embodying the skills. You can think about this in another, more fruitful way if you want. You can let that feeling of discomfort be *your* signal that the learning process is actively taking place – the various neurological connections have sprouted and begun to lay down the pathways that lead to seamless skill.

NLP is an accelerated learning methodology. It is therefore quite possible to find yourself going directly from stage 1 to stage 4 with little conscious awareness of your arrival. After all, this is merely the learning and changing process we used unconsciously as children. You can rest assured that I have structured this book in such a way that you can more rapidly acquire the various skills as you progress through it.

Your goals and outcomes

You have already picked up this book and started to read through it. Yet before you go any further I would like to ask you a question. What is it that you really want to get out of *Changing with NLP?* As you think about that question, and before you fully answer it, I'd like you to step back for a moment and consider a few things. Why are you reading this book? What is your overall purpose in studying it? What is important to you about what you are currently doing? What is it that you want to achieve?

In the modelling of excellence by NLP, one thing came up time and time again with achievers in all fields of activity – they began with the end in mind. They set up very specific, evidence-based goals so that they would know they were actually achieving their outcomes. And they did this not only for the 'big' things in life, but also for more routine day-to-day matters – and everything else in between. Even with something as simple as reading a book, they set themselves aims, goals and outcomes before starting off. They looked on it as a way to format their mind so that they would automatically pick up on all the things that were important to them. And rather than limiting themselves to one or two goals, they set as many as they could possibly think of, in the knowledge – from previous experience – that a large number of them would actually be achieved.

You are now about to spend some time reading this book and acquiring a set of new skills. I assume that you want to make as effective use of that time as you possibly can while enjoying yourself in the process. To this end I suggest that you complete the following exercise modelled from NLP trainers David Shephard and Tad James.

Exercise 1:   My goals and outcomes

1   What are my goals and outcomes with regard to reading this book? What exactly would they be such that, having successfully finished the book, successfully completed all of the processes and successfully gone beyond my expectations, achieving all my goals, I would have to say 'That was the best book I have ever read on developing and improving my change management skills'?

2   Now write down as many goals and outcomes as possible that come to mind. Take at least 5–10 minutes right now. Aim to have at least 10 goals ... maybe even 20! You can keep adding to this collection as you read through the book.

3   Now take each of your goals in turn and sit back in your chair and begin to contemplate. Imagine what it would be like to have successfully completed the goal. Imagine how you would look, walk, talk, stand, sit, breathe and move differently. How would others know, just by seeing you, that you had achieved it, and more? Allow that picture to become brighter, closer and more colourful, until it feels just right.

4   When you have done this with all of your goals, imagine that every single one of them coalesced together into one giant integrated outcome. What would it be like to achieve all of this? Enjoy the feelings of success.

This is the kind of exercise that you can come back to time and time again. Whenever you decide on a new goal, you can run it through this process. The more often you do it, the more quickly it will streamline and become an automatic accompaniment to your everyday life.

There is only one more thing that we need to address before you cut loose and fully engage in the rest of the book. And that is ...

Your learning state

Whenever you want to learn something easily, it is important to be in the right state or frame of mind. How much learning do you do when you are angry, frustrated, fearful or sad? Do you remember the times of ritual humiliation that went by the name of 'consultant's teaching rounds'? These states are not conducive to learning – well, certainly not the kind of learning I have in mind here. Educationalists now agree that because learning is a state-dependent phenomenon, it is important to be in a state that is relaxed and open to learning. So let us see what kinds of other states are useful.

What is it like when you feel *fascinated* by something? The kinds of times when you are watching, listening to or doing something that completely holds your interest. Times when your full attention is taken up. Perhaps when you are watching an elegant performer flow through their moves. When have you felt this way before?

What about *curiosity*? Have you ever wondered what that feels like in your body? Times when you are not entirely sure about what is going to happen next, yet you have a sensation of pleasant anticipation. A bit like the feeling you get when you have been in a queue and it's your turn next!

Have you ever *surprised yourself*? Perhaps there was a time when you thought you couldn't do something because it was too hard or difficult – yet you ended up succeeding anyway and surprising yourself in the process. Maybe there was a time when you did something against the odds – and you enjoyed the result immensely.

What about *playfulness*? Think of those times when you were having fun simply for fun's sake. Maybe you don't have too many of those as an adult! Perhaps you can think of times spent playing with children in a silly game. Maybe there were times when you were younger and you were simply doing what you enjoyed best.

And what about those times when you are using an *automatic skill*? Perhaps this involves driving a car or cooking a meal. Times when you are displaying a particular skill without thinking about it – in a flow state. You are here in the present moment and at the same time you are able to respond to any new stimulus that comes along.

All of the above examples can be thought of as individual building blocks of the kind of learning state that allows you to gather up and organise new information almost by osmosis. I suggest that you identify times in the past when you have been in each of the constituent components before doing the last exercise in this chapter.

Exercise 2:   Building your learning state

1   Find a quiet spot for the next 5–10 minutes and allow yourself to relax. Make sure that you have examples of the states of fascination, curiosity, surprise, playfulness and automatic skill.

2   For each state in turn, take each individual memory and imagine being right back inside it again, reliving it once more. Make the pictures in your mind's eye brighter, more colourful and closer. Turn up the volume of the sound until it feels just right. Really luxuriate in the feelings. Do this for all of them now.

3   Now imagine mixing all of the feelings from each state and coalescing them into one. You can imagine a pictorial collage of all the memories at once – you don't have to see them clearly, but just know that they are there.

4   Once the feelings have coalesced, you can imagine being in this kind of state as you read *Changing with NLP* – or as you are doing any other activity you wish to learn more easily. You can wonder what would happen if you were in this state each and every time you were learning something new.

We have now arrived at the jumping-off point for reading and assimilating the rest of this book. The foundations have been laid for you to gain as much from this experience as you possibly can. We shall touch base again in the final chapter to ensure your continuing skills development.

CHAPTER 2

Models of learning and changing

Introduction

In this chapter we are concerned not so much about the end product, *what* has been learned, as about the actual process itself, *how* learning has actually taken place. Would it surprise you that seemingly dissimilar events, such as learning mathematical formulae and being cured of a phobia, share many similar underlying processes? They really do work in much the same way. In fact, a great deal of the history of psychology has been focused on elucidating the various mechanisms of learning and changing.

These mechanisms would appear to operate on a kind of continuum, from an apparently passive response to environmental events on the one hand to an active synthetic cognitive approach on the other. *Classical conditioning*, which was much researched by Ivan Pavlov in the early 1900s, defines learning as the pairing together of two stimuli that occur in close succession in time. A dog salivating in response to the sound of a bell is the archetypical example. *Operant conditioning*, which was championed by BF Skinner in the 1940s, showed how the reinforcers that operated as a *consequence* of the behaviour played a large part in determining its recurrence. In lay terms, we are talking rewards and punishments, carrots and sticks.

This behaviourist approach was increasingly challenged by the *cognitive theorists*, such as Jerome Bruner, who believed that there was a gap between stimulus and response which allowed thinking, especially in relation to past experiences, to modulate the subsequent reaction. And of course *cognitive therapy*, developed by Beck in the 1970s, has become one of the most useful treatment modalities for the distorted thinking patterns that are prevalent in conditions such as depression.

Social learning theory, promoted by Albert Bandura from the 1960s onward, has focused on the learning that takes place by *observation* of a model. We have probably all come back from courses and seminars and found ourselves using language and displaying skills that we had not consciously set out to learn. Somehow we assimilated them as an unconscious process from covert modelling of the trainer. Bandura's theory of *self-efficacy* (whether we believe we can succeed ... or not), which we shall explore in depth throughout this book, is probably one of the most important determinants of behavioural change.

As we come from the late twentieth into the twenty-first century there has been much focus on *state-dependent memory and learning*, with additional inputs from *complexity and chaos theory* applied to the life sciences. Briefly, the state of mind and body that you are in at the time of learning (e.g. happy, sad, joyful, depressed, drunk) plays an important part in the later recovery of the information which is laid down. This is a vital component for ensuing behavioural change.

So just exactly how are learning and changing connected? It seems that you cannot have one without the other. Learning is usually defined as a *relatively permanent change in behaviour due to past experience*. We can get a little more pedantic by calling it a change in *behavioural potential*. This apparent play on words acknowledges the fact that learning (behavioural potential) can occur, but that performance (actual behaviour) is a distinctive expression of that potential which can fluctuate depending on the context. You may not have known just exactly how much you had learned prior to your Finals, but your performance in the exam itself was a test of that learning. And the vagaries of pre-exam nerves, a good night's sleep beforehand (or otherwise) and your confidence levels determined the results.

As this chapter unfolds, then, we shall explore each of the various approaches to learning and changing, and build them into a unified model that serves as the foundational base upon which we shall subsequently map across the relevant NLP processes and techniques. None of these approaches stands alone as the 'one right and true way to learn and change'. We shall see that they are all merely ways of describing the same complex learning process from different yet more simplifying perspectives.

Classical conditioning

The essential feature of Pavlovian *classical conditioning* is that a specific, initially neutral environmental stimulus becomes linked to a particular behavioural response. Dogs naturally salivate at the sight of food. Prior to conditioning, a bell is a completely neutral stimulus which evokes no response at all. During the conditioning process the bell is repeatedly rung *only* at times when the dog is salivating in expectation of food. Within a short period of time, ringing the bell by itself *without* the production of food causes the same response.

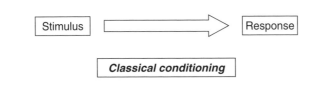

Figure 2.1:   Conditioned responses.

This is a simple yet at the same time profound model of learning which, as we shall explore in subsequent chapters, is at the root of many illnesses and recovery from them. For example, in the expanding field of cancer chemotherapy, many patients suffer increasing bouts of nausea and vomiting not only as a direct result of the pulses of drugs themselves, but also as a conditioned response coupled with anticipatory anxiety about the next dose. This can be effectively managed by a counter-conditioning process.

Usually, to pure behaviourists, conditioning stimuli are thought of as originating in the outside world. You only have to think about the sound of a cardiac arrest bleep or see a blue flashing light to get that all too familiar feeling. Yet, as we shall discover in the various case histories that follow, *internal* thoughts, sounds, images, evocative words and tactile sensations can all act as conditioning stimuli. This, we shall see in due course, gives far more scope for therapeutic interventions.

In a separate experiment, Pavlov conditioned dogs to a neutral non-salivatory response with a metronome. When he later paired the metronome with the bell (the previous conditioned salivatory response), firing both off at the same time, it completely cancelled the effect. No salivation took place! *Counter-conditioning* was thus born, and this has major therapeutic implications that we shall consider shortly.

Systematic desensitisation and aversion therapy

In the 1950s, Joseph Wolpe began to use classical conditioning techniques in the treatment of fears and phobias. Essentially, in *systematic desensitisation*, fear (a sympathetic arousal state) was paired with its opposite, relaxation (a parasympathetic state induced by deep muscular relaxation techniques). Patients were encouraged to think of their fears and phobias in a hierarchy from least to most fearful experiences *while remaining in the relaxation state*. This led to a high degree of problem resolution. Variants of this technique are still widely utilised today.

Psychologists then began to experiment with other competing (counter-conditioning) responses, such as pleasant thoughts, humour, laughter and even sexual arousal. Research has demonstrated their effectiveness in many conditions. One interesting example is that of blood product phobias, which usually involve fainting or passing out. Pairing with deep muscular relaxation actually worsens the response by further lowering blood pressure. However, inducing muscular *contraction* instead, in a more highly charged dynamic state, while simultaneously thinking about the specific phobia, not only keeps the blood pressure up but can also lead to a one-session cure of the problem! In this way, *many* different states can be creatively paired with the original problem to facilitate resolution. We shall examine various novel approaches using this principle in the chapters to come.

The principle in *aversion therapy* is to associate a noxious experience with a maladaptive behaviour. The idea is that the patient is prevented from performing the behaviour by the aversive feelings which are engendered. A classic example is use of the drug Antabuse in the treatment of alcohol abuse, which pairs severe nausea and vomiting with taking an alcoholic drink. Other uses include utilising evocative visual imagery of vomitus, and pairing the feeling engendered with smoking a cigarette. Aversion has mainly been used in the treatment of addictions and sexually deviant behaviours.

Of course, aversion can also develop in ordinary life situations. Consider the child who has been sick in a car and who subsequently associates all car travelling with sickness. In this case, however, we would want to use different counter-conditioning techniques to relieve the aversion stimulus! You can probably think of many other similar types of situations. And the astute reader will by now be recognising that there are an infinite number of ways to pair together unique patient experiences to produce myriad results. In fact, you may well be wondering just which aspects of psychological, psychosomatic or even physical illnesses have inbuilt conditioning and counter-conditioning elements. Hold on to that thought as you continue reading.

We can now update our evolving model as shown in Figure 2.2.

There are many specific nuances of systematic desensitisation and aversion which we shall cover in depth in the relevant chapters.

Operant conditioning

BF Skinner is the person most linked to *operant conditioning*. Indeed, it has often been called Skinnerian conditioning! He showed that the *consequences* of a behavioural response could predict the future likelihood of that behaviour's recurrence. In this way the consequences could act as a *reinforcer*, providing

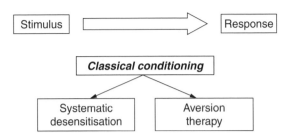

Figure 2.2:   Desensitisation and aversion.

motivation to perform in the same way again. Reinforcement can be either positive or negative, and both forms are different from punishment. The following examples will demonstrate this.

Reinforcement *always* increases the frequency of a particular behaviour. Positive reinforcement tends to move towards what you want more of – for example, the promise of a toy as a reward for a child's good behaviour, praise and approval for a job well done, or the relaxation that follows smoking a cigarette.

Negative reinforcement is *not* punishment, although it is often confused with it! Negative reinforcement moves you away from what you don't want – for example, taking a painkiller is reinforced by relieving pain, smoking a cigarette is reinforced by relieving anxiety or withdrawal symptoms, and eating smaller food portions is reinforced by avoiding weight gain.

Avoidance behaviour is a form of negative reinforcement. The social phobic who is anxious about an imminent dinner party and relieves her anxiety by making an excuse not to attend experiences immediate feelings of relief flooding over her. This actually increases the likelihood of future repetition of avoidance, thus making the problem seem even more insurmountable. Facing up to one's fears is a common-sense dictum that has many parallels in behaviour therapy treatments.

Let us add this to our developing model as shown in Figure 2.3.

Think of one of the recurring issues in general practice in terms of operant conditioning, namely the prescription of an antibiotic for self-limiting minor illness. For the doctor working under constraints of time and pressure, giving a prescription can quickly bring a consultation to an end. However, the patient receives the positive reinforcer of getting what is wanted – the prescription. And as the symptoms of the self-limiting illness recede over a few days, the antibiotic is erroneously thought to have cleared the problem. Thus it acts as a negative reinforcer.

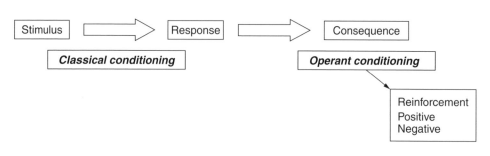

Figure 2.3:   Adding operant conditioning.

How many patients do you know who say 'It always takes two courses of the antibiotic to get better, doctor'? The same principle is in action over a longer time frame. The pulling effect *towards* what you want, joined to the pushing *away from* what you don't want, is very potent. This powerful combination working together ensures that the patient quickly learns that all such episodes of illness require a prescription of medication!

Reinforcement is often at the heart of some of the most challenging chronic behavioural problems to change. For example, gambling is a behaviour that is reinforced by a variable ratio schedule. Winnings come in variable amounts, from small to very large, and over variable time frames, from short to long. You never really know just when the next big win will occur. It might be just around the corner – the very next bet! The longer you go without a win, the more likely it is that your number will come up. Or so the gambling logic goes. This kind of pattern can be very resistant to extinction.

Consequential deceleration therapy

This long, seemingly complex name is given to those interventions that aim to reduce the target problem behaviour. Given that all behaviours are maintained by reinforcement, if the reinforcers are withheld, *extinction* occurs. The classic example is the crying baby whose crying is maintained by parental attention. 'Checking' to see that the child is 'all right' paradoxically keeps the behaviour going. However, leaving the child to cry and withholding attention usually causes a fairly swift resolution of the problem within 3–10 days. Occasionally an *extinction burst* occurs when the crying initially gets worse prior to improving.

Extinction is one of the processes that underlies 'facing your fears'. Remaining in a fearful situation *while the fear peaks and subsides* at the same time as being prevented from using your normal avoidance behaviours can quickly lead to useful change. This is called *exposure therapy*.

Physical aversion can also be used as a consequence, *after* the behaviour has occurred. Rubber bands that are 'snapped' on the wrist, noxious odours and mild electric shocks have all been used to treat maladaptive behaviours such as hair pulling, self-mutilation and nail biting, among others. These are less commonly used nowadays because of their punitive connotations.

Although we shall discuss the finer details in specific chapters, let us now further update our model as shown in Figure 2.4.

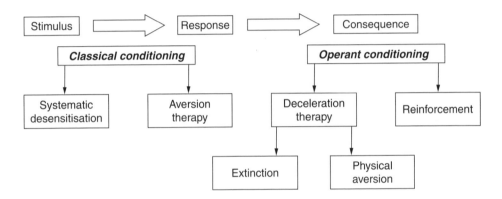

Figure 2.4:   Adding deceleration therapy and reinforcement.

Cognitive theories of learning

The cognitive theorists felt that the behavioural models, although important, did not fully explain all the mechanisms of learning and changing. An emphasis solely on observable behaviour failed to take account of thinking processes – the unseen thoughts, emotions, beliefs and prior experiences which modified the gap that came between stimulus and response. One prominent cognitive developmentalist was Jerome Bruner.

Bruner studied the way in which children's cognitive abilities matured through three main stages. The *motor* stage involves, for example, how we learn to tie our shoelaces, ride a bike, etc. We come to know the world through our actions, which are then represented as 'muscular memory'. The *imagery* stage consists of our internal mental pictures and sounds, which have been built up through repetitive encounters with objects in the external world. The *language* stage occurs when we develop our capacities for naming and abstract thought, which allows us to further manipulate our internal and external worlds by means of word labels.

Of course, each aspect is used to a greater or lesser degree, as an adult, in everyday situations as we move through life. For example, suppose that you wanted to get directions for travelling from A to B. Someone who knew the way could physically take you there (the *motor* mode). Or they could draw a diagram of your route for you to take with you on your way, the *imagery* mode. Or they could give you verbal directions, such as turn right here, left there, straight on, etc. (the *language* mode). Each set of 'instructions' becomes increasingly complex, and all of them in some way involve retrieving and making available our past experience and knowledge to bring them to bear in the here and now.

An outline of this model is shown in Figure 2.5.

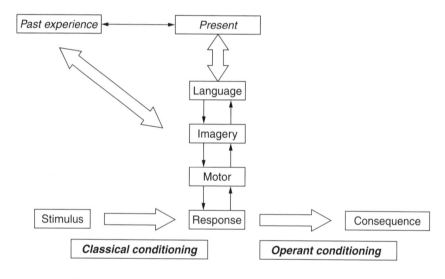

Figure 2.5: Adding cognitive factors.

This model begins to open up possibilities for learning and changing in numerous ways. A stimulus occurring here and now may be first *compared* with past experiences, beliefs, concepts and abstractions *before* a response occurs. This of course happens at the speed of thought which, if you think about it, is pretty fast! Maladaptive past experiences may form a template for present un-wanted thoughts and behaviours. We can thus begin to manipulate the motor actions, internal imagery and self-talk which produce unwanted responses, and start to create the behaviours that we want instead.

Dealing with thoughts in this way is called *cognitive–behavioural therapy*, which became the increasingly dominant psychotherapeutic discipline in the latter stages of the last century, and for which much empirical and evidence-based research of efficacy exists. There are essentially two ways to deal with problems in the cognitive domain, although each has its subsets of differing approaches and methodologies. These are *cognitive restructuring* and *cognitive skills training*.

Cognitive restructuring assumes that faulty thoughts and imagery prevent patients from responding in the way they would like to at the present moment. People who are depressed may tell themselves over and over again that they are a failure, in an internal voice that sounds sad and gloomy. They may make dark foreboding pictures of what is likely to happen, based on their past experiences. They make many cognitive distortions, such as black-and-white dichotomised thinking about events, over-generalising from single negative experiences, and erroneously personalising neutral statements made by others. Therapy involves identifying such distortions, and restructuring and updating them accordingly. Although historically functioning to a larger degree by modifying and changing internal self-talk, we shall find that changing visual and auditory images can also have profoundly beneficial effects.

Cognitive skills training, on the other hand, is really about teaching patients the thinking skills that they lack in particular contexts – skills which they have failed to develop. Someone might become depressed not necessarily because of faulty cognitions, but perhaps because they do not have the assertion skills necessary to have their needs respectfully met. Perhaps they lack problem-solving skills or relationship-building skills. By *modelling* people who can do these things effectively – utilising thinking, language and behavioural skills and strategies that work in the real world – we can use the derived model as a template for change. This overlaps to some extent with Bandura's social learning theories in the next section. Although a large part of this work has also focused on internal self-talk, there is much to be gained by adding appropriate visual and auditory imagery.

We can add this to our model as shown in Figure 2.6.

Social learning theory

Albert Bandura's name is the one most associated with *social learning theory*, which was in its early stages of development in the 1960s. While not denying the importance of classical and operant conditioning, social learning theorists believe that they did not adequately account for the development of new behaviours. They proposed that *observational learning* – whereby learning

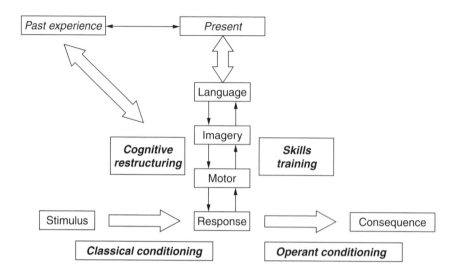

Figure 2.6:   Cognitive restructuring and skills training.

occurred by watching a model perform a particular task – was quite distinct from conditioning.

One of the interesting things about this kind of learning, which has become known as *modelling*, is that it takes place spontaneously, outwith conscious awareness. This is usually at an unconscious level, often without the learner making any deliberate effort to learn or the 'model' doing any teaching as such. This is one of the ways in which children seem to automatically copy parental language, emotional expression and behaviours. Of course what is modelled spontaneously in this way can be beneficial ... or not, as the case may be!

In a classic example of modelling at work, Bandura exposed children who were phobic about dogs to several videos. These showed age-related peers, some of whom initially seemed to be apprehensive, approaching, playing with and cuddling dogs, while remaining completely safe throughout. Following this intervention, without any other 'therapy', there was a high rate of phobia cure.

Models can be of many different shapes and sizes. They can be live (appearing in the flesh), or symbolic, appearing indirectly (such as television characters, and heroes in books and in oral descriptions like stories and metaphors). You can even imagine in your mind's eye a model performing the task you are going to do just before you do it, thus enhancing your own performance. In a more complex intervention you can *self-model* by videoing yourself performing a task, and by re-editing you can put together an improved version which enhances future performance. Peter Dowrick, a pioneer of video self-modelling therapy, asks his patients to create *video futures* which show them coping and adapting successfully in imminent challenging situations. All of these processes have been validated by research.

Modelling happens vicariously in everyday situations. For example, I remember seeing two children and their mother waiting at a bus-stop. One of the children shouted at and hit the other on the arm. The mother turned round and yelled 'Don't yell and hit your sister like that' as she simultaneously hit him on the arm! Which message do you think won through? The verbal or the non-verbal? There is a lot of truth to the saying 'Example is the most important form of teaching and learning'.

The degree of expertise of the model is also significant. A *coping model* is one who may initially display some anxiety, yet still – over time – learn to perform the task well. A *mastery model* is an expert who is competent from the outset. Coping models are better matched to patients who display initial fear and anxiety. Mastery models are better for precise skills training in the absence of fear and anxiety. This is common sense really. We have all marvelled at how an expert skilfully achieves his outcome and at the same time thought we could never become so good at the skills. We gave up trying! Yet seeing a peer who started off 'just like us', and who developed the skills over time, allows us more easily to imagine doing the same.

This brings us to Bandura's second and possibly more important theory – that of *self-efficacy*. This can be stated in lay terms as follows. If you think you can, you're *more* likely to succeed – if you think you can't, you're *less* likely to succeed. In other words, our expectations and our beliefs about how possible it is to achieve our future outcome are the main determinants of whether we in fact do so.

According to Bandura, a person's perceived level of self-efficacy will not only determine whether they actually begin a task, but will also modulate the amount of effort and the length of time they will spend on it. In essence, the greater the perceived self-efficacy, the greater the degree of perseverance in the face of any obstacles. In fact, Bandura postulates that *all* behaviour change therapies work by strengthening a patient's belief that they will succeed in the task.

Nothing succeeds like success, and direct experience of successfully performing a task or achieving a goal is a very powerful source of self-efficacy. Think back to a time when you accomplished something that you were initially unsure you could do. How did that feel? How did that modify your future attempts? Self-efficacy is also strengthened by examples such as seeing peers succeed at a similar task, the utilisation of therapists' verbal persuasion skills, and the reduction in over-arousal that accompanies relaxation training – a feature of many interventions.

So let us add Bandura's insights to our model as shown in Figure 2.7.

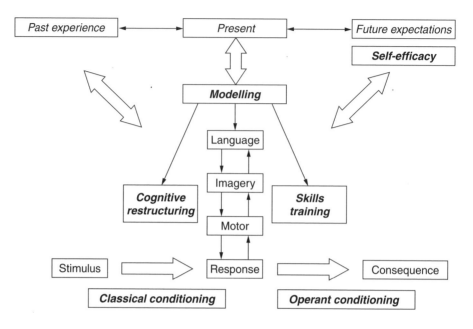

Figure 2.7: Modelling.

State-dependent memory and learning

The last decade or so has seen the emergence of much research detailing the neuroendocrine basis of memory and learning. Although all of the 'big players' are involved, such as dopamine, serotonin, noradrenaline, gamma-aminobutyric acid (GABA), etc., there are literally hundreds of neuropeptides which are thought to modulate the information transduction that takes place as experiences are changed into memory in and around the limbic–hypothalamic–pituitary system. Fear not, though, we shall not be exploring any complicated neuroanatomy or molecular biology! (For a detailed discourse on this and chaos, complexity and self-organising systems, considered in the next section, the reader is referred to *The Symptom Path to Enlightenment* by Ernest Rossi.)

Our internal state of mind and body (happy, sad, joyful, depressed, fearful, angry, relaxed, etc.) can be thought of as being inextricably intertwined with the different mixes of neuropeptides and hormonal influences that are prevalent at any one time. We can think of each state as having an individual 'signature' with differing emotions and states that vary in the type and amount of substrate present. It seems that when learning takes place it is *state dependent*, in the sense that recall and retrieval of the information are most complete when we access the original state in which it was encoded.

A classic experiment that demonstrates this is to have a group of people drink enough alcohol for them to be on the verge of being intoxicated. Then give them some specific facts to remember. When they are sober again, they will fail to recall the facts. However, give them a few alcoholic drinks again and – hey presto – they remember once more, because the information is only retrievable in the state in which it was originally encoded.

Other studies have shown that the external context can also play a part in learning and recall. Two groups of students learned the same information. The first group was tested in the same room in which they learned. The second group was tested in a different room. The first group consistently outscored the second. The same study has been performed with the first group being examined both in the original learning room and then in another room. They still recalled more in the original context, with the external cues providing greater access to the state-dependent information.

These two studies shed some light on problems such as post-traumatic stress disorder (PTSD). War veterans who have been exposed to severe battle conditions lay down traumatic memories when they are in extreme physiological states in the war zone. After returning home they find that external cues such as a car backfiring or a firework exploding are enough to precipitate them back into the original memory, with the full physiological effects, such as tachycardia and profuse sweating, also recurring. This can also be thought of as a form of classical conditioning, with the external cue eliciting the state. A similar series of events takes place with phobias.

One way to think of this is to imagine that the response is encapsulated within a *neuronal network* – a series of hundreds if not thousands of neurons which fire off as their encoded memory is triggered. As this excitation pattern spreads across the brain it releases large quantities of neuropeptides which mediate the physiological response. Entrainment and streamlining occur such that the response can not only strengthen but also become functionally separate from, and thus inaccessible to, the influence of other neuronal networks. In effect, if the maladaptive behaviour is also learned in a state that is considerably different from the patient's normal everyday reality, it can become functionally autonomous and outwith conscious control.

However, we already know that this is the case – our patients tell us every day! They say things like 'I just don't know what came over me', 'I felt like I was completely out of control', 'It's just a habit I can't break', 'I've tried so hard to do something different, but I can't seem to' or 'It seems so easy for other people, but not me'. In effect they are saying that they are being 'run', at times, by state-dependent neuronal networks which are triggered and function autonomously in certain contexts.

And yet in other contexts of life these very same patients may have many resources available to them which they are as yet unable to bring to bear in order to change the 'problem' situation. They may have other neuronal networks that encode memories, states, skills and behaviours such as determination, relaxation, humour, patience, motivation, etc. Unfortunately, because the problem is state bound and autonomous, they have not yet been able to integrate these neuronal networks together in a way that leads to resolution. In fact, one could say that the whole process of *learning and changing is really the operation of accessing differing state-bound neuronal networks and bringing one to bear on the other.*

As we add state-dependent memory and learning (SDML) to our model we can envisage it as a boundary condition within which each of the other elements is embedded (*see* Figure 2.8).

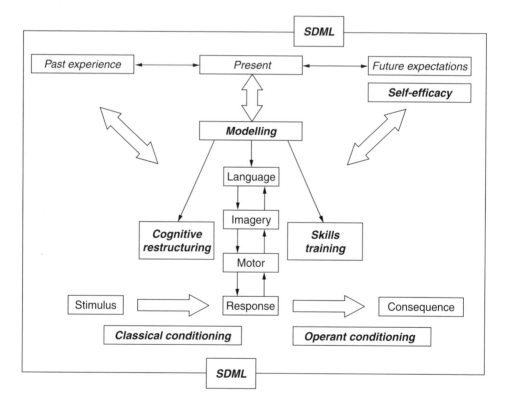

Figure 2.8:   State-dependent memory and learning.

Chaos, complexity and self-organising systems

Chaos and complexity theory is the 'new kid on the block' in theories of learning and changing. We live in a complex, rapidly changing world, and a fundamental feature – indeed requirement – is our ability to creatively adapt to novel situations. And we are each faced with novel situations both psychologically and physiologically as we negotiate the various phase transitions of life from childhood to adolescence, adulthood, mid-life and old age. We start off single, perhaps get married and adapt to life as a couple, have children, they fly the nest, perhaps we change jobs or move to a new area, parents die, or a spouse dies, to name but a few circumstances with which we must come to terms. In a sense we are always living on the edge of chaos, organising our internal and external world to adapt accordingly. We are indeed *self-organising systems.*

One way of thinking of physical and mental health is in terms of our ability to manage the critical transition points and crises – big or small – in a creative and adaptive manner. If we deal with these events with a flexible display of appropriate behaviour, previously learned or newly acquired, then our system is 'healthy'. However, symptoms arise when we persist in using fixed, rigid, inflexible behaviours on a repeated basis, that maladaptively fail to achieve the outcome we really want. We remain stuck, and our system is 'unhealthy'.

Chaos, complexity and self-organising systems theory is a branch of mathematical thinking that has been increasingly applied to the social and life sciences. It deals with non-linear systems where the apparent chaos can actually be described by some fairly simple differential equations. Don't worry, though, we won't get into any complicated mathematics here!

Linear systems display cause-and-effect characteristics, such as A causes B causes C causes D, etc. They are relatively simple and straightforward. However, non-linear systems suggest that A, B, C and D are dynamically linked together such that changes in one element can cause simultaneous changes in one or all of the others – including, of course, multiple positive and negative feedback loops. This is a truly complex system, and much more akin to life as we know and live it.

Systems such as the weather, water turbulence in rivers, biochemical reactions, the human heartbeat, oscillations in predator and prey numbers in natural ecosystems, relationship dynamics in both humans and animals, and the psychology of personality, emotions and behaviour are all non-linear. They are more than the sum of their individual parts, and their emergent properties and behaviours display characteristic patterns that are underpinned by *attractors.*

An *attractor* is the underlying pattern which holds the apparently chaotic elements of a complex system in a fairly stable pattern over time. Consider a patient who is depressed and has the belief 'I'm a failure'. This belief acts as an attractor around which all incoming information is self-organised. If he tries something new that fails, this will corroborate the belief: 'I told you so! I'll never get better'. If you point out something that was a success, it will be written off as a 'lucky fluke'. Our beliefs – our perceptual filters – act as self-organising attractors for life's experiences.

Attractors are often thought of as 'basins' (*see* Robert Dilts' website at www.nlpu.com). The depth and breadth of the basin relate to the attractor's intensity and ease of access. A deep, wide basin may be easy to access and relatively intense in experience (e.g. depression), or the basin may be deep and narrow, accessed infrequently, yet extremely intense (e.g. a phobia).

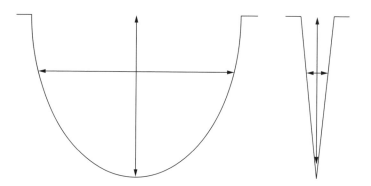

Figure 2.9:   Types of attractor basins.

Perhaps the basin is shallow and wide – a state that is experienced frequently although not so intensely (e.g. irritation or confusion, or perhaps even recurring mild anxiety). Maybe it is shallow and narrow (e.g. the occasional sharp jab of a fleeting doubt!).

Of course, this can apply to 'good' states, too, such as a moment of intense joy (narrow and deep), the confidence that you can handle whatever life throws at you (wide and deep), a glimmer of hope (shallow and narrow) or a neutral state of mind when driving your car (shallow and wide).

So how does all of this fit with learning and changing? Attractors can be thought of as the *reference points* around which information is organised. New learning is self-organised for ease of recall and application in terms of thoughts, emotions and behaviours. However, this learning can be adaptive or maladaptive, useful or problematic, helpful or a hindrance, with the underlying mechanism of acquisition being the same in each case.

You may be asking how change occurs with this model. Let us imagine a problem, such as depression, with a wide and deep basin, and a ball resting at the centre, representing the core issue that requires change. Most of the time we expend a lot of energy trying to push the ball as far as we can up the curved side wall in an attempt to escape this basin and come to rest in another, which we call the 'solution'. All too frequently, however, the effort is too great and we slip back down to the centre again. After a few futile attempts we give up, resigned to little hope of things getting better.

According to attractor theory, the attractor itself needs to be destabilised *first*, prior to change occurring. Once it has been destabilised it will spontaneously begin to reorganise into a different configuration with a different attractor pattern. In change therapy, this is known as a *pattern interrupt*. There are many things that can serve this function, including humour and laughter, confusion, sudden surprise, shock, spontaneous trance states, conversational non sequiturs and verbal reframes, to name but a few.

Following destabilisation the system is poised for permanent change to occur by the addition of a new attractor. Various skills and resources, different thinking patterns and behaviours are all examples of different types of attractor which can reorganise the existing architecture, allowing reconfiguration in a 'solution'. We can envisage our problem states, or desired states, and the resources to go from one to the other, as an *attractor landscape* of life that we navigate on a daily basis.

In fact, all of the different models of learning and changing that we have encountered so far can be explained in these terms. In *classical conditioning*, two opposite states (attractors), namely fear and relaxation, are brought together. In *operant conditioning*, we move towards what we want or away from what we don't want (attractors again). In *cognitive theory*, the beliefs (attractors) that hold problems in place are restructured and updated. In *modelling*, the model of excellence serves as an unconscious attractor for that particular skill. In *self-efficacy*, a strong expectation of future success (attractor) becomes a powerful motivator for change. In *state-dependent memory and learning*, an external cue, such as a firework (attractor), can revivify previous emotionally intense experiences.

Thus if we put all of these models together, we can envisage attractor basins as the landscape through which learning and changing take place (*see* Figure 2.10).

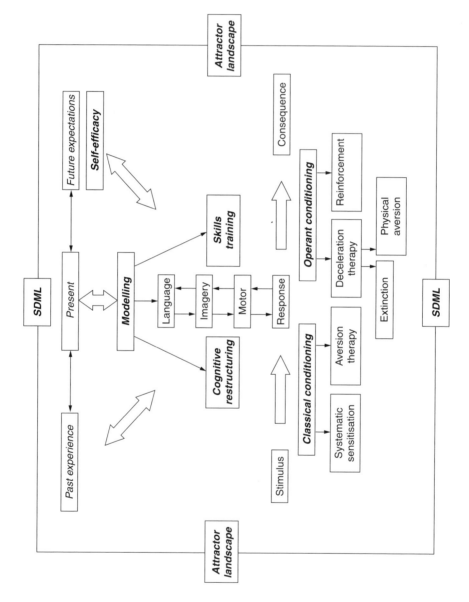

Figure 2.10: Overall map of learning and changing.

Concluding

This chapter has run fairly swiftly through the major theories of learning and changing. For those of you who might wish to study the material in more depth, you will find ample resources in the Bibliography. In subsequent chapters we shall be exploring each of these areas through the lens of NLP, further expanding our knowledge by analysing specific day-to-day clinical encounters. This will lay bare the various mechanisms whereby each of the NLP techniques achieves change.

Of course, none of these mechanisms for change stands alone. It is possible to take a single learning event and make sense of it by adopting each of the above perspectives. There is no one right way, and learning and changing are in reality such complex processes that gross simplification runs the risk of mistaking a single tree for the whole forest. The forest itself, to continue the analogy, is home not just to trees. It supports not only a variety of different tree species but also a complete ecosystem of interdependent life forms whose fortunes may vary in a cyclical manner. It is a truly self-organising system.

In ending, perhaps for simplicity's sake we should highlight the basic theme that seems to recur in all forms of learning and changing. This is that in some way, by one process or another, *we must access different state-dependent neural networks and bring one to bear on another*.

Keep this in mind as you continue to read on ...

CHAPTER 3

Basics of changing with NLP

Introduction

This chapter will introduce the fundamental aspects of NLP change processes and allow you to see how easily they map across on to the models of the previous chapter. Subsequent chapters will flesh out the skeleton developed here, going into each change process in much more depth. So in effect this is an overview of the NLP approach to learning and changing which you may find similar, yet at the same time intriguingly different, to what you already know. And as Dr Milton Erickson said, because *there are many things that you really don't know that you already know*, you may find yourself intuitively making sense of it all as you read along.

The roots of NLP were firmly planted in the therapeutic encounter. Bandler and Grinder were intensely interested in the process of learning and changing. And they were interested not only in *how* various therapeutic wizards achieved their results, but also in *how* clients were doing things differently after the intervention had taken place. By utilising the tools of the modelling approach, which we shall come to shortly, they systematically investigated the subjective structure of experience. They worked out just *what* specifically people were doing in their internal thoughts, imagery, beliefs and external behaviours that represented the pivotal points for change.

Yet their approach and thinking style were somewhat unique. When they were investigating various types of phobia, they felt that mainstream psychology was holding the wrong end of the stick. Rather than trying haphazardly to find a cure among those who were still afflicted, they did something quite different. They advertised in the newspapers for people who *had had* a phobia which had 'spontaneously' resolved. To a client, they all reported some variation of 'looking back on it now, it's as if it had happened to someone else'. From their modelling of how the subjective structure of their inner experience had changed, Bandler and Grinder developed the much-vaunted NLP fast phobia cure (*see* Chapter 10 for details).

On another occasion, Bandler was impressed by how patients who were depressed actually maintained their condition. He found that many of them were good at discounting positive experiences by immediately picturing how it would all go wrong. They would literally see themselves failing in their mind's eye. Bandler modelled the mental process they were going through and realised that by *reversing* the pattern, generative change could be enabled to occur. The Swish pattern was thus developed, and has since been successfully applied in many different areas (*see* Chapter 9 for details).

This is the kind of thinking that pervades NLP. We want to elucidate the *structure* of someone's internal experience. We want to find out *how* they maintain their problem state. We want to find out just *which part* of a pattern holds a problem in place, which when subsequently changed – by one of the techniques that you will learn in this book – allows a reconfiguration to occur, such that we are left with the structure of the solution instead.

In this chapter, then, starting with the basic building blocks of the structure of internal experience, we shall cover the principal mechanisms of learning and changing with NLP. Of course, NLP is an unashamed plagiariser of many fields of excellence, elucidating and distilling the patterns of successful intervention – patterns which work effectively. And as we go on, we shall show just how NLP has taken, utilised and refined the various validated models of the last chapter, building them into a coherent *NLP model of change*, which you will increasingly find can be easily applied in day-to-day consultations and other situations.

The structure of internal experience

How do we make sense of the myriad experiences that bombard our everyday senses? How do we know what to pay attention to and what to ignore? How is it that we ascribe significance to *certain* things, but not others? If we were literally able to attend fully to the countless thousands of stimuli that occur every second, we would probably find this a recipe for madness!

Figure 3.1 illustrates a simple NLP model of what happens to external information as we apprehend it.

Our experience of the external world is composed of the things we see, hear, feel, smell and taste. In NLP talk these are visual (V), auditory (A), kinaesthetic (K), olfactory (O) and gustatory (G) modalities. As we take in this information via our senses, it passes through various filters. Because we can only pay conscious attention to a small portion of all the available information, we *delete* large quantities of it from our experience. What is left is further organised by our internal rules – that is, the *generalisations* that we live by. Then we *distort* the

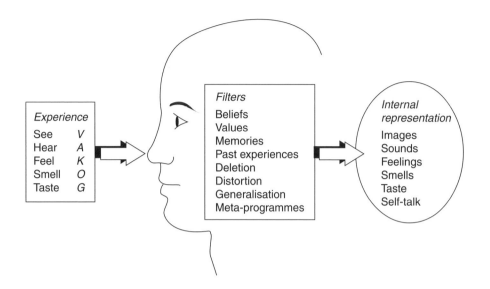

Figure 3.1:   NLP model of communication.

remainder to fit with our other filters, especially our beliefs, values, memories and past experience base.

In a sense, then, these filters act as self-organising *attractors* for all incoming data. What we end up with – our *internal representation*, what we *think* is going on 'out there' – is coloured by the many facets of our unique individual lives to date. These representations are therefore at least one step removed from the reality they seek to portray. And further self-talk *about* that representation, with increasing layers of added abstraction, further removes us from direct sensory experience.

So how do we actually structure that internal representation? Is it simply an amorphous thought or does it have form and substance? When you think of something you like, how does your mind know that it is different from something you dislike? Likewise, what is the difference between something you firmly believe and something you disbelieve? Certainty and uncertainty? Past and future? Pleasure and pain? Good and bad?

In the following exercise it would be useful for you to think of yourself as a cinematographer, with the ability to notice the finer details of both the pictorial imagery that is projected on to the screen and the accompanying soundtrack, and also the ability to identify just what feelings this engenders in you.

Exercise 3:   Exploring mental perspectives

Think of a really good pleasant memory from the past. Perhaps a time when you achieved something of importance at work, in sport, etc. Maybe a memorable holiday, a place you visited or a dramatic sunset. Perhaps a time when you were having fun with family, friends or relations. When you have the memory, think about the following.

Visual
- Create a mental picture of the event. If you can't yet see it clearly, pretend that you can. Perhaps it's almost invisible, like the one I'm picturing now.
- Is it in colour or black and white? It is like a movie or a still framed photograph? Is it close at hand or far away? Fuzzy or in sharp focus? Framed or unbounded? Are there single or multiple images? Are they two-dimensional or three-dimensional?
- Imagine it projected out in visual space around you. Do you see it straight ahead, up, down, left or right?
- Are you inside it, seeing it as it is happening (associated)? Or are you outside it, watching yourself from a distance (dissociated)?

Auditory
- Now listen to the soundtrack of the experience. If you cannot yet hear it clearly, just pretend that you can.
- Is the volume loud or soft? Does it come from close by or far away? From which direction? Up, down, left or right? Point to it.
- Is the sound 'surround sound' or more easily heard in one ear? If it is the latter, which one?
- Is it clear or muffled? Soft or harsh? High or low pitch?

Kinaesthetic
- How does this experience feel in your body? Pay attention to the feeling. Where is it located? Put your hand on it. How intense is it? Does it feel light or heavy? Does it start in one place and move to another (e.g. from abdomen to chest)? How quickly does it move? Is it hot or cold? Continuous or discontinuous?

You have just explored the structure of an experience, the building blocks of a thought. If the visual, auditory and kinaesthetic senses are the modalities of that experience, then the finer details are the *submodalities*, which vary according to the thought itself. You can repeat the above experiment with a neutral or more negative experience and notice the differences. Check out like and dislike, certainty and uncertainty, etc. You will find some subtle and not so subtle changes. We shall explore these in more depth later.

Anchoring

Anchoring is the name that NLP gives to *Pavlovian classical conditioning* whereby a certain stimulus elicits a certain response. Whereas classical conditioning is concerned with an external stimulus causing an observable behavioural response, NLP has expanded this notion markedly to include internal thoughts and responses, too.

We are well used to external stimuli changing our states of mind and body. Everyone has had the experience of a certain tune being played which immediately transports them back to a memorable experience in the past. Hearing our name said by a loved one in *that* particular tone of voice may bring feelings of love *or* irritation! Seeing a beautiful sunset may elicit feelings of peaceful serenity. The feeling of a hug can change a negative emotion completely and instantly.

Yet internal stimuli can also do exactly the same thing. Picture in your mind's eye the person you love having fun. Remember again the sound of their laughter. Imagine feeling their touch in *that* particular way! These internal visual, auditory and kinaesthetic stimuli can all fairly quickly change our states – for good or ill.

In the same way, we can think of our other internal thoughts and symbols – our beliefs, values, attitudes and concepts – as being the anchoring stimuli that elicit different sets of responses. In fact, NLP expands the whole conditioning concept to suggest that *everything is an anchor for something.*

Where Pavlov used mainly auditory and visual stimuli as conditioning agents, much of NLP therapy and change work uses kinaesthetic stimuli – mainly touch – to anchor responses. When someone is in an intense state (confidence, joy, fear, anger, etc.) touching them in a particular place (e.g. a knuckle) in a particular way at the peak of the state will condition the response such that touching again in the same way will re-elicit the state. This is known as *kinaesthetic anchoring* and, as we shall see in due course, it can be used to effect profound change.

Kinaesthetic anchors are one of the most important NLP additions to mainstream psychology. The ability to elicit a particular state and anchor it in a reproducible way effectively gives us a handle with which we can add resources to problem states with a great deal of precision. We can be just like a chef, mixing and adding together different ingredients for change.

For example, a specific simple phobia (e.g. fear of spiders) can be anchored to one knuckle, while resource states (e.g. confidence, strength, laughter, humour, etc.) can be anchored to the knuckles of the other hand. Firing them all off simultaneously can significantly modify the original response, leading to problem resolution. This counter-conditioning process is termed *collapsing anchors* (*see* Chapter 7), and although it appears to be very simple, it can be powerfully therapeutic.

Various noxious aversive stimuli (e.g. vivid mental imagery of vomitus) can also be paired directly with behaviours such as smoking, etc. However, this is often operationally achieved by a slightly different procedure, termed *chaining anchors* together, which we shall encounter in the next section.

Let us now map this process across on to our original model as shown in Figure 3.2.

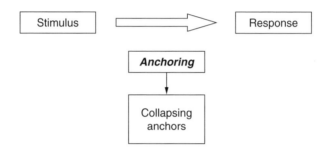

Figure 3.2:   Anchoring.

With this concept in mind, we can readily see how various psychological and psychosomatic symptoms can be approached and resolved. Yet what if we were to consider that physical symptoms of pathological disease processes (e.g. allergy, various cancers, autoimmune conditions, rheumatoid arthritis, neurological degenerations, peptic ulcer, etc.) might all, in principle, be anchored and tackled in the same way? Although the evidence is as yet mainly anecdotal, NLP has reported many 'spontaneous remissions' using the above methodology via the various techniques you will read about in due course.

Motivation direction

NLP has always been interested in people's motivation strategies – how they actually get themselves started doing something. And not only that, but also how they complete what they have chosen to do. Despite the apparently myriad ways in which different people motivate themselves to perform different tasks, the fundamentals recur time and time again. They either move *towards* what they want, or *away from* what they do not want (or a combination of the two).

One way to find out someone's motivation direction is to ask them what achieving their outcome will do for them. For example, the question 'What will stopping smoking do for you?' may get the answer 'prevent lung cancer or ischaemic heart disease' (away from) or 'the breath to play with my grandchildren and save money for a great holiday' (towards).

What we do *always* has consequences of one kind or another. Performing a behaviour brings with it both potential gains *and* losses. Moreover, *not* performing a behaviour likewise has consequences. Whether or not we engage in a particular task over and over again depends on the consequences of our previous actions – positive and negative reinforcement in operant conditioning terms. The benefits of continuing smoking (e.g. relaxation, time out, relief from stress, etc.), which occur in the here and now, may outweigh the benefits of stopping, which are not seen until a much later date.

So how can we use this knowledge of 'towards' and 'away from' motivation to encourage behavioural change? Let me ask you something. Have you ever tasted dog faeces? Could you imagine now having some stuck to your teeth or in your nose? How do you feel right now? When vividly imagined, this is quite a noxious stimulus!

Let us continue with our example of smoking. We could set up, on our patient's various knuckles, anchors for a noxious stimulus, another pleasurable behaviour that they enjoy (not smoking!), and a big bright compelling picture of them as a non-smoker. Ask them to imagine reaching for a cigarette, and then fire off each anchor in turn.

What does this do? The act of reaching for a cigarette is paired to an aversive experience. As this peaks and then moves to relief, the anchor for another pleasurable behaviour is fired off, followed by the one for life as a non-smoker. This causes an initial moving *away from* motivation to be paired with moving *towards* what is wanted instead. *Chaining anchors* is a process that can be used in a variety of ways in a number of conditions (*see* Chapter 8). It can be thought of as a *propulsion system*, whereby there is an almost simultaneous *push* away from what is not wanted and a *pull* towards what is wanted.

In this way, in operant conditioning terms, we can decelerate unwanted target maladaptive behaviours and positively reinforce adaptive ones. Our model now becomes that shown in Figure 3.3.

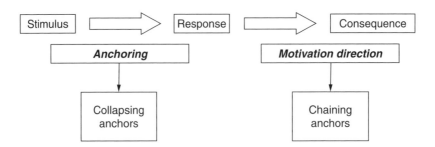

Figure 3.3:   Adding motivation direction.

Logical levels of experience

In the early days of NLP, the components of experience that were the target points for interventions were external behaviour, internal state (i.e. affect), and cognitions. This was referred to as the *Mercedes model* because the diagram representing it (*see* Figure 3.4) looks like the car symbol!

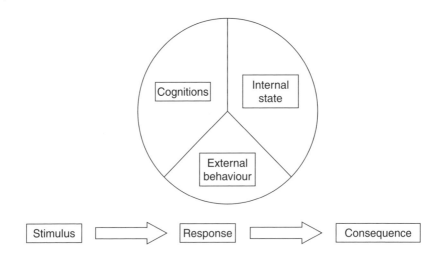

Figure 3.4:   Interaction of cognitions, state and behaviour.

This was the basis on which the early NLP interventions were devised, in particular the various anchoring procedures and the phobia cure. Responses could be modified by changing external physiology (different postures, gestures, etc.), accessing a different state and restructuring thought processes. More and more emphasis was placed on cognitions, especially the *strategies*, the internal sequencing of thoughts that predicated observable behaviour. These strategies were the various combinations of visual, auditory and kinaesthetic modalities that were the drivers of behaviour.

For example, someone might motivate him- or herself by making an internal image of a successfully completed task (V), telling him- or herself in an excited tonality about how good it would be to get finished (A), and having an internal feeling drawing him or her towards actually beginning the task (K). In this way the strategies for processes such as effective decision making, learning something new, becoming convinced, etc. were elucidated. The discovery of submodalities helped to refine the process further, with more detail and specificity about the pivotal drivers of change.

However, it became clear that there were more levels of experience which could be usefully delineated and whose processes of change differed from simple strategies. This led Robert Dilts to devise the *logical levels model*, which is one of the most widely utilised models today. Although many would now agree that the model is neither 'logical' nor hierarchical as first described, it is a most useful pragmatic map for organising the contents of the various categories of therapeutic interventions. I prefer to use it in a circular format, as change in one area can lead to self-organising reciprocal change in any of the other levels.

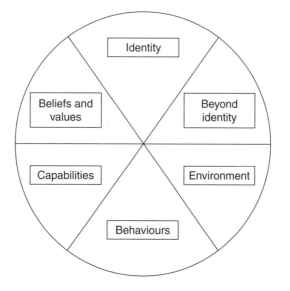

Figure 3.5:   Logical levels model.

Let us consider each of them in turn.

- *Environment.* This is the *where* and *when* of a problem's occurrence. Some problems may occur in specific locations but not in others, or perhaps only within a particular time frame. Where and when they do *not* occur can provide valuable information for change.
- *Behaviours.* This is *what* you actually *do* in that environment. An external observer of a problem would notice what you were doing at that time, including your posture, gestures, voice tone, breathing rate, movements, etc. This is a sensory-specific description. What would you actually be doing if you no longer had the problem?
- *Capability.* This is *how* you do what you do. It includes the internal thinking skills and strategies that can keep a problem in place (e.g. depression, phobia), and also the strategies which, when applied, can lead to a solution. How would you be thinking differently when the problem is solved?
- *Beliefs and values.* This is *why* you do what you do. Values are our prime motivators, and beliefs are the operational rules that express our values in action. Much learning and changing can usefully take place by making an intervention at this level. *Cognitive therapy* specifically addresses this level, too. What would be a more useful belief to acquire and utilise in that particular situation?
- *Identity.* This consists of our core beliefs about ourselves – *who* we really are. This sense of self pervades our everyday situations, our everyday roles, and we may like it or loathe it. This is the area of self-worth and self-esteem – which may be high or, as is more usually the case in problems such as depression, may be low. Who will you become once this issue has been solved?
- *Beyond identity.* This level is about how we connect with the outside world – how we relate to other people, the *who else* involved in the situation. This is a prime area of intervention in *interpersonal therapy.* How will you be relating differently in this situation when you have made the changes?

The *logical levels model* is a very useful expansion of the territory normally encompassed by cognitive–behavioural therapy. *Every single problem* that your patients bring to consultation can be fruitfully considered from each level. There is no one 'magical' level that enables lasting learning and changing to occur. Because we are speaking about a whole person – a self-organising system – an intervention at any level may be the catalyst that unlocks the door to the solution. Sometimes this can happen after one simple applied technique. At other times, in more health-challenging situations, interventions are required at all levels, simultaneously or sequentially, the sum total overcoming the system's inertia and allowing the emergence of a stable and lasting solution.

Our continually updating model is shown in Figure 3.6.

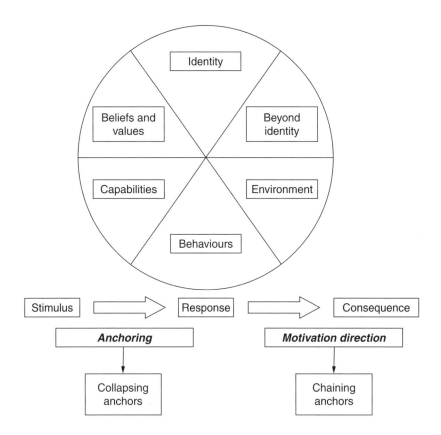

Figure 3.6: Expanding levels of cognition.

Modelling

Modelling is the engine that drives NLP, and is the process whereby the many techniques you will find in this book were elucidated. Albert Bandura showed how change can occur by vicarious modelling, with neither the 'learner' nor the 'teacher' being consciously aware of their roles or what specifically was being learned. NLP has taken the whole topic and usefully further subdivided it, adding many tools which flesh out the details, the specifics and the *how to's* of modelling excellence.

Bandura was concerned with *unconscious* modelling – the kind of learning that children normally engage in as they mimic their parents and identify with role models and peers. Because there is little discrimination in unconscious modelling, you may acquire more than you bargained for – not only their specific behaviour, but their warts and all! *Conscious* modelling occurs when we pay special attention, like an outside observer, to the *structure* of what the model is actually doing. We may deliberately focus down on a particular skill, a thinking strategy or a small part of a larger set of behaviours.

We can elicit information from each of the *logical levels*, building the bigger picture out of each accumulated piece. We can explore a model's thinking patterns – the various strategies that it uses to achieve results – in terms of visual, auditory and kinaesthetic modalities and submodalities. We can take note of language patterns, beliefs and attitudes, and how they inform the modelled behaviour. We can pay special attention to physiology, postures and gestures, especially eye and other accessing cues (*see* Appendix 4).

Modelling is fundamental to effective and ecological change. We can model just exactly *how* our patients experience and maintain their problem states, whether those be phobia, depression, anxiety, physical symptoms or a disease process. From modelling those who have successfully overcome similar states, we can devise an intervention using the *logical level* categories, applying leverage at the pivotal point for optimum systemic influence. Whether we are utilising *cognitive restructuring* or *skills training*, modelling is the sine qua non of learning and changing with NLP.

We can add this to our model as shown in Figure 3.7.

Outcome setting

NLP is an outcome-focused, solution-centred behavioural technology for change. From the early days it was clear that if a patient did not have a detailed, specific sensory-based goal in mind, then effective change would be less than easy. One of NLP's major contributions to the field is the exploration and setting of well-formed outcomes.

You will recall from Bandura's theory of self-efficacy that a major determinant of successful change is the *clear expectation* not only that it will take place, but also that the patient believes they have the necessary capabilities to ensure the outcome. Robert Dilts has expanded Bandura's work into the model shown in Figure 3.8.

Let us examine each area in turn.

- *Desirable*. The agreed outcome must be something that you definitely want to have – something that is sufficiently motivating for you to want to move towards.
- *Possible*. The outcome must be possible to achieve and not simply a pipe-dream. It needs to be couched in realistic terms.

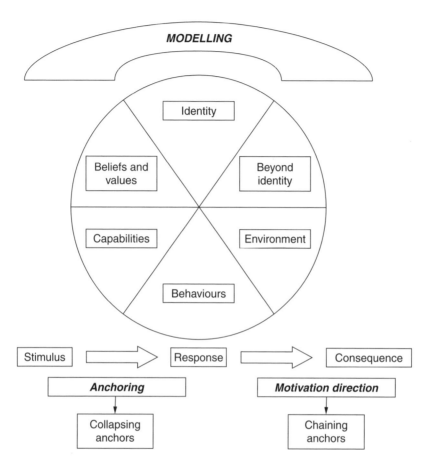

Figure 3.7:   Basic NLP modelling.

- *Capable.* The person must either have or be able to acquire the necessary skills to enable them to achieve their outcome. This is often the area where most learning and change take place.
- *Ecological.* The achievement of the outcome must fit with all of the other personal, work and relationship goals that are already in progress. If they conflict in any major way, the chances of achieving the outcome are greatly reduced.
- *Deserving.* The person must believe that they deserve to achieve the outcome. This is intimately linked to self-worth and self-esteem which, if poor, may reduce their chances markedly.
- *Responsible.* Who is responsible for achieving the outcome – self or others? Failing to take ownership of an outcome to 'see it through' abdicates responsibility to someone else, usually the health professional. This is not a recipe for success!

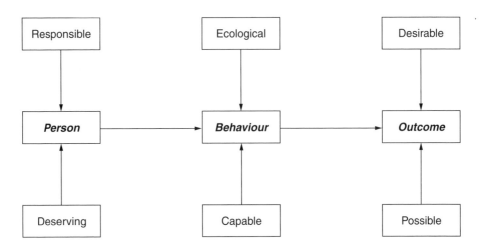

Figure 3.8:   Self-efficacy and expectation.

If we can say a resounding *Yes!* to all the above then we believe that we have all the necessary resources for reaching our goal. Some areas may be stronger than others, and some may be weaker. This gives us the opportunity to perform a mini-inventory and see where an intervention will pay dividends. We can also incorporate material from each of the *logical levels* to ensure that the outcome we build acts as a powerful *attractor* and is truly compelling. We shall deal with the specific details of outcome setting in Chapter 5.

Our updated model is now as shown in Figure 3.9.

Time for a change

How do you distinguish in your mind's eye between something you have already done and something you are going to do? What is the mental difference between the holiday you enjoyed previously and the one you are looking forward to next? We all have an internal mental structure for time that separates past, present and future so that we can make sense of ongoing experience, plan ahead and utilise past resources in fruitful ways.

So just how do *you* structure time? What does your personal internal map look like? The following exercise will allow you to notice and begin to make use of your own personal timeline.

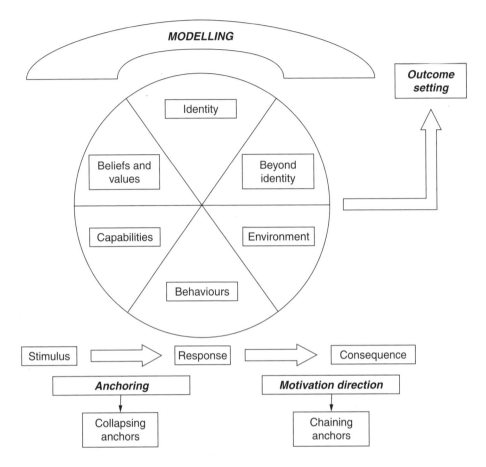

Figure 3.9: Adding outcome setting.

Exercise 4: Eliciting your timeline

Think of a behaviour that you do every day, such as cleaning your teeth, reading a newspaper, driving a car, etc. Use this experience as you go through the exercise.

1   You know that you did this today, yesterday, last week, last month and last year. Get a sense of each of these five inner representations. Even if you can't see all of them clearly in your mind's eye, pretend that you can.

2   Imagine that you can reach out and touch each one individually. Notice which images are closer and which are further away. Imagine a thread connecting them all together. In which direction does it run?

3   Now imagine that you are going to perform this behaviour tomorrow, next week, next month and next year. Again, if you can't yet see them clearly in your mind's eye, pretend that you can.

4   Notice which images are closer and which are further away as you imagine reaching out to touch each one. If a thread were to connect them all together, in which direction would it run?

5   Now join up the past to the present to the future, and as you do so, survey your timeline and get to know what you have already used without knowing.

Although everyone may have their own unique way of organising their timeline, there are certain generalisations that usually apply. For many right-handed people the past is seen as a diagonal line off to the left, often at a 45° angle. The future may be at a similar angle off to the right. For others, the future is straight ahead and the past is directly behind.

If you think about it, you know this intuitively by what people say. Some always have 'time on their side', while others can 'put the past behind them'. Some have had 'a colourful past', while others are 'looking forward to a bright future'. It's interesting that children's fairy tales often start with the words 'once upon a time'. What if each of these statements was a literal representation of each person's internal structuring of time?

Some people are 'inside' now – they are fully in the present moment and feel the feelings associated with current events, for good or ill. They may get 'lost' in time, and become so engrossed in what they are doing that the past and future are forgotten about. NLP calls this 'in time'. Although you can experience the pleasure of many events in this way, it is also the structure of problems such as addictions – an intense need which must be satisfied 'right now', with no thought of past problems or future consequences.

Some people have the present moment just ahead of them – 'outside' them-selves and somewhat dissociated and disconnected. They can see the past and future quite clearly, which makes this a great position for short- and long-term planning. They experience feelings *about* the event, not *of* the event itself, and may therefore miss out on pleasure in the here and now. They are busy thinking of the next thing on their list that needs to be done. NLP calls this 'through time'.

A person's view of time correlates closely with certain clinical conditions. Those who are depressed are past oriented, imposing all of their perceived 'failures' and short-comings on the here and now, and disconnecting from past resources. Those who are anxious focus on the future, imagining how things can go terribly wrong, feeling the intense feelings of trepidation in the present. Problem magnification tends to shut down avenues of access to coping skills (*see* Chapter 17).

The NLP discovery of timelines has opened up far more opportunities for both remedial and generative change. In a sense, our personality – who we are today – is the sum total and product of all that has happened to us in our lives so far. Witness the disintegration of personality that occurs in conditions such as Alzheimer's disease, when we literally forget who we are and what we have done on a day-to-day basis. Since many people believe that what has happened in the past creates our responses today, changing the internal structure of problematic past memories can profoundly alter those responses for the better. We can also use this technology to create the kind of future outcome expectations that optimally enhance self-efficacy.

You will recall from the section on state-dependent memory and learning (SDML) that certain external (or internal) contextual cues can precipitate a physiological response today that has its origins in the past. These autonomous neuronal networks, spontaneously fired off, seem to have a life of their own which is difficult to consciously override. By using an *anchor* for the negative event occurring in the here and now, we can utilise timelines to find the root cause of the issue – the original template as it were – which when updated by new resources using NLP techniques can lead to speedy problem resolution (*see* Chapter 15).

Our continually updating model is shown in Figure 3.10.

States

NLP places a great deal of emphasis on a person's state, but just what do we mean by this? A state is more than just the emotion, the affect that it displays. People may describe and label their state at any one time as happy, sad, joyful, angry, peaceful, upset, ecstatic, etc. However, states are more than that. We can think of a state as a container that encompasses all of our thought processes, feelings and behaviours in a particular context, in a particular time and place.

If we use the *logical levels* of experience as a template, we can see that our state is the sum total of all the neurological and behavioural activity that is going on at each level. At the *identity* level we will be in a particular role at the time – father, mother, doctor, son, daughter, shopper, holidaymaker, etc. Each of these roles has a particular set of *beliefs* and *values* attached to it which will vary

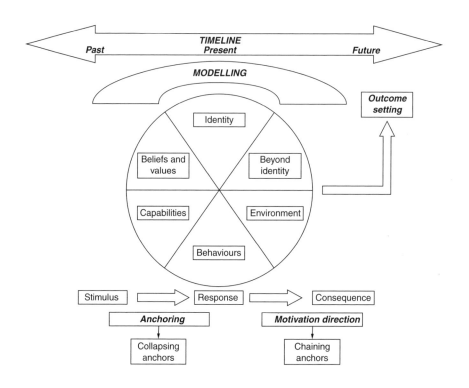

Figure 3.10:   Timeline perspectives.

according to the circumstances. We will adopt particular thinking strategies and ways of processing information – our *capabilities*. And all of these will inform our *behaviours* as we interact with the significant other people in our lives (*beyond identity*).

In many ways, our states are also the containers for the particular skill sets that we use on a daily basis. It is difficult to feel depressed when you are happy. It is hard to feel happy if you are depressed! Neither state easily supports the other's thinking strategies, beliefs and behaviours. If you are at ease with your-self, flowing with the task, it is easy to establish rapport with patients. However, if you are angry, upset, running late, anxious, etc., then difficulty in establish-ing a good connection increases exponentially. You need to *be in the right state for the task at hand.*

One way to think of this is to consider that each state and its incorporated skill sets has its own *neuronal networks* which, when triggered contextually, allow the utilisation of certain behaviours. Over time, these become habituated and autonomous, and we tend to inhabit certain states far more frequently than others on a daily basis. We are generally not conscious of all the inner activity that is going on in each state, and perhaps up to 90% may be outwith our everyday awareness at any one time.

States tend to run us, rather than vice versa. We often operate out of states which were initially set up in the past from significant emotional events that we lived through and learned from. All well and good if these were positive learning events, but not so good if they were negative (e.g. phobias, abuse, humiliation, pain, separation, etc.).

NLP operates on the principle that we can choose which state we want to be in – appropriate for the situation – whenever we want. We can exhume recurrent problematical neuronal networks and update them with the resource states that we want instead, learning, updating and changing as we go along. We can take times in the past when we have excelled and bring these resources into the here and now, using them today and tomorrow. In accordance with SDML, we can view the landscape of our evolving model as a series of *differing states which can be brought to bear on each other for both problem resolution and generative change.*

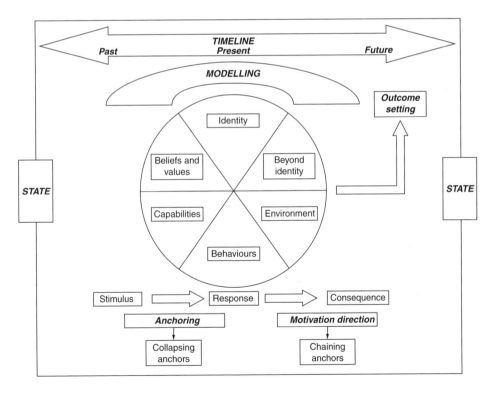

Figure 3.11:   NLP model of learning and change.

Changing with NLP

As an outcome-focused, solution-centred behavioural technology, NLP has always been concerned about results – how to get from problem state to solution state. Seminal NLP contributor Robert Dilts formulated the *general change model* (*see* Figure 3.12) on which a large part of NLP change processes is based.

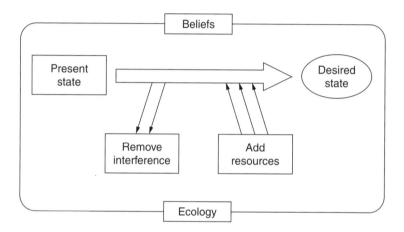

Figure 3.12:   NLP model of change.

The *present state* is the existing problem as formulated, which for most people is a recurrent issue which they have as yet failed to resolve. The *desired state* is what we want instead – the solution – and we have already gone through the general principles involved in enhancing self-efficacy in this area. Usually there are one or more blocks which are the *interferences* that prevent the solution from easily occurring. These must be removed. We then have to *add resources* at the various logical levels, and these will involve one or more of the diverse techniques you will read about shortly. The existing problem is framed within the twin pillars of the patient's current *beliefs* on the one hand, which may need updating, and *ecology* (the study of consequences for the whole system) on the other.

NLP is very much a systems-based approach, and it fits well with the *self-organising systems theory* that Dilts has previously elucidated. Pushing too hard for an outcome without removing interferences is like driving a car with the accelerator and brake applied simultaneously. Often the most important systemic question is 'What prevents the change from having already occurred?' Removing the brakes allows for smooth acceleration to your destination.

Both problem state and solution state act as system *attractors*. The problem state attractor must be destabilised in some way while simultaneously ensuring that the solution state is sufficiently compelling to move towards. Because the *attractor basins* of problems such as depression and phobia are markedly dissimilar, different types and intensities of resources will be required for each. The NLP *fast phobia cure* (*see* Chapter 10) is a good example of how traumatic memory attractors can be easily destabilised by altering submodalities. The various techniques utilised in the succeeding chapters will show you how reconfiguration can occur around a stable solution attractor.

Meta-pattern for all NLP techniques

Trainers John Overdurf and Julie Silverthorn have spoken about the meta-pattern of all NLP techniques – the common pathway by which the various processes bring about change. This is essentially a five-step model, and every single one of the techniques you will read about here can be viewed through this lens. You will find a general outline here, and some useful questions for each stage in Appendix 5.

1   *Associate to problem state*. The patient needs to bring the problem with him or her into the therapy room! Specific questioning techniques will ensure not only that we understand the structure of the presenting issue, but also that we will have a behavioural demonstration as the patient associates into the problem state. Failure to ensure this initial step may mean that they only talk *about* the problem in a disconnected way, which may actually prevent resolution. We shall use many different types of questioning to obtain the necessary information.

2   *Dissociate from problem state*. Once we know the problem's structure and have anchored the state in some way, we must then distance the patient from it to enable the search for resources to take place. Because it is difficult to solve a problem from within the existing thinking and behavioural patterns, we must dissociate the patient sufficiently, usually by interrupting or changing their state in some way, prior to performing the intervention. This can be done by simply asking the outcome question 'What do you want instead?', although we shall use many other methods as well.

3   *Access resources*. Knowing the structure of both the problem and the solution we are heading for allows us to search for the right kind of resource(s) that will destabilise the situation and allow reconfiguration to take place

in a more beneficial way. Resources may come from the patient's own personal history or be added from examples of successful modelling of thinking and behavioural strategies in that particular situation. We shall explore many ways of accessing resources in each chapter.

4 *Apply resources.* Having decided on the most appropriate resources for effective change, we can now apply them to the problem situation and observe the results that we obtain. We can test whether the specific changes required have actually occurred. If not, we can add additional resources. The rest of this book will cover, chapter by chapter and problem by problem, the specific change techniques that you can choose for successful application.

5 *Future pace.* This is an NLP term which deals with ensuring that the changes made in the consulting room are actually actioned later, outside in the real world. This mostly involves, by various means, projecting the patient into their imagined future having successfully made the changes, and noticing what is different now. We shall use anchoring and timeline techniques to reconnect the stimulus that used to cause the problem when triggered to cause the solution to occur instead.

Although every single NLP technique can be examined from the perspective of the above five core elements and applied therapeutically, there are two other precursors which need to be in place in order to enhance your results. These are your *own state*, and having an appropriate level of *rapport* with your patient.

How effective do you think you are when you are feeling rushed and harassed? Compare this with times when you are in the 'flow' – a relaxed yet attentive state, focusing easily on the other person, with the right skills for the job in hand arising almost intuitively. Using the various anchoring techniques that you will be learning in due course, you will find it easier to reaccess *consulting flow states* for catalysing effective change.

One thing that all change therapies have in common is the ability to develop an empathic therapeutic alliance – a good working relationship. Along with patient expectations of treatment, this is one of the main factors that predicts a successful outcome. *Rapport* is the NLP term for working together 'in sync' in this way. The behavioural elements include *matching* and *mirroring* of body language, together with the cognitive ability to discern and utilise patients' thinking patterns. This subject is dealt with in depth in *Consulting with NLP* (by Lewis Walker, published in 2002 by Radcliffe Medical Press).

Therefore, if we piece these seven elements together, we can formulate a model for change that is applicable to each situation, as shown in Figure 3.13.

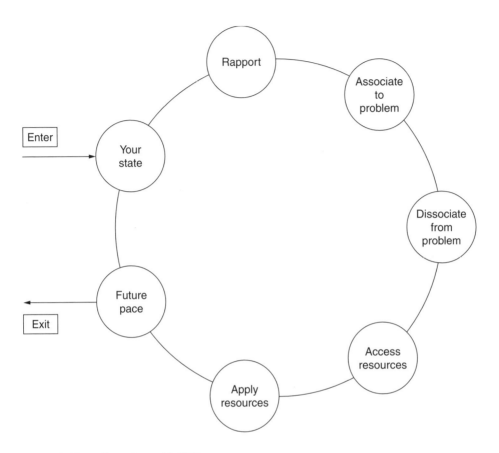

Figure 3.13:   Changing with NLP.

Concluding

This chapter has elucidated the fundamentals of the NLP approach to learning and changing, mapping across the various key elements on to the previous chapter's well-validated behavioural and psychological models. We have seen how NLP relates to classical and operant conditioning, cognitive modelling and self-efficacy theories, together with complexity, chaos and self-organising systems.

There is no doubt that, in a sense, NLP is a plagiariser of many fields of study. The best examples of learning and changing are modelled with various NLP tools, stripped back to their bare essentials, and streamlined to provide a sensitive, elegant, simple yet powerful process for profound change. NLP may not obtain any better results than standard therapy approaches, but it certainly achieves the results within a much shorter time frame. Although it is possible to argue that NLP therapy has not been subjected to validated process and outcome studies, the approaches that it has modelled certainly have been, and their proven efficacy is undoubted. In many respects, therefore, NLP can be seen as simply another set of strategies for performing cognitive–behavioural interventions.

In the chapters to follow we shall, step by step, build up from basics an NLP toolkit which you will be able to use effectively with many patients. Each chapter will highlight one of the various change processes with multiple examples taken from successful case studies. We shall further elucidate the different sections of our overall model for change, going into more depth about the mechanisms – *how* the processes actually work. In each case we shall link this to the validated cognitive–behavioural therapy processes, showing *why* change has occurred. And in all of this we shall be utilising the seven stages of *Changing with NLP*. You cannot not learn!

CHAPTER 4

Anatomy of change

Introduction

Until relatively recently the currency of change – thinking and behaving differently – was confined to both a changed thought and an examination of external behaviour. The intricacies of the brain and its neurobiological functioning have at times been viewed simply as a 'black box'. We knew that somehow, somewhere, something inside that black box facilitated the change – even caused it to occur – although the details of just exactly what was happening remained sketchy at best. Whilst neuroanatomists have delineated multiple brain pathways over the years, until the last decade or so we have been relatively blind to most of their functional aspects.

The explosion of brain research that took place in the 1990s has changed all of that. We now have sophisticated *real-time magnetic resonance imaging* (fMRI) scanners which can take upward of four images every second. We can see far more clearly the flux of brain activity as it undertakes different tasks – just as it happens. Rather than simply knowing about the various anatomical pathways, we are beginning to gain a sense of just exactly how they interact with one another in the dance of activity that is involved in thinking and behaving. We can almost see where a thought arises from and the journey that it takes through cortical and subcortical structures.

Neurologists have learned a great deal by using these sophisticated techniques to map out where a particular lesion has occurred in patients who present with different clinical conditions. For example, in the visual pathways alone they have been able to investigate patterns of rare cerebrovascular accidents giving rise to obscure syndromes, and have found that specialised areas of the visual cortex deal specifically with movement, recognition of faces, colour and black-and-white imagery, etc. They have found that some syndromes that were previously considered to be psychiatric have a distinct neurobiological basis – with both a location and a pathway. Perhaps it is not too far-fetched to speculate that in the not too distant future neurology and psychiatry will join together again as they did a century ago. Rather than thinking in terms of purely mental or physical disorders, we may have a discipline that is simply called 'brain disorders'.

This explosion in research has also led to major discoveries in the anatomy and physiology of the emotions. Fear in particular, and its lesser derivative anxiety, have been extensively studied by renowned researcher Joseph LeDoux. We know how phobias are formed and the pathways that the incoming information takes in the brain. We know how the biochemical actions of adrenaline and other stress hormones play a part in disorders such as post-traumatic stress disorder and panic attacks. These studies have shown both the importance and the functioning of the limbic system, especially in the area of non-conscious memories.

Learning and memory are interdependent processes that are key to any sustained behavioural change. We have now elucidated areas of the brain that deal explicitly with motor skills, as well as those involved in conscious and non-conscious memories. We recognise that both memory and imagination involve the same neurobiological mechanisms, and how easy it is to install a 'false memory'. The more we find out about these systems, the more we recognise how malleable memories really are – good news for those in the change business!

In this chapter, then, we shall look in more detail at some of the important brain mechanisms involved in learning and changing. You can rest assured that I will keep the neuroanatomy as simple as possible.

Sensory systems

All incoming information – whether it be visual, auditory, kinaesthetic or gustatory – is handled in a very similar way by the brain. With few exceptions (olfactory being the prime one), information from the right half of the body, eye and ear crosses to the left side of the brain, and vice versa. Portions of the electromagnetic spectrum 'out there' in the real world travel through a series of neurological pathways before finally being assimilated in a conjoined *representation* of the world at large.

Each of our five senses deals with a finite range of that spectrum, so even at our first point of contact with the outside world, the information to which we have access is already subtly limited – even before we start processing! In fact, you may not have fully recognised until now that you can never be truly aware of all that is at large about you – does that make sense? Although we shall look in more detail at the visual system, the same principles and processes hold true for the other pathways as well.

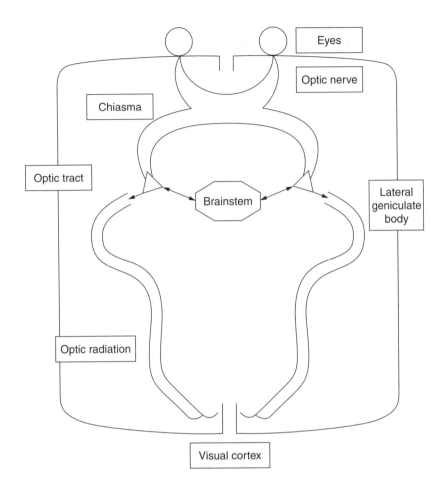

Figure 4.1:   Visual pathways.

Light from a visual stimulus passes through the lens of the eye to form an inverted image on the retina. These electromagnetic impulses are transformed by the rods and cones into electrical energy which is transmitted via the optic nerve, optic chiasma and optic tract to connect to the lateral geniculate body. During the process, information from the right half of the visual field crosses over to the left half, and vice versa.

The lateral geniculate body is part of the thalamus, which is one of the major relay stations of the brain. All incoming information from the senses passes through one or other of its nuclei en route upward to the cortex or downward to the brainstem. The thalamus is part of the limbic system, which as we shall see later plays a large part in emotions and memory.

The lateral geniculate body has a two-way connection to the brainstem, so even at this early stage of visual processing, before we are even consciously aware of what we are seeing, there is a huge amount of important non-conscious activity going on. We shall return to this again shortly. Having made the connection to the lateral geniculate body, a new set of nerves – the optic radiation – takes the further transduced information on to the visual cortex in the occipital lobe of the brain.

When it arrives at V1 – the area on the visual cortex where we have our first conscious image of what we are seeing – the information is quickly shunted to areas that deal with depth and distance, colour, motion, stereo vision, etc. In fact, it seems that what we described in the last chapter as *submodalities* actually have physical correlates in and around the visual cortex. Stimulation of one or more of these centres can literally change how we see what we see *as* we see it.

However, even at this stage, the 'picture' that we have on the visual cortex, even though we are conscious of it, is still only raw data – we have yet to make sense of it. Further neuronal relays take the information into the temporal and parietal lobes. The so-called 'what' pathway in the temporal lobe is concerned with the recognition of objects. We have subdivisions for animate and inanimate objects, facial recognition and human body parts, among many others. We are still not finished, because the act of recognition also requires an emotional input via the amygdala in the limbic system before it is eventually passed to the frontal lobe, where full recognition takes place. Of course, these are two-way systems with much information being passed back and forth and modulating the final visual product.

There is also another visual pathway – the so-called 'how' pathway. This conveys the visual data to the parietal lobe, which is concerned with spatial functions such as navigation, movement, grasping, etc. Interestingly, in the condition known as blindsight, the patient is unable to see in the normal sense because of destruction of V1 on the occipital cortex (e.g. by a stroke). However, because the 'how' pathway still has connections to it via the brainstem, the patient may still catch a ball that is thrown to them, even though they do not consciously see it – they can 'see' it non-consciously!

Therapeutic implications

'Seeing' what is out there is clearly a tremendously complex task. The impoverished set of information that our senses gather from the world is further transduced and transformed by several neurological connections, and similar data from the other senses is treated in exactly the same way. By an as yet poorly understood mechanism, the product of the input from each sensory channel is synthesised together like a holographic projection, so that the image produced by our occipital lobe appears as if it is a full sensory experience of the 'real world'.

Then, of course, we perform yet another transform – we add language. We use word labels, symbols and icons together with metaphor, poetry and mathematics, etc. to describe what our senses portray. And these descriptors – these linguistic representations – include our judgements (good and bad, better and worse). Yet all the time we are unaware that this is simply the product of a play of neuronal impulses – the theatre of our mind creating a virtual reality.

And that, of course, is the key to all this – 'as if'. We do not experience reality out there. We simply have our *interpretation* of what is going on – an interpretation of our own internal *representation*. The evidence points to the fact that 50% of the input into the occipital lobes comes from other parts of the brain, not only the eyes. Language, emotion and sensation are mixed together in ever-changing ratios. The same pathways are active when you close your eyes and remember back to your last pleasurable holiday or other such event, picturing how it looked and who was there with you. 'Seeing' is an active, synthetic, creative process. The mind is not a mirror that truthfully reflects reality.

So where does this fit with therapeutic interventions? Well, the good news is that if it is we who create the representation, then it is also we who can change it. And that is exactly what therapies such as cognitive–behavioural therapy and NLP do. They find out just how someone represents their current problem issue – their 'reality' – and then manipulate the structure of those representations (both sensory and linguistic) to facilitate learning and changing. And from a neurological point of view there are many, many points and places of intervention.

Emotions and the limbic system

When we feel an emotion such as pleasure, disgust, joy, fear, guilt or shame, we are really at the conscious end of the spectrum, explaining in cognitive terms what has actually happened non-consciously moments before. Emotion researchers such as Joseph LeDoux have found only a few primary emotions, from which the more complex ones are textured. They arise in the limbic system, a subcortical structure that includes several brain nuclei which are intimately connected – the amygdala, thalamus, caudate, putamen and hippocampus. We shall focus in due course on the fear system that resides in the amygdala.

Most researchers have suggested that the primary emotions are fear, anger, disgust and love. They do not require consciousness to act, and in fact are best thought of as primitive defence and survival mechanisms that turn us away from danger – fight or flight – and impel us to move towards areas of benefit.

Interestingly, there are more 'negative' ones than 'positive' ones! They are very much like a basic operant conditioning system that triggers automatically. Although there are two-way cortical connections, the bulk of the information flow is from the limbic system to the frontal cortex. The higher-level brain has great difficulty trying to dampen down these primary emotions when they occur. We cannot simply 'think' them away.

More complex emotions, such as guilt, shame, delight, sullenness and even anxiety, tend to involve far more of a cognitive input for their construction. They require comparisons with previously learned responses, and are synthesised from combinations of the basic emotions laced with thoughts and memories. Messages are then sent back down to the limbic system, which communicates with the hypothalamus, causing it to send neuroendocrine messages to the rest of the body.

The release of adrenaline, noradrenaline, corticosteroids and various peptides has effects on blood pressure, respiratory rate and muscle tension. In fact, each emotion has its own 'signature' of chemicals. Of course, for the primary emotions this neurohormonal cascade happens automatically – unconsciously – and we become aware that 'something is up' only by the feedback of our bodily reactions.

It is difficult to stop an emotion when it is going full steam ahead. Emotions demand action of one kind or another – that is their main purpose. Whether you hit someone, run away, scream angrily or simply have a hint of sarcasm in your voice, the message has been expressed. Higher cortical functions do not dampen down emotions terribly well. Yet actions such as repetitive handwashing in obsessive-compulsive disorder are part of a mental and physical ritual to attempt to displace the anxious feelings that are engendered. Working hard on non-emotional mental tasks tends to inhibit the amygdala, so in a sense keeping busy is a good maxim to follow. However, whenever you stop being busy, the emotions may well arise again.

Fear and the amygdala

Fear and its related construct, anxiety, are both found in many of the clinical issues that patients bring to consultation. Although fear has a useful protective function, in many of these cases (phobias, post-traumatic stress disorder, anxiety and panic attack) it is actually triggered as a conditioned response. The anatomical pathways that connect to the amygdala become very important in these situations.

All incoming sensory information travels first to the thalamus, from which it is relayed to other brain areas. There are two main pathways to the amygdala

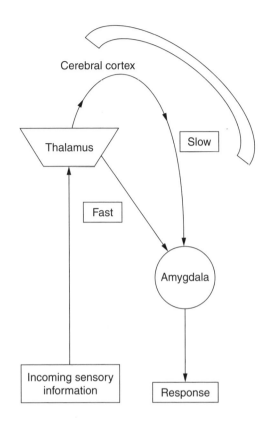

Figure 4.2:   Quick and slow pathways to the amygdala.

– the nucleus that is responsible for fear and also anger. The first, somewhat tortuous pathway goes via the thalamus to the cerebral cortex, where it further relays with information-gathering and recognition systems prior to connecting back with instructions to the amygdala. In neurological terms, this can take a considerable period of time.

The second pathway is much quicker yet less discriminatory. From the sensory input that goes to the thalamus (e.g. from the visual pathway) there is a direct, one-stop connection to the amygdala. This can trigger an immediate fight or flight reaction via the release of hypothalamic hormone. Movement along this pathway is so quick that it happens before you are consciously aware of the stimulus – you have not even consciously registered what you have 'seen'. Conditioned fear responses seem to take this pathway preferentially. For example, if you have a phobia of an insect (e.g. a bee or wasp), then your amygdala will already have 'seen' it and initiated the phobic response *before* you actually register it consciously on your visual cortex.

So how does this conditioning arise? It seems that the amygdala can store non-conscious memories in much the same way that other parts of the brain register conscious memories. Phobias arise through Pavlovian conditioned responses in a similar manner to dogs salivating in response to the sound of bells. Exposure to a situation with the concurrent triggering of a fear response causes the two to be inextricably linked. In post-traumatic stress disorder, the memory may literally be 'burnt' into the amygdala with the simultaneously high circulating levels of stress hormone and neurotransmitter acting like photographic plate fixatives.

During periods of high stress and anxiety, these hormonal responses not only make the amygdala more sensitive to laying down unconscious memories, but also interfere with the normal processing of conscious memories. Therefore in a traumatic situation (e.g. rape) the conscious memory of the event may be very fragmented, yet the unconscious memory may trigger reactions to other environmental stimuli (VAKOG) that were present yet peripheral to the action. Sometimes the memory can even be completely unconscious. Patients may then find themselves becoming uneasy in certain situations and contexts for no 'apparent' reason. Because the amygdala is sensitive to the circulating levels of stress hormones, other causes of stress may inadvertently trigger the original anxiety-provoking memory.

A standard and time-honoured intervention for this type of problem is exposure therapy with extinction of the fear-related response. However, LeDoux's evidence (albeit mostly with rats!) suggests that this effects a 'cure' by cortical over-riding of the amygdala. In times of extreme stress produced by other events, the previously treated problem may then flare up again. This is not altogether surprising, as in 'live' exposure therapy the patient has to endure enough anxiety for it to peak, cross the threshold, and then develop into a neutral response, while remaining in the fear-provoking situation.

Other approaches may be more beneficial. *Counter-conditioning* uses another emotional response – ranging from complete relaxation through to pleasure and sexual arousal – to compete with the original stimulus. Pleasure in particular has a strong inhibitory effect on the amygdala. Rather than cognitively 'thinking' the problem away, one emotion can neutralise the other.

Newer techniques such as eye movement desensitisation and reprocessing (EMDR) and the NLP phobia cure are also very useful and powerful. It may be that they allow processing of the unconsciously stored memory in the amygdala so that it becomes consciously stored via the hippocampus instead. Then it can be safely rerouted into long-term memory, now coded as a 'past' event with much less emotional significance.

Memory and learning

Memory and learning are not quite synonymous, yet they are inextricably linked. Most people think of memory as one type of 'compartment' in the brain, where everything we 'know' is contained. However, there are four main types of memory storage, depending on the kind of experience it involves.

Motor skills – the habitual things we do everyday, including the oft-repeated statement 'you always remember how to ride a bike' – are stored both in the putamen (limbic system) and in the cerebellum. They require little conscious activity for their re-enactment. Instinctual reflexes, and very deeply ingrained habits which may have a genetic component, are stored in the caudate.

What we usually think of as memory is divided into two components, namely semantic and episodic memory. Semantic memory is like our general knowledge about the world – facts and figures. We know the name of the capital city of our own country, yet we have no real recollection of when we first learned that fact. We know many thousands of words in our native language and what they mean, but we cannot recall just exactly when and where we were or who else was present when we learned them. It is an *atemporal* memory system – it does not require time for expression. Our values – the words that express the things that are highly important to us – fit here, too. This type of memory is stored in the temporal lobe, and retrieval is assisted by the frontal lobes of the brain.

Episodic memory is our personal past memory, filled with details such as when the event occurred, who was there, the sights and sounds, the prevailing mood and even the smells and tastes. This is the kind of memory that is stored with a film-like quality so that remembering involves conjuring up the whole experience – it is *temporal* in nature. This type of memory is heavily state dependent – the more positive or negative the state, the more likely it is that we will remember the event. In fact, recalling the event will bring back the prevailing state of mind you were in when the memory was laid down. Trivial past events that have little or no attached emotion are easily forgotten. What did you have for your Friday tea three weeks ago? Episodic memory seems to be stored in fragments throughout the cortex, and once again the frontal lobes are the key to its retrieval and reconstitution.

We have already discussed the fourth memory system, namely the amygdala. This stores all fear-based memories, such as phobias and flashbacks, and includes a large non-conscious element.

Encoding memories

Organisation and consolidation of memories take place in the hippocampus. If the latter has been destroyed (by a rare stroke or, as in one famous case, by neurosurgical procedures), the person cannot learn anything new from that moment onward. They remain frozen in time. The hippocampus has links to virtually every part of the cortex, and it acts as a sorting and relay centre for information. It seems to synthesise all of the sensory data from the various parts of the brain into a holographic representation which it 'glues' together into an event or 'episode'.

Consolidation of this episode into a memory takes place during sleep, when the events of the day are replayed over and over. This repetitive regeneration is akin to laser etching on a compact disc. The more emotion there is involved in the event, the deeper the etching. Full consolidation may take as long as two years. Then the encoded memory is deposited in various parts of the cortex to be reconstituted by the frontal lobes. Because they are 'glued' together, remembering only one of the original elements of the event (sights, sounds, smells, etc.) brings up the whole memory holographically. This, of course, is the basis of the NLP anchoring techniques that we shall encounter shortly.

Consolidation can be affected by stress hormones and lack of sleep. Although a short burst of stress hormones is required as a photographic fixative, too much can have different effects. In chronic long-term stress, the encoding process may simply not occur – events are not laid down, so there is little or no recall. However, with very high circulating levels of stress hormones, not only is there poor laying down of hippocampal memory, but the amygdala will lay down non-conscious memories instead. This can give rise to feelings of dread for no 'apparent' reason.

Remembering

Memories are not objective facts that can be replayed in much the same way as the home-made video of your summer holiday. They are highly subjective and malleable. The act of remembering is an active, synthetic process. We create and recreate our memories every time we bring one to mind. Depending on which part of the memory we focus on, the experience may be different each time we remember it. And not only that – how we remember it also depends on our current state of mind when we conjure it up again.

Each time we recreate the memory, there is a possibility that we can add nuances to it which can change it a little – or a lot. We can be so creative in our remembering that the memory may bear little resemblance to what 'actually' happened. This is not entirely surprising, since we learned in the section on the visual system that we can never know reality 'out there', only our representation and interpretation of it 'in here'. We may re-edit a memory of what someone said, add in what we should have said or done in reply but did not, run that version over and over again, and end up with our own personal 'contamination' of the event. In fact, all memories are potentially contaminated in this way.

We can also selectively enhance certain events so that we are more likely to remember them over the course of time. Since strong emotional states are correlated with long-term recall, we can manipulate our state at the time of learning so that it facilitates easy recollection of the material. For example, we can deliberately evoke positive emotions prior to a learning event. Or, when remembering an event, we can enhance it by the addition of evocative associations – the basis of many mnemonic-type techniques.

The structure of a memory can change over time. A person who is in the acute stages of grief over a bereavement remembers the deceased in a very different way once that grief has been resolved. Usually this involves the passage of time, as memories naturally fade a little. Furthermore, being in different states of mind when doing the remembering (e.g. happy or some other positive emotion) will change the emotional tone of the original memory. This is like counter-conditioning done slowly over many months. The NLP grief resolution process (*see* Chapter 12) can markedly speed up this process.

It is also entirely possible to install false memories of events that never even occurred. The false memory syndrome can be brought about by well-meaning therapists insisting that some long-forgotten episode of abuse is the cause of today's symptoms and must be recovered. In a trance-like, emotionally charged state, it is actually quite easy to unwittingly lead a patient to 'remember' a non-existent event.

Although it can be difficult to sort this out – as the courts in the USA know only too well – it is possible that brain imaging can shed some light. It may be that different areas of the brain are activated with a false memory and that the 'unconscious' knows the difference even if the patient is not consciously aware of it. Given that memories are state-dependent phenomena, it is possible that two differing memories of the same event or time span may coexist separately – kept apart by the different encoding states.

Happiness, pleasure and addiction

Happiness is a state of mind that has several components. We are usually aware of the feelings of physical pleasure, the absence of negative emotions and a sense of meaningfulness and connection. It is mediated by a wave of dopamine spreading through different neurological pathways. The state only lasts for as long as the dopamine continues to flow. In this strong sense of well-being there are powerful inhibitory effects on the amygdala that prevent the expression of fear-based reactions. Dopamine-induced states can act as powerful counter-conditioners, as we shall see in the chapters to come.

Dopamine activates the ventromedial area of the prefrontal cortex. This is the frontal lobe centre that gives us an increased feeling of cohesiveness and meaning as we relate to everyday life. Too much stimulation can lead to mania – with everything and everyone being connected in a grandiose way. Too little leads to the senseless and fragmented meaninglessness of depression.

Too much or too little dopamine in other parts of the brain is associated with a variety of clinical conditions. Too little dopamine in the basal ganglia gives rise to Parkinson's disease, which is characterised by difficulty in initiating voluntary movements, with accompanying rigidity and tremor, whereas too much dopamine is implicated in Tourette's syndrome, with uncontrolled vocal and motor tics. In the pathways that lead to the frontal cortex, excess dopamine is associated with the florid visual hallucinations of schizophrenia, and hypomania. Deficiency is linked to depression and the so-called negative symptoms of schizophrenia such as lethargy, catalepsy and withdrawal. There are important connections to the orbital cortex (the part of the frontal lobes that is just above the eyes). This area is concerned with planning various actions, and overactivity here is implicated in obsessive-compulsive disorder.

Dopamine is intimately connected with the brain's reward system. In fact, the rush of dopamine that occurs when we get what we want leads to a sense of relief and satisfaction. This occurs when an external (or internal) stimulus causes changes in the limbic system that gives us our 'urges' of desire which are registered consciously. We then set in train a series of actions that result in getting what we want – achieving our goal and deriving the satisfaction that goes with it. However, when we are thwarted or frustrated the dopamine levels fail to rise, and we are left with a dysphoric feeling.

Increased levels of dopamine in the nucleus accumbens (limbic system) are the key to mediating both the reward and positive reinforcement of the various drugs of misuse (with the exception of benzodiazepines). Dopamine levels increase in response to certain cues which have become conditioned reflexes associated with the addiction (e.g. syringe, needle, public house, cigarette advert, etc.). Thus seeing the cue triggers a dysphoria that increases the drive to obtain the drug. This may be a particular area where varieties of counter-conditioning by anchoring can have a therapeutic effect.

Drugs of addiction cause binding and therefore reduced availability of dopamine receptor sites. This in turn increases the drive to take more of the drug to give the same feelings of satisfaction by releasing more dopamine. This is a major factor in withdrawal, as low levels of dopamine are associated with increased craving, drug seeking and relapse. The release of dopamine provides relief from withdrawal symptoms and therefore acts by operant conditioning as a negative reinforcer. Interventions could be targeted by inducing those states that release dopamine, linking them by classical and operant conditioning methodologies to various points along the addictions pathway.

Executive functions

The frontal lobes are the executive parts of our brains. They deal with our many ideas, plans and strategies, and they host our short-term memory – we can keep things in mind as we work on them. They are the seat of self-awareness and help us to focus attention, control impulses and attend to our subjective feelings. We can arrange incoming material into concepts, bind various perceptions together, make meaning of the world and use all of these to construct feedforward predictions about the future.

It is from our frontal lobes that our individual personalities emerge, and damage to them (both gross and subtle) can lead to major changes in personality expression. It is not surprising, then, that conditions such as schizophrenia, hypomania, depression, attention deficit hyperactivity disorder (ADHD) and obsessive-compulsive disorder (OCD) are linked to frontal lobe dysfunctions. The frontal lobes may also be overwhelmed from time to time by floods of emotion that arise from the many connections from the limbic system. There are fewer connections travelling in the reverse direction, although thinking hard about certain concepts (e.g. mathematical formulae) or getting active and doing something physically can both reduce the emotional overwhelming. These strategies are often used as distraction behaviours to counteract anxiety.

The orbito-frontal cortex (above the eyes) is important for the perception of pleasant and unpleasant odours, the representation of the reward value of a stimulus, and the guiding of goal-directed and normal social behaviour. The insula (an area where the frontal and temporal lobes meet) is important in conditioned taste aversion, anxiety, nausea and pain perception. These higher functions can be used both in goal-setting processes and in planning aversive stimuli to be used in counter- and operant conditioning.

The incidence of conditions such as depression seems to be increasing exponentially decade by decade. In general medical practice, approximately two in every five patients have this either as a presenting condition by itself or linked to another clinical problem. Various brain imaging and scanning studies have clearly shown the reduction in activity of many parts of the frontal lobes. Other parts of the parietal and temporal lobes that usually mediate external attentional focus are also underactive. This shows that people who are depressed are generally internally focused and shut down.

The anterior cingulate cortex lies a few inches directly behind the eyes on the inside edge of the invaginated folds of the frontal cortex. It has many rich connections with the limbic system, and may indeed be a type of emotional control centre. High levels of activity in this centre are associated with mania – an overwhelming feeling of connectedness to all things and significance in every little detail. However, it seems that in depression it is active in a different way. The prefrontal lobes pull out sad memories from the past, the amygdala summons up the requisite negative emotion, and the anterior cingulate 'glues' them together, further locking attention into a spiral of depressing thoughts and feelings. This shows the importance of interventional strategies which can distance the sad memories and replace them with ones associated with positive emotions to lock on to instead.

The anterior cingulate cortex is also involved in pain perception. Scans show that it 'lights up' strongly both when we consciously experience pain and when we are mindful of strong emotions. Interestingly, in patients who have silent angina (i.e. are consciously unaware of their cardiac ischaemia) this region is quiet. Pain is a complex constructed perception in much the same way as our conscious appreciation of underlying emotions. As such we can engage in various mental distractions initiated by the frontal lobe (e.g. mental arithmetic, imaging the view of a room from a different perspective, etc.) which can diminish our perception of discomfort.

Pain is also reduced by opioid painkillers such as morphine, which block the receptors in neurons that are normally filled by endorphins and enkephalins. These are the body's natural opiates which are produced in response to acute pain stimuli. They dampen down activity in the anterior cingulate cortex, mediating a reduction in conscious pain perception. It is possible to increase the level of circulating brain endorphins by employing vivid imagery of pleasurable experiences. This can be used as an effective mental technique that is entirely within the patient's control (*see* Chapter 17).

Concluding

In general, all of the information in this chapter is extremely useful to any therapist who is attempting to work with patients who have disturbing cognitions, emotions and behaviours. We have seen that reality is 'really' a construct – something we make up in our minds in order to interpret and explain the outside world. We do not act directly on this world – only on our thoughts about it. The act of sensing is a complex mix of neurological transforms of incoming stimuli combined with our own internally generated data.

Much as we like to think of ourselves as rational beings, more often than not we are driven by the many emotional responses that arise in the limbic system, responses of which we only become aware *after* the event – as they are generated unconsciously. Cortical processes can help to modify this activity, yet when the emotions are overwhelming (e.g. as in fear) the effect can be highly intrusive at best, and paralysing at worst. The non-conscious memories that are stored in the amygdala are the target of many of the therapeutic endeavours that will be described throughout this book.

We have found that memory and imagination operate with the same neural circuitry. There are different methods of storage for each of the specific memory types – procedural, semantic, episodic and fear based. Yet for some of these, particularly episodic and fear-based memories, their structure has enormous malleability such that therapeutic change becomes eminently possible. And that change is possible in both the representation of the memory itself *and* its semantics – changing the *meaning* of the event.

We have seen that too much or too little of a brain chemical, namely dopamine, can create widely differing scenarios ranging from Parkinson's disease to mania. It is also strongly implicated in addictive disorders. Knowledge of these pathways can provide clues for intervention strategies. Higher cerebral functions arising in the frontal lobes can at least to some extent modulate and co-ordinate activity in other parts of the brain – both for good and for ill. It is becoming increasingly clear that the various parts of our brain work together synergistically to produce an emergent holographic pattern – a pattern that is amenable to change via many different approaches.

The great message of neurology is that we have constructed our interpretation of reality. Changing the construction will not change external reality – far from it. Bees and wasps will still fly around! However, what will change is *how* we deal with that reality. The rest of this book will introduce you to the methodologies and techniques of NLP that will show you *how* to radically alter those interpretations for therapeutic gain.

Practice

CHAPTER 5

Getting what you want

Introduction

Before we plunge headlong into the various techniques and clinical applications of NLP in the following chapters, there is something that we need to address first. Something that makes the process of the therapeutic encounter more productive. Something that sets both ourselves and our clients up in a way that increases the likelihood of a successful session – getting what we both want. And that, of course, is effective outcome setting.

There is no point putting to sea and setting sail without knowing our destination, our journey's end. Otherwise we shall be tossed on the waves of both prevailing wind and current, at the mercy of the elements rather than utilising our seamanship skills. All of the validated cognitive–behavioural therapies recognise the importance of setting goals for therapeutic outcomes. This is an area which NLP – an outcome-focused, solution-centred approach – has studied in depth, making a considerable impact on the formulation of realistic, achievable aims and expectations.

But first, from your own experience, how easy do you find it to set yourself a behavioural goal, and not only to stick to it, but also to achieve the desired outcome? Have you ever successfully (and deliberately) lost weight? Or stopped smoking? Or taken up and adhered to an exercise regime? How are your problem-solving skills? Do you find it easy to size up a situation and know what to do in order to effect a resolution? Have you ever personally had a clinical problem such as anxiety, depression, a phobia or a panic attack? How did you resolve it? Or do you find it easier to help patients get their outcomes met rather than your own?

And what about the converse? Have you ever been certain that you were going to fail at something? You just knew beforehand you would not be able to do it. It was an insurmountable task, even impossible looking. Yet you succeeded, against your expectations. You delightfully surprised yourself as you rose to the occasion. You found yourself, in retrospect, utilising skills that you never knew you had in the first place, or utilising existing skills in completely new ways.

Just what is going on in these examples of success and apparent failure? Are they just simply random events, a 'lucky day', simply a fluke? Or are there some underlying reasons – a process, a structure – which determine whether or not we get a result? Because we all want to increase our chances of successfully achieving our goals and having our outcomes met, NLP has elucidated the process, the structure that underlies the formulating of goals in such a way as to enhance our chances of getting what we want.

The great golfer Arnold Palmer once hit a shot off the fairway that seemed to rise only six feet or so into the air, then scuttle along the ground, running on and on, and finishing a foot away from the pin. A spectator shouted 'That was just a lucky fluke!' And Palmer replied 'Yup, and the more I practise, the luckier I get'. The art of repeatedly ensuring the setting of good clinical outcomes and determining where we want to end up, rather than merely focusing on the process of getting there, can allow us to achieve our goal by a variety of means – occasionally in unexpected ways.

Steps to successful outcomes

In this section we shall go through each of the steps required for successfully setting the kinds of outcomes that increase our patients' chances of getting what they want. In each of the succeeding chapters, the following process is implicitly utilised in each clinical situation. We shall go through each step formally here, and later in the chapter you will see how this can be used conversationally, almost casually, yet still ensuring that each base is covered adequately.

1 Stated in positives

Too many of us, when asked what we want, give our answers in the form of something to move *away from*, rather than what we want to move *towards*. We are clear about what we want to avoid or get rid of, but not so clear about what we want instead. If I ask you *not* to think about a kangaroo with wellington boots on, what happens? *You cannot not think about what you don't want to think about without thinking about it first!*

Here are some patient examples:

- *'I want to stop feeling irritated, down and depressed.'*
- *'I just don't want to be tired all the time.'*
- *'I don't want to panic when I'm in the supermarket.'*
- *'I don't want to have to go round the house continually checking that all the plugs are out.'*

- 'I want this pain to go away.'
- 'I want to stop wheezing as much.'

The difficulty with all of the above is that they focus either generally or in more specific detail on what is *not* wanted. In so doing, however, they run the risk of more of the same. So what can we do instead? How do we turn this around? The most important question to ask is **'What do you want instead?'**

And keep on asking it until what is said is stated in the positive – the direction you want to go towards.

- 'I want to feel more of the joys of life, be happier in myself.'
- 'I want to have more energy.'
- 'I want to push my trolley calmly round the supermarket aisles.'
- 'I want to go out of the house with a clear mind.'
- 'I want to feel more comfortable more often.'
- 'I want to feel that I can get a deep enough breath whenever I want.'

The most important part of this section, that will benefit all aspects of your developing communication skills, whether they be with patients, friends, colleagues or family members, is to *get into the habit of saying things in the way you want them to turn out.*

2 Started and maintained by you

When confronted with health challenges, many individuals leave their outcome in other people's hands, allowing themselves inadvertently to become victims of a developing situation, with the resolution being outwith their control. If we set up our outcomes such that other people have to make changes before we can get what we want, then we are significantly reducing our chances of success, leaving things more and more in the lap of the gods. This in itself is both stressful and further debilitating to health.

One patient was suffering such increased job stress that she came to see me requesting to be 'signed off' work. She had been experiencing increasing difficulties with her immediate superior, who was not 'pulling his weight'. More and more of the administrative burden of the department was falling on her shoulders. She was not sleeping well, could not focus clearly on her day-to-day tasks, and was continually on the verge of tears. 'If only he would change, do more of his own tasks, live up to his responsibilities, then I would feel much better', she bewailed. She felt that she could not confront him without breaking down. The only solution, it seemed, was to avoid going to work.

Clearly her superior needed to make changes. Yet in reality she herself had little control of that particular outcome. When we explored the situation in more depth, we found that there were certain things that she could do for *herself* to ease the situation. She learned to prioritise her own tasks within her job description, leaving undone those tasks that were his responsibility. She remembered a time when she had calmly and successfully confronted an angry man who had bashed into her car in a car park. She began using the same skill with her superior in this new situation. She also wrote down her concerns about his continued poor performance and brought them to the attention of *his* superior. In effect, she did the very things that were within *her* control.

The question to ask here is **'What resources can you personally bring to bear on this situation?'**

Of course, these resources may be the very skills you have already been utilising in other contexts in the past. In a sense these skills may be dissociated from the current situation, and in some way need to be revivified, amplified and connected to the place where they are needed. Sometimes the resource required is actually a particular skill that is lacking and has not yet been developed. From modelling what works in that particular context for other people, the skill can be learned, rehearsed and applied appropriately. You will find many ways to do this in subsequent chapters.

In order even to start heading towards a particular outcome, another important question we need to ask is **'What would having that outcome do for you?'**

This 'chunks up' to the larger benefits of achieving the goal, and in so doing provides a higher degree of motivation to continue doing what is necessary to achieve your aim. I asked the patient in the above example what would be the *benefit* of effectively confronting her superior. Her answers were 'a feeling of relief, the satisfaction of knowing I'd done the right thing, and an increase in my confidence and self-esteem'. These benefits became the continuing embedded motivators that helped her to put the specific skills into action.

Ultimately, we are only potentially in control of ourselves – our own thoughts, feelings, behaviours and outcomes. The converse also applies – we are not responsible for another person's behaviours, feelings and actions. However, we can develop the capacity to *influence* them appropriately in some way, developing a 'win–win' outcome so that both sets of needs are respectfully met. We may be able to change our own behaviours in a way that encourages others to help us to get what we want. By imagining ourselves in their shoes, we can ask ourselves the following additional questions:

- **'What do I need to do to ensure that they want to help me to achieve my outcome?'**
- **'What are the most persuasive elements from their perspective?'**

3 Sensory-based evidence

One of the main problems in setting outcomes is being too vague about what is really wanted. A goal of 'feeling better in myself', 'I just want to be happy' or 'to have more self-esteem' is really too abstractly conceptualised to allow for meaningful accomplishment. Accepting patients' aims that are so general almost dooms the ensuing consultations and interventions to failure. We need to express outcomes in far more specific and detailed terms.

Cognitive–behavioural therapies in general and NLP approaches in particular focus very much on obtaining a clear, specific, sensory-based, behavioural description of what the patient really wants. We ask them to imagine having successfully achieved their goal, and to specify what is *different* in their ongoing sensory experience now.

The following questions are useful:

- *'How will you know when you have your outcome?'*
- *'What will you be seeing, hearing, feeling, smelling and tasting?'*
- *'If someone else saw you achieving your outcome, what would they be noticing?'*

We need to target the particular behaviour that the patient will be doing *instead*. The more the outcome is vividly imagined 'as if' it was real, and the more detailed the sensory description, the more likely it will be that you can build the kind of positive expectation that fuels self-efficacy. Often it is useful to imagine that someone has video-taped the patient's success and now you are both looking at it from a comfortable distance – an outside view, as it were. This 'believed-in' future representation acts as a powerfully compelling *attractor* for directionalised change.

Some examples include the following:

- *'I can see myself running upstairs breathing easily, my inhaler in my pocket.'*
- *'There's a crowd of people at the supermarket and I'm feeling calm inside, simply focusing on my shopping list.'*
- *'I've checked the plugs once, forgotten all about them now I'm outside, and am playing with the kids, hearing their laughter.'*
- *'With all the energy I've got, I've taken up jogging again. I look so fit and trim!'*

When we look at the *miracle question* shortly you will see how this sensory-based description can flow in a simple conversational format.

4 Consider consequences and by-products

Many of the perceived difficulties and challenges involved in either making a successful change or simply staying the same are all about the potential consequences that arise when we contemplate doing something different. We indulge in consequential thinking when, having imagined successfully achieving our outcome, we notice the knock-on effects, for better or worse, that may also occur as a result. Sometimes getting what we think we want may have unlooked-for negative effects that quickly become apparent. We may lack a safety net. Furthermore, choosing one particular course of action means choosing *not* to pursue other avenues – in effect leaving them closed off. Every choice has an upside (the potential benefits and gains) and a downside (the potential drawbacks and losses).

Of course, there are also consequences of remaining the same and choosing not to make changes. The saying 'better the devil you know' typifies this form of thinking where there is a certain comfort, security and perceived benefit in staying exactly as we are. This is sometimes (often pejoratively) called the *secondary gain* of a clinical problem, a typical example being the care and attention we receive from loved ones because we are 'ill', which evaporates as soon as we are better! It is important to identify any positive intention underlying a troublesome recurrent behavioural pattern, and to make certain that this is then incorporated within the solution. This helps to ensure that subsequent change fits ecologically with current systems. Of course, the downside of staying as we are is the stagnation that accompanies failing to open ourselves to learning and developing new skills, further tightening the often self-imposed straitjacket.

We therefore need to weigh the consequences of achieving any outcome against those of remaining the same. Exploring these issues with the following questions can help to tease out the directional motivating dynamics, whose energies we can then realign more appropriately.

- *'What will you gain/lose by achieving your outcome?'*
- *'What will you gain/lose by remaining the same?'*

I once had a patient with a social phobia. He wanted to be more comfortable in social gatherings of more than a few people. He felt that his self-confidence would increase, he would make more friends, develop new interests, and possibly even meet 'Miss Right'. However, he recognised that one of his solitary pleasures was 'losing himself' in great literary works, which he could do for hours at a time. Consequently there might be far less time available for doing the things he currently enjoyed. He also began to understand that his present avoidant strategy had the aim of keeping him safe, secure and comfortable. Although he was initially daunted by the fact that there were several social skills he needed to learn, he knew that failing to act and staying as he was would prevent the longer-term deeper satisfaction of developing a more intimate relationship.

Teasing out the various consequences in this way – what insurance companies call upside and downside planning – flushes out the more significant variables, which when fully attended to allow for more balanced outcome setting and increased potential for actual achievement.

5 Identify limiting factors

Sometimes accessing the specific resources that are required and applying them to our goal is all we need to do to ensure our outcome. However, there may be particular obstacles that get in our way and current limitations that we need to deal with first, before the path to our destination is clear. Failure to attend to these is like driving a car with one foot on the accelerator and the other simultaneously on the brake. Our self-imposed 'drag' holds us back. This is a classic self-organising systems problem whereby the main intervention is to remove the limitation, rather than stepping harder on the 'gas'.

The first question to ask is '**What prevents you from achieving your outcome?**'

You can examine the answers to this question in terms of the *logical levels* categories. Some obstacles may be on an *environmental* level, such as lack of money, materials, information or some other external resource. Perhaps you think you lack a particular *behaviour* or *capability* (skill). Maybe the limiting factor is at the level of *beliefs*, *values* or *identity*. You may believe that you just cannot develop a particular skill or response. Perhaps there is a values conflict – an internal debate about what is more important in this situation. You may think that you are just not the kind of person who can succeed, or worse still that you do not deserve to. Identifying the level at which the blockage takes place will help you to decide which specific NLP tool is required for change. The following question will further elucidate what is needed: '**What resource(s) do you need instead?**'

Often we find that the specific skills required are actually present in our lives in a completely different context, yet because we have coded them differently in our minds, it is as if we have forgotten that they exist.

Pauline came to consult about feeling 'tired all the time' and stressed out from work. She had been promoted to a manager's role a few months earlier, and felt that she was not coping with her staff. She was finding resolving conflict between two staff members especially difficult. What stopped her was 'I'm just no good at sorting out people problems'. What she needed instead were 'negotiating skills', but despite reading books on the subject she still felt bemused. We examined various contexts in her life, and it became clear that she was actually pretty good at sorting out the various arguments and territorial disputes that took place between her 11-year-old daughter and 9-year-old son. She had never thought of these as negotiating skills before, just a 'knack' for keeping the peace in a win–win fashion. With these practical examples suitably revivified and recontextualised in her mind, she went on to use the same skills successfully at work.

6 Ecology concerns

An ecology check ensures that your current aims, aspirations, goals and outcomes fit not only with yourself, but also within the wider systems to which you belong, such as family, friends, work, social system and the larger community. When outcomes fail to materialise, it is often because ecology has been violated in some way.

Take the problem of serious drug addiction – for example, to heroin. Getting off heroin is actually relatively easy, but staying off is a different matter altogether. Just consider this. If your whole way of life has been concerned with getting enough money by various means to obtain your next fix (often illegal *and* exciting), if all of your friends and social acquaintances are part of the drug scene, and if the neighbourhood in which you live is already run down with high unemployment to boot, then unless you have a complete social transplant, the current system will tend to prevent lasting change. This is not to negate the good work that is already being done by drug counsellors, but simply to widen the perspective to include all of the salient factors.

Of course, an individual can also have internal ecology concerns, when the attempted solution itself becomes the problem. This is like having two parts of yourself embroiled in inner conflict. A patient with asthma was also a smoker. She smoked to calm herself down, to ensure her personal space and to 'have time for me'. Unfortunately, this made her asthma worse. Part of her wanted to stop smoking in order to improve her overall health, yet another part wanted to continue in order to obtain the above-mentioned gains. This kind of incongruency needs to be both recognised and respectfully dealt with in order to ensure a solution that fits the whole person.

Watch out for responses that start with any of the following:

* *'Yes, but ...'*
* *'On the one hand ..., yet on the other ...'*
* *'Well, part of me wants to ... but another part ...'*

We shall deal more fully with the mechanisms for resolving more major degrees of incongruency in Chapter 16.

Specific questions that check for ecology and which can be used at any time in the outcome-setting process include the following:

- *'How will this outcome fit with the rest of you? Your family? Your friends? Your business? Your job?'*
- *'How will getting your outcome benefit the other people in your life? Is it a win–win approach?'*
- *'Is it worth the cost to you?'*
- *'Does it fit with your sense of self?'*

It has become clearer to me over the past year or so that specifically incorporating how *others* will benefit from your outcome is a very important, yet often over-looked aspect. It seems that by widening your thinking to include the positive effect that achieving your outcome will have on others, you cause a ripple effect in the systems to which you belong that appears to allow a more pervasive degree of change. It also helps to fit smaller outcomes into the larger frames of patients' health beliefs and expectations, ensuring a greater degree of leverage, motivation and the commitment required for success in any endeavour.

Figure 5.1 shows a useful *aide-mémoire* (adapted from Ian McDermott) for setting outcomes. Photocopy it and have it visible when you are consulting.

Unconscious caveats

The outcome process we have just considered can be a very powerful tool when used to achieve clinical goals. Yet it can be too rigidly 'conscious' and logical in its application if we fail to calibrate effectively to the non-verbal communication of parallel unconscious processing. Non-verbal messages accompany all aspects of communication – and can be at variance with the spoken word. And occasion-ally the solutions of our conscious mind are actually keeping the problem going by their rational attempts to resolve it – the attempted solution *is* the problem. During outcome-setting processes, then, it is important to have a mechanism that allows us to ascertain the patient's congruence (conscious and uncon-scious agreement) about the desired goal. In this respect, NLP co-founder John Grinder would rather turn most of the outcome setting over to the unconscious mind.

There are (at least) two ways in which we can ensure this degree of con-gruence in the chosen outcome. One way is to develop our calibration skills so that during conversational elicitation of the patient's goals we can look for their 'yes-set' (*see Consulting with NLP* by Lewis Walker). These are the minimal cues

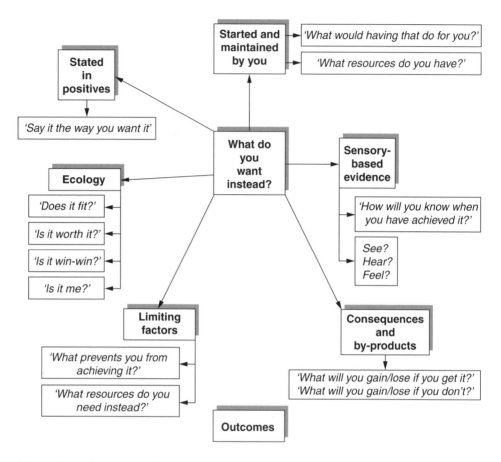

Figure 5.1:   Outcome setting.

and non-conscious responses that are apparent in unequivocal agreement. If these signals are reliably present with the chosen outcome, then we can move forward with confidence. If not, we need to backtrack and sort out any incongruency.

In Chapter 13 you will be introduced to a method that allows both you and your patient to calibrate more effectively to unconscious mechanisms for change. You will learn how to engage unconscious processes so that the patient can have a direct and clear internal signal for 'yes' and 'no'. These signals can be used to ratify or even choose outcomes that are ecological for the whole system. In this way, then, you can bring the formidable resources of non-conscious processing to bear on the current situation for more effective goal setting.

The miracle question

We have discussed the various underlying principles and questions which can help to elucidate just exactly which outcomes our patients may want instead. In one respect it can seem quite formal to ask about each facet in this way. Yet the above is merely a guide – an internal map if you like – to help to ensure that you cover all of the bases. It is quite possible, even desirable, to elicit outcomes in a more conversational format that fits with the ebb and flow of ordinary consultations. So just exactly how can you do this?

Steve de Shazer, an exponent of solution-focused therapy, believes that *noticing differences* and putting them to work is a key element of any change process. Too many people, as we have seen above, focus on what is wrong. By asking the *miracle question*, de Shazer conversationally opens up a solution space to contemplate what life would be like if the problem had simply disappeared. Here is the question.

> ***'Imagine that you went to bed tonight and while you were asleep a miracle occurred, such that when you awoke your problem had gone. You do not know how or why, because you were asleep. You only know that it has gone. Tell me what would be different now.'***

Let's look at this further in action. The patient is a 53-year-old binge drinker. These days he is more often under the influence of alcohol than not. His long-suffering wife, who has her own problems with anxiety, barely tolerates him now. His married daughter often gets a call to come over and help to clean him up. At times he recognises that he 'needs to do something about it', but he rarely gets around to this, having had a few failed encounters with Alcoholics Anonymous in the past. Unexpectedly, having rarely consulted about this problem, he turns up sober for today's appointment. Given all that has been going on for him, I ask him what he wants instead.

> Patient: *Well, it's like I just don't seem to be able to say no to drink ... I want to, but I can't ... I can't see how it could be different ... (looks off into the middle distance) ... believe me, I've tried ... I just seem to always give in to the urge.*
> Doctor: *Yeah ... and I understand it's not easy to simply tell yourself not to (nods head). ... Could I ask you a question ... and it might seem a bit daft ... initially ... but sometimes it helps people think differently ... ?*
> Patient: *I suppose so ... (looking at the floor).*
> Doctor: *OK, here goes. ... Just imagine you go to bed tonight ... like you do most nights ... but this night is different ... tonight when you're sleeping ... a miracle occurs ... the kind of miracle that when you wake up in the morning ... your problem's gone ... completely ... resolved.*

Patient: *Fat chance, doctor ... have you been drinking? ... (we both laugh).*

Doctor: *Yeah ... seems a strange thought, doesn't it? Yet, what if ... maybe if we pretend ...*

Patient: *You mean imagine?*

Doctor: *Yeah ... imagine that you don't know how ... you don't know why ... all you know is that for some reason ... a quirk of fate perhaps ... and you're better ... it's all over ... gone ... what's different about you then?*

Patient: *Different ... (thinks long and hard) ... well ... I suppose my tongue doesn't feel stuck to the roof of my mouth ... and I'm not bursting to pee!*

Doctor: *So if it's not stuck ... and you don't need a pee ... what are you noticing instead?*

Patient: *I suppose I feel a bit more human ... not like the dregs of humanity ... (laughs).*

Doctor: *Suppose you go the bathroom ... and look in the mirror ... what do you see?*

Patient: *What do I see? ...* **well me**, *of course!* (note the linguistic ambiguity).

Doctor: *Well ... so how do you look different?*

Patient: *Well, my eyes ... they're not red and scary like!*

Doctor: *So what do you see instead?*

Patient: *(contemplatively) ... it's like ... and this might sound a bit daft ... it's like I used to look like 10 years ago ... younger ... my hair's tidy ... even my nostril hairs are clipped! (straightens up in the chair, head rises, shoulders go back)*

Doctor: *So, imagine ... like this ... you go downstairs ... for breakfast ... how would Mary know ... without you telling her ... you're different now ... changed now?*

Patient: *She'd have a fit ... I never make it to breakfast!*

Doctor: *Yet if you did ... make it, that is ... what would she notice that was different?*

Patient: *Well ... (takes a big breath)... I'm clean-shaven ... got clean clothes on ... she'll never believe this!*

Doctor: *And when you speak ... how does she know in your voice ... you're better now?*

Patient: *(cracks up laughing) ... well, the fact we're even speaking is a minor miracle ... especially at that time of day ... it's been such a time (wistfully).*

Doctor: *So ... being this way ... what are the benefits?*

Patient: *Well ... I'm healthier for a start ... Mary and I ... well, things are better between us ... a bit more money as well.*

Doctor: *Tell me about Gill (daughter) ... how would she know you've changed now?*

Patient: *Well ... she wouldn't have to come across and get things cleaned up so much.*

Doctor: *So what's different? ... What does she notice instead?*
Patient: *I'm not sure ... probably just that I'm clean ... doing more for myself.*
Doctor: *So what sort of things would you be doing to occupy your time?*
Patient: *Hmm ... well the chances of a job are not great ... I dunno ... I used to be a dab hand at building doll's houses, cribs ... that sort of thing ... I was always good with my hands ... I do need something to occupy me.*
Doctor: *And you know ... being realistic ... there are bound to be times you get that urge ... what happens then? ... how do you get round that?*
Patient: *(thinks long and hard) ... I'm not sure about that ... I've slipped up so many times ...*
Doctor: *Well ... maybe ... in between now and our next consultation ... it might be an idea to ponder a bit more about that question ...*

We have just begun, conversationally, in a short consultation, to elicit the important parts of a well-formed outcome. You can check just which of the bases we have covered and which ones remain. Binge drinking is a challenging problem, and there are no 'one step and you are free' solutions. Yet thinking in this way, about *what you want to have happen instead,* can be quite liberating, and it can form the early building blocks upon which you can add many of the change techniques described in the following chapters. As a sequential incongruity, this kind of problem is often best managed by a parts integration process (*see* Chapter 16). Yet at the same time, de Shazer himself reports finding that many patients have already improved substantially after two or three conversational sessions like the one above *(see Words Were Originally Magic by Steve de Shazer).*

Concluding

I cannot really over-emphasise the importance of setting well-formed outcomes. They are the foundational aspect on which therapeutic success is built – regardless of the underlying clinical concern. Ensuring that your patients consider these questions carefully, by constructing a detailed, sensory-rich picture of what they really want, unleashes powerful forces for ecological change work. It markedly increases self-efficacy, that believed-in ability to not only know that the outcome is possible, but also that they have the capabilities and the overarching sense of self-worth for successful achievement. In self-organising theory terms, they have carved out a compelling *attractor* symbol which, every time they think of it, begins to draw them inexorably and almost magnetically towards the realisation of their goal.

So as this chapter ends, and you contemplate moving on to the next section of clinical encounter, namely the successful application of various NLP skills, I would like you to take a moment to consider the following. If you were the kind of doctor or health professional who was adept at setting outcomes in this way, what is it that you would be doing differently? If you could picture yourself using this skill, what would you look like and sound like, and how would it feel to act in this way? What would your patients notice that was different about you, as they are on the receiving end of respectful outcome questioning? Just how many benefits can you conceive of right *now* being this way? And if there are any obstacles to your achieving this task, you might like to think about which of your many other resources you could bring to bear in order to smooth your path. As you continue your reading, you can begin to allow this whole process to become an integral part of your consulting style, so much so that it fits you like a glove!

CHAPTER 6

Building resources

Introduction

When our patients come to see us they are usually in the throes of one problem or another. In the further telling of their tale they may find themselves drawn inexorably into its greater depths. This may be a place from which it is not easy to climb out unaided. It is generally an unresourceful state of mind and body, and the type of thinking and physiology that accompany it make it difficult both to generate solutions and to gain access to the kinds of behavioural patterns and past experiences that can make a difference for the better.

You may even have experienced this for yourself. Perhaps you have had (or currently have) a particular issue about which you ruminated excessively – one that preoccupied your thoughts, distancing you both from the present moment and from any skills that you may have had lying dormant in an unreachable inner recess of your brain. What did it feel like to be in that state? What kind of thoughts did you have? Try to remember your posture, your physiology and your gestures. There is no doubt that when people feel stuck in this way, going over and over an issue repetitively yet being unable to find the way out, solutions are hard to find.

So what is it that we need to do? Well, the simple yet non-simplistic answer is to have a mechanism which can begin to reconnect us to the kinds of powerful states that we can reaccess at will. A light which can guide us out of the tunnel. A map of the maze indicating the exit points. We need to uncover potential solutions wherever we can find them.

Solution-focused therapists are those who *find and build on patients' strengths*. They look for *what is already working* for them in their lives so far. They uncover the kinds of skills which may have lain dormant for some time, stored in the attics of people's memories. Sometimes they have to be quite creative in turning a past event into a current resource. Nevertheless, their goal is to dust off these memories, bring them into the light of day, and utilise the skills therein in the here and now.

Because finding and building resources are such an integral part of NLP, it will repay you many times over to immerse yourself in the kinds of skills that this chapter describes, in the knowledge that you will reap dividends in the pages to come.

Alex and the scanner

Alex was 28 years old when he was first diagnosed with Hodgkin's lymphoma, a type of cancer of the body's lymph glands. He had always appeared a little anxious even before that, and had been bothered by mild asthma. However, on this occasion, antibiotics and inhalers had not done the trick, and a subsequent chest X-ray had shown marked mediastinal enlargement. A lymph node biopsy confirmed the diagnosis. In order to stage the disease spread, Alex had had a CT scan from chest to abdomen.

During the procedure, which required him to lie still for several minutes while passing through a rotating tunnel that sounded like a washing-machine gone mad, he felt claustrophobic, with increasing feelings of panic and breathlessness. He had managed to survive the experience, but now that his radiotherapy and chemotherapy were over he had to undergo another scan to check his body's response to treatment. Although he wanted to go through with it, he definitely did not want to experience those feelings again. I saw him at the health centre to discuss what else we could do to help.

'Well, Alex, I know that was a difficult time you *had* had back then' I said, as I gestured in the direction of the past, to his left. 'What I'm interested in is how you want things to be different next week', gesturing to his right. 'How do you want to feel instead?'

'Well, comfortable, I suppose', he said, looking anything but comfortable! 'I just don't want to have any of these feelings surface again.' He took a sharp in-breath and furrowed his eyebrows as his eyes darted off furtively to his left. You will find that, like Alex, many patients who have memories which still have a negative emotional charge will often project them out into the space around them. By observing their direction of gaze you will get a glimpse into their personal coding and organising system.

'OK, let's do this slightly differently. Let's pretend that a miracle had occurred through the night ... the problem is magically gone ... you don't know how or why ... only that it's the day of the scan and you're feeling fine. Talk me through what's happening.'

'That sounds a bit of a tall order!' he said, as his eyes widened and his head moved back simultaneously. For some people, all you need to do is to reframe the question slightly as you ask it again. 'I know, and so do you, that it's not really real', I replied, 'but what if you just went ahead and pretended anyway, like make-believe.' It's interesting how many people will go ahead and suspend their critical reality with the words *pretend* and *make-believe*.

As his breathing slowed, he seemed to look into the middle distance, his pupils dilating. 'Well, I'm lying on the scanner bed, there's a radiographer adjusting things around me, and ... surprisingly ... I look fine, quite relaxed even!' He scratched his head. I asked him to give me more details about his facial expression, his breathing and anything else he noticed. 'Well, my eyes are closed, and I'm smiling a little, like I'm having a private joke inside my head.'

This time I asked him to see himself through the eyes of the radiographer, to imagine things from her perspective. 'It's like he's just another patient, going through the same old routine, with no fuss or bother. In fact it's like he's somewhere else, not paying any attention to what's happening', he said almost nonchalantly. We continued to imagine how things would look, sound and feel as he continued through to completion of the scan. Building up a description of an outcome in this way can seem like an ordinary conversation, and can be used regardless of the presenting issue.

'That all looks good in theory, doc, but I can't believe that just thinking it through like that will *really make it come true*.' Like many people, Alex was just a little sceptical at this stage – a common occurrence. And of course, outcome setting is simply the first part of the process of getting what you want. I reminded him that we had a few more things to do first before he could leave the room confident of success. (And you, the reader, can think about what is presupposed in that last sentence.)

I asked him 'What is it like when you *feel comfortable* in your body in that way?' He replied that it was a *relaxing* kind of feeling. I told him that for me, *relaxing* in that way reminded me of summer days, lying on the beach, not a care in the world. 'What gives you that relaxing feeling ... you know, when it feels so good?'

His head tilted slightly as he looked up. Then a grin spread across his face. 'I had a full body massage last year when we were on holiday. My muscles had been quite tight ... it was great ... like drifting into inner space.' I asked about the sights, the sounds and the smells, to deepen the experience of that memory. It seemed as if this would be a good one to build into a useful resource state. I asked if anything else gave him the same kind of feeling. 'Yes. Occasionally I treat myself to a steaming hot bath and just lounge in it, with some music playing softly in the background.' So fairly quickly and easily we had unearthed two past experiences in different contexts which could be utilised to his advantage in the approaching encounter with the scanner.

Because these experiences had both occurred in a recumbent position, and his forthcoming scan would be in a similar position, I suggested that for the next part – actually *building the resources* into a usable form – it would be a good idea if he lay down on my couch. I explained to him that I was going to lead him back into each memory in turn, revivifying and deepening the experiences, and that as they peaked in intensity of feeling I would anchor them by touching his knuckle. I said something along the following lines.

'As you think about your massage, and the *relaxing feelings*, you can start by picturing the room you were in ... the masseuse ... the sights ... the sounds ... and the smells. As you *go there now* ... you can go more *deeply inside yourself* ... adjusting your internal pictures and sounds so that it *feels just right*. And with each breath you take you can *deepen the experience* ... allowing the *comfort to spread ... all over ...*'

With another two or three breaths his face had gone flaccid and slightly flushed, and on a deeper exhale I reached over to touch his knuckle, saying 'relaaaxiinng ... nowww' in a longer drawn-out way. In NLP terms, I had set a kinaesthetic anchor, a Pavlovian conditioned response, so that touching his knuckle in the same way would re-elicit the state. I asked him to clear his mind and then repeated the same process, both to deepen the relaxed state and to intensify the connecting anchor.

We did exactly the same thing with the 'bath-time' scenario, manipulating the pictures, sounds, feelings and smells so that he felt profoundly relaxed. I anchored the experience to the *same* knuckle in identical fashion. One caveat when doing this is to ensure that *you access the same kind of feelings* in yourself so that your state changes, too, and you flow in synchrony with your patient. This maintains and deepens the rapport appreciably. In fact, failure to do this not only makes you appear 'wooden', but actually seems to reduce the intensity of the state for the patient!

Having set the anchor, the next step was to give Alex personal control so that he could trigger the feelings at will. I asked him 'When you're on the scanner bed, what pictures, words, sounds and gestures will allow you to *reaccess this state* whenever you need to? What is it that you see yourself doing there to remind you to *use this?*' He decided that while lying on the scanner bed he could pinch his thumb and ring finger together as he said the word 'relaaaaxxx' in a soft drawn-out tone. He would also picture the bottle of oil that the masseuse used, which he had found quite evocative.

I led him into the state again by triggering the anchor that I had set on his knuckle, and as it peaked, he practised his own visual, auditory and kinaesthetic cues. Every time I mentioned the scanner, the radiographer and the procedure itself, I touched his knuckle so that the feelings permeated his thoughts about the various aspects of the procedure to come.

With his own personal triggers set, he went off home to practise, developing an increasing sense of self-mastery as he began to relax on cue. Afterwards he reported that although he was a little apprehensive just before the scan, he found that when he lay down he went even more deeply into the relaxed state than he thought he would. He ended up with a satisfied smug grin which drew comment from the radiographer 'I know just what you're thinking, son!' His yearly check scans since then have been untroubled.

Margaret and 'the son-in-law'

Margaret, a grandmother in her fifties, came to see me about an altercation with her son-in-law, Derek. He and her daughter Lesley had been separated for a few weeks, and both Lesley and her two children (both under five) had been staying with her. On the previous Saturday, Derek had turned up late at night to the house, worse the wear for drink, aggressively demanding to take the children away with him. Although they had both been quite frightened, the women had managed to get him out prior to calling the police. Margaret had initially 'frozen with fear' and, feeling that she had dealt with the situation inadequately, wanted help with developing a more resourceful response. She wanted to be prepared for any future occurrence.

I asked her 'So given what's happened, how would you rather respond instead? What does *being resourceful* mean for you? What would be different about you if you were resourceful in that way?'

'Well, I want to be strong ... feel determined that I can stand up to him ... say clearly that enough is enough.' We explored the consequences of acting in that way. I wanted to ensure that although she could feel more confident in dealing with future situations, she would also take all of the necessary steps to ensure that her safety and that of her family came first. I did not want her to put herself unnecessarily in the firing line with false bravado.

I asked when in her past she had experienced the feeling of *'enough is enough'* – to identify a time when she had gone over the threshold and vowed *'never again'*. About five years previously she had given up smoking, for the first and only time. She had remained a non-smoker and could clearly recall the time she had given up for good. In her mind's eye, I asked her to step inside that memory again – the moment when she went over the threshold – to relive it fully again, seeing what she saw, hearing what she said, and feeling the feelings fully again.

To help revivify it more intensely, I told her to 'make the pictures *bigger, brighter, closer* ... turn up the volume of the sounds, making it *surround sound* ... intensify the feelings, allowing them to *spread all over* your body.' We repeated this again even more intensely, and as the state peaked she said forcefully *'enough is enough'*. She glowed from the inside out as I anchored the state on her knuckle.

I asked her to think of a time when she was *absolutely determined* to do something and she had done it. A time when she had committed herself 100% in pursuit of a goal in which she had succeeded. A time when she had focused completely on the task in hand, pursuing it to the end.

She recalled a time when she had gone on a 20-mile sponsored walk for a cancer charity. By the time 15 miles had elapsed, her feet were badly blistered and bleeding. She was determined to finish and steeled herself to continue. We concentrated on 'that determined feeling' as we vividly relived the memory, anchoring the feeling on a second knuckle.

For *'being strong'*, the kind of resource she meant was that of mental toughness rather than physical prowess. The kind of inner strength that told her she could endure anything. Three years previously her mother had died after a long drawn-out battle against breast cancer. Towards the end she had moved in with her, looking after her day and night. Although it had been a struggle initially, she had surprised herself by tapping into a wellspring of mental and physical energy that carried her through. In rising to the task in this way, the memory became a symbol of her fortitude. Suitably revivified, we anchored it on a third knuckle.

Margaret decided that squeezing her right hand into a fist, saying the words 'be strong', and picturing a stamped-on and crushed packet of cigarettes would be her internal cues to recreate a powerful state of being. As I fired off each anchored knuckle in turn, she used her own cues at the peak of each state. After a little practice, she found that the three original states had merged together into one highly energised yet resolute 'super-state'. In NLP terms we had *stacked* the anchors one on top of another.

As an added extra I asked her to make a picture of Derek. While she did this I fired off her anchors and she did the same. She looked rather puzzled just afterwards, and I asked what had happened. She said 'He seemed to just shrink in size, before my very eyes! And the closer he got the stronger I felt.' The very thought of Derek had now become its own self-reinforcing anchor for strengthening her resolve.

There were two further incidents of confrontation with Derek after this, both of which she coped with well. And although Lesley and he never did get back together again, Margaret felt that in subsequent meetings he was far less demanding and headstrong, much more subdued, and even at times quite docile. She was happy with the final outcome!

Building resources

In this section I shall give you the specific steps – the format, the how to's – for building effective resources so that you can anchor and reaccess them at will, both for your patients *and* for yourself. You can experiment with a whole variety of different states and experiences, and to help you I have included in the appendix a list of *great states* (*see* Appendix 1).

You can practise the following exercise by yourself or with a colleague, anchoring some powerful resources for future use. In doing so you will find that you can use it far more easily with patients. It will simply flow.

Exercise 5:   Building resource states

1   Choose a particular resource or state that you want to anchor. Giving it a name, a label, will help you to begin to *search your memory banks* for examples.

2   Find *a specific example* from your past, no matter whether this was a recent event or one previously long forgotten but just returning to mind now. Choose one which can *reconnect* you strongly to the feelings you were having back then.

3   Now imagine yourself *fully back in that experience* as if it is happening here and now. *Step right into it*, wrapping it all around you. See what you are seeing in the experience, hear what you are hearing, and allow the feelings to grow and spread all over your body with every breath that you take. It may help to imagine the picture being *bigger, brighter, more colourful and closer*. Adjust the volume of the sound until it feels just right.

4   Now you can *set your anchor*. While you are fully in that state:
  •   choose *a word* or phrase that best typifies the state – for example, 'enough is enough' – saying it in a way that fits the state
  •   choose *a visual trigger* – something that is either always in that situation or reminds you strongly of it
  •   choose *a kinaesthetic trigger* – something you don't usually do, such as squeezing the tip of your index finger or knuckle with your other hand. Time this to coincide with the peak of the feeling.
  You can *repeat all of the above several times*, ensuring that you are fully associated into the memory each time. This will *condition the response* even more fully.

5   If you are using this format with a patient or client, you can replace step 4 with the following. As the intensity of the state peaks, choose a kinaesthetic anchor, such as a touch on their knuckle or shoulder, a squeeze of their elbow or upper arm, etc. Press slightly more firmly as the feelings intensify.

> 6 Once conditioned, you can *mentally rehearse using your anchors* just prior to the next time you will need them. *Imagine being in that situation*, triggering your anchored state, and *noticing the differences* in your response. The more you and your patients practise this short ritual, the more easily it will become second nature, *happening automatically* in the situation, without thinking about it consciously.

You can utilise this more readily by consulting the *great states* list in Appendix 1, anchoring different states to different fingers. You can literally have your resources at your fingertips! Towards the end of this chapter you will have a chance to use this technology to enhance your abilities to deal more effectively with any situation that arises by *being your best self.* You might like to begin now to think in just what way this will benefit both you and your patients.

Trouble-shooting tips

Having completed the above exercise, you may have some questions about the process if it has not *yet* had the desired effect. Like any new behaviour, it is worth practising to get it right. So what are the important caveats about anchoring processes?

1 You and your patient must choose a memory or event that has *sufficient emotional intensity.* The stronger the elicited state, the better the effect. Ensure that you have stepped fully inside the memory and are not simply watching it from the outside, like an observer.
2 You must also ensure that you do *enough repetitions*, usually three to five, to build a strong, stable state. It gets easier and quicker with each one.
3 Your *timing* of the trigger may have been either too early or too late. Too early and there is not enough emotional intensity. Too late and the state has reached a plateau and faded (*see* Figure 6.1).
4 Ensure that you are both starting from a relatively neutral state. Residual negative emotions such as fear, anxiety, anger and sadness may actually overwhelm the positive state you are attempting to build. It may be useful to 'shake off' residual negative emotions by standing up and moving around a little first.
5 Anchoring techniques require *rapport* to achieve the best effect. It is really important that you go into the state that you are eliciting in your patient

as well. By going there first you will lead them much more deeply into the experience.

6   Different states may require you to modify what you say. States such as calm and relaxation are impossible to generate if you are asking the patient to make their pictures bigger and brighter, adjusting the volume of the sounds as you speak fast and excitedly in their ear! In these situations, access the relaxed state yourself, and ... speak ... more slowly ... asking them to adjust the pictures and sounds so that it feels just right.

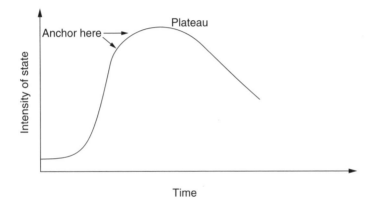

Figure 6.1:   Anchoring states.

Stacking anchors

Stacking anchors is the NLP term for putting more than one state on to the same kinaesthetic trigger. The result is a more powerful combination of states which can be very useful in the collapsing anchors process described in the next chapter. Often the summation is far more effective than a single state when brought to bear in potentially tricky or difficult situations. The process seems to integrate all of the states such that recalling even a single one gives simultaneous access to all of the rest.

One approach is simply to stack all of the states on to one anchor. Initially you can set a kinaesthetic anchor on a knuckle, elicit each state one by one, and as they peak add them sequentially. As you trigger the summated states together, you can also add an evocative word and a pictorial symbol, which can serve as additional anchors to use in varying circumstances.

Another approach is to anchor each state separately on several different knuckles. Then you can trigger them in various combinations together, initially two at a time, building up so that eventually you trigger them all simultaneously. Personally I find that this seems to give a better blending of the individual states into one 'super state'. Again you can add evocative words and pictures together with a separate, single, kinaesthetic anchor (e.g. a clenched fist) for easier one-step access.

It is far easier to do this with states that share a similar energy level, such as *powerful, dynamic, energised, enthused,* etc. If you pair excitement and calm relaxation together you will definitely feel the unusual internal feelings of push–pull around the solar plexus area, as if both are 'fighting it out'. Of course, you can have a separate stacked anchor for calm, peaceful, serene, etc. You will get a chance to do this for yourself later in this chapter.

This kind of anchoring can also be used as a 'break state', so that several times in the course of a day you can give yourself a time-out and luxuriate for a few moments in resourceful feelings. If your day has not been going as well as expected, it can pull you out of negative thoughts and feelings, giving you a platform from which to do things differently.

How anchoring works: connecting theory and practice

As we learned in Chapter 3, anchoring is the NLP equivalent of Pavlovian *classical conditioning.* Also, in *operant conditioning* terms, because success breeds success, this in itself can act as its own positive reinforcer. However, although we have used an external stimulus – a touch – to condition the state, we have also gone much further than the behaviourists. We have added *cognitive* aspects, such as internal pictures, sounds and words, using them as conditioning stimuli as well. Broadening the conditioning application in this way opens up a variety of therapeutic manoeuvres which we shall explore in due course.

In a sense, using anchors like this allows for both contemporaneous *cognitive restructuring* and *skills training.* Associating past resources to current areas of concern favourably changes the perception of these events, allowing a new response to replace old behaviours. The submodalities of the experience will spontaneously restructure themselves in a different way. This kind of skill, *modelled* from those who can successfully bring positive aspects of their life's experience to bear on today's events, is packaged in a simple, easily learnable and transferable way. By teaching patients how to do it for themselves, you increase their opportunities to apply this skill in other everyday contexts – generative learning.

Anchors elicit *state-dependent* memories which in themselves are powerful *systems attractors* for the knowledge, learning, skill sets and behaviours that are contained within their specific *neural networks*. Reconnecting, amplifying and entraining the networks via stacking anchors, and at the same time associating them to future events, allows for the kind of *self-efficacy* expectation that Bandura believes is one of the main hallmarks of sustained behavioural change. This is the ability to give a masterful response to a situation that may previously have held low expectations, or indeed the passive assumption of a victim's role. Of course, this kind of self-mastery is extremely potent in fuelling future, believed-in, achievable outcomes.

Going round in circles

Because the elicitation and anchoring of states are a fundamental component of virtually all NLP techniques, we are going to consider an additional way to achieve this. Although those whose preferred way of taking in information is visual will be at home with the standard building resources format, others who process mainly kinaesthetically may find that the following fits them better. However, before going into details about the *circle of excellence*, I shall first describe some brief demonstration cases.

Brenda and the bully

Brenda, aged 15 years, could not cope with the bullying tactics of a girl in her year at school. Although there had been no major physical violence, she felt psychologically intimidated to the extent that her self-esteem had slumped, she felt increasingly nervous while in school, and she was concerned about the effect that this was having on her schoolwork. Her mother, for whom NLP techniques had worked successfully some time previously, suggested that Brenda, who initially appeared somewhat shy and introspective, should 'come for a session'.

Brenda told me a little about how she felt, but rather than have her reassociate to obviously painful feelings, I asked a fairly standard solution-centred approach question: 'Tell me what's actually going well in your life at present'. At this point her demeanour changed completely as she waxed lyrical about her dancing classes (tap, ballet and disco) and her longer-term aim to go to a performing arts college and follow a career in dance. Her favourite was disco dance, and she had recently reached a high position in national finals. She was quite animated during the telling of the tale.

Getting back to the matter in hand, I asked her, if she had a magic wand, how she would like to be different around the bully. (As an aside, I do keep a magician's magic wand in my desk drawer – just in case!) 'Well ... I'd like to be confident ... able to go wherever I want in school ... and to know that even if she's there I can still feel OK.' We built up a picture of just exactly how she would look, sound and feel if she were acting in the way she really wanted.

'What was it like at the end of your nationals performance, when you knew you'd done the best you could, you'd been flawless, and the audience appreciated your talent?' I asked. She lit up as she told me about how great it had felt being in the spotlight, with the audience clapping, her friends cheering wildly and the huge grin she had on her face. We decided that this would be an excellent resource to use.

I asked her to imagine a circle on the floor just ahead of her, in her favourite colour, which was orange. 'In that circle, I want you to see *that you* going through the performance again. And it doesn't really matter whether you *really see it clearly* or simply pretend that you do ... *see it clearly*, that is ... a life-size Brenda ... doing it all again ... and just before she reaches the best bit ... all the applause at the end ... *all those great feelings* ... I'd like you to step into the orange circle ... step right into Brenda ... and enjoy it all again.'

When she was in the circle, reliving it all, her eyes closed, with small, unconscious movements of her arms and legs, I said 'And with every breath you take ... make the pictures *bigger, brighter, more colourful* ... turn up the volume of the sound ... make it *surround sound* ... and *double* those feelings. Let your orange circle really grow big and bright so that it's *enveloping* you ... and at the peak of the feeling ... step out of the circle.'

We did this twice more, really building up the intensity, and I also anchored the state kinaesthetically with a touch on her shoulder. The next time she stepped into the orange circle and began to glow, I touched her shoulder and added 'And as those feelings peak, just notice that girl who *had* given you all that trouble previously ... notice how you *feel differently* ... notice how you can *keep this good feeling* ... no matter where you go ... no matter what you do ... no matter what she says or does ...'.

Initially she was a bit sceptical about how this would work out in the real world of school. I suggested that she should spend some time at home, stepping in and out of her circle, deciding where else in her school life she would attach the feelings (and any other contexts), and then let me know how she was getting on.

A few weeks later I asked her how things were going. She said that she had not really had a chance to try it out with the bully as, for some mysterious reason, the girl now left her alone and no longer troubled her! In her own parlance, she was now 'putting out different vibes'. Brenda has now completed her schooling and enrolled at performing arts college.

Pat's presentation

Pat, who was in her late thirties, had enrolled for a further education course at the local college. Unknown to her at the time of paying her fees for the year, she later found out that she would have to give several presentations to her class of 20 or so colleagues. With the first one due in a week's time, she felt a rising degree of nervousness and trepidation. A friend had suggested that she might get a beta-blocker drug, which she herself had found had helped her be calmer during her driving test. However, Pat, an otherwise accomplished woman, was not too keen on taking medication, and wondered about alternatives.

We went through the standard outcome-setting process first, establishing that she wanted to feel calm and confident, have a strong voice, and look as if she was enjoying herself. She knew that her performance would also depend on preparing her material adequately so that she had a full grasp of it all and could focus on presenting it well.

We decided that her love of cooking and giving dinner parties matched the kind of resources she needed. Deciding what to cook, buying choice ingredients, following the recipe with a few ad libs, and finally presenting the finished product for her guests to savour was a similar process to preparing and giving her college presentation. Because the best part was the pleasure she felt at the admiring glances and comments when she was unveiling her creation, we used this as the main resource in her *circle of excellence*, connecting it strongly to looking out at her audience as she presented her prepared material confidently.

By relating the tasks involved in the presentation to something for which she already had a strategy and that she could do well, she felt much more confident in the lead-up to the event itself. She sent me a note afterwards telling me that it had gone well. The best bit was the room in which she did the presentation. The carpet was lilac – exactly the same colour as her resource circle!

Mary's music

Mary, aged 32 years, had been depressed on and off for nearly two years. She was on her second course of antidepressants, but after two months still had a flat affect, and was low in energy and poorly motivated to do her household tasks. She was not keen on the idea of referral to the mental health team consultant, feeling that this was a stigma she could do without. Although low in spirits, she was not suicidal, and said that her three-year-old daughter gave her something to live for.

I told her that there was another approach which I believed would help within two weeks, provided that she gave me a commitment to stick to the task. I would only tell her what it was once she had agreed to do it. This is a strategy I sometimes use to engage a patient's commitment, and it intrigued Mary so much she said yes!

I asked to go through her various music CDs and choose six songs with the following characteristics. They had to be upbeat, dance-type rhythms and songs that were personally meaningful to her in some positive way. Lasting 20 minutes or so in total, she had to record them on to one CD, entitled 'Getting Better'. Every morning she had to play the CD with headphones on, dancing vigorously to the music. I asked her to think about her favourite colour and imagine that this was shining on her like a spotlight as she danced, following her every move.

She thought I was a bit mad, but agreed to do it anyway. She said she would close the living-room curtains because she did not want the neighbours looking in and thinking that she was as daft as me! The upshot was that she didn't do it for 20 minutes a day. She actually did it several times a day, using her personal CD as she vacuumed the house, washed and ironed. Within two weeks her energy levels, mood and motivation had improved significantly. Interestingly, while dancing in her 'golden circle' she began to think quite differently about her numerous problems, the physiological state change affording various useful perspectives that seemed to arise spontaneously. She is now off medication and maintaining her gains.

Circle of excellence

This way of building resources adds a stronger kinaesthetic component to the process, and is often useful for accessing a whole-body physiological response, especially in those who are not so good at visualising. If you think about it, many memories involve movement, and replicating this in any revivification process can make the state easier to access and also deepen the accompanying feelings. The use of spatial locations in this way is part of many of the exercises that you will encounter later in this book.

For the following exercise (adapted from British trainer Ian McDermott) you could use one of the resources you used previously for comparison, or find a completely new one.

Exercise 6:   Circle of excellence

Choose a resource that it would be useful for you to have in an upcoming situation. Consult Appendix 1 for many more choices.

1   *Imagine a circle*, in your favourite colour, placed on the floor at a point of your choosing.
2   As you think about a time when you had that *particular resource*, imagine you are seeing it *happening again*, inside the circle. Even if you can't see it clearly, pretend that you can, making sure that you appear life size.
3   Now *step inside* the circle, fully into that you, so that you are *reliving the experience*, seeing what you are seeing, hearing what you are hearing, feeling all of the feelings again. It may help to make the pictures bigger, brighter, more colourful ... turning up the volume of the sound ... doubling the intensity of the feelings with every breath.
4   As the *feelings reach a peak*, notice the colour of your circle glowing, and then step outside it. Imagine that those resources remain within the circle, ready for use when you step inside it again.
5   You can *repeat the above steps* both to intensify the state and for any additional resources you may require.
6   Now *think of the trigger* – the very first thing you will see, hear or feel in the upcoming situation. As you do this, *step into your circle, reaccessing all of your resources*, and letting the colour glow. Take these resources to where they are needed and *notice how things are different now* – how things have *changed for the better*.
7   If any negative feelings still remain, *recycle through the process*, adding different resources to get the result you want.

As with all anchoring processes, when you do this with a patient it is important to step into your own resourceful states, too, so that you both keep in rapport and you lead the patient in the right direction, too. When people do not experience a strong state, it is usually because they have remained dissociated. They are still 'outside' themselves watching like an observer. To ensure that they really do step 'inside', use present-tense language to keep them associated.

Being your best self

In *Consulting with NLP*, I introduced the concept of having access to the many times in the past when you had been in the flow of life, enjoying yourself and living up to the best of your expectations – the various times, places and contexts throughout your life (work, family, friends, etc.) that stand out as positive resources. As we consider this now, it seems to me that there are certain 'generic' resources which we have all had from time to time, and which would be extremely useful to have to hand. In the following paragraphs we shall consider the kinds of states that I often get my patients to think about, not only at consultation but also as 'homework'. Jot down the experiences that come to mind.

Think of those times when you have *achieved something of great importance* to you – something that you were delighted about, that had major significance. It may have been winning a golf competition, or passing a driving test or some other examination. Perhaps, like one of my patients, you planned the holiday of a lifetime, and actually went on it, savouring the achievement. Maybe, like another, you started up your own business. Both you and your patients can take a note of these occasions.

A state linked to this is a time when you were absolutely *determined to do something* and you did it – a time when you committed yourself fully, focusing completely on the task in hand, brushing aside any obstacles that stood in your way. George decided to run the London Marathon for a cancer charity. Although his asthma initially seemed to be an obstacle, as he wheezed during and after each training run, his determination carried him over the finishing-line. What things have you been determined to do *and* completed?

However, there are times when you think that you cannot possibly succeed. Times when all the odds are stacked against you – a seemingly impossible task. Times when you *thought you couldn't do it, yet you succeeded anyway* – you rose to the occasion, surprising yourself in the process. Alan remembered when he was at the gym with his mates. They challenged him to bench press 90 kg, which they had all done. At the time his best was 80 kg, and he was sure that he would fail. As he started the lift he felt strangely galvanised, with a sense of inner strength surging through him as he surpassed his expectations. What similar memories do you have?

Have you ever said *enough is enough* and meant it, following through with a behavioural change? Perhaps you stopped eating chocolate as part of a healthier lifestyle. Maybe, like Anne, you got fed up with being abused in a relationship and finally plucked up the courage to leave. Or even, like Margaret, you stopped smoking for good. Think of the times when you have crossed the threshold in a particular context and said *never again*, and didn't. Write them down now.

An interesting resource is a time when you *went somewhere new and arrived safely*. Jean had gone to London for the first time on a training course. Lodgings had been organised for her with people she didn't know. She felt some trepidation beforehand, but followed the instructions, managed to find the right place, and ended up having a great three days. I remember going out on an urgent house-call and getting lost. I spied a local postman who gave me exact directions. What do these examples have in common? They are both about *staying on track*, about having a destination in mind and doing what it takes to get there. This is the kind of resource that many patients need as they embark on a course of treatment which may prove difficult, or even hazardous, yet they must keep the outcome in mind, and keep going.

What things are you *really passionate* about? What fires you up, makes you excited and gets you so interested that you lose all track of time? What subjects do you get animated about so that you can't stop talking about them? What are your hobbies and interests – the things that really enthral you so that you lose yourself in them? When you immerse yourself in this kind of memory (whether it is a particular sport, collecting toy cars, do-it-yourself, cooking, painting, music, etc.) you enter a *flow state*, where time ceases and you activate the best in yourself. These are great states to revivify and use in other contexts.

When you have found examples of all of these in your own personal history, use the anchoring techniques to build them up, either attaching them to separate knuckles or even joining them all together in one large circle of excellence. Then ask yourself 'In which particular upcoming situations would it be useful to have all of these resources to hand?'.

These situations do not necessarily need to be of major significance. What if the ringing of your alarm clock triggered off those resourceful feelings? Would that be a useful way to start your day? What if you attached the state to seeing yourself in your bathroom mirror, the feeling of the hot shower against your back, or the smell and taste of breakfast-time coffee? You can add many other seemingly minor occasions, such as getting into and starting up your car, crossing the threshold of your health centre, the faces of your staff members and fellow colleagues (yes, a definite stretch!), the door to your consulting-room and myriad more. In this way your state can be constantly 'topped up' as you progress through your daily activities.

When both you and your patients start to view currently challenging situations through the lens of these particular resources, really *being your best self*, you may find that previously unlooked for, even unseen solutions begin to materialise.

Building resourceful conclusions

This has been an in-depth chapter – an important chapter, perhaps one of the most important ones in this book. Why is this? Well, the ability to *find and amplify personal strengths* is a fundamental skill that underpins all of the other approaches you will read about in due course. This is why I have given so many different examples. It is a way of stating, quite emphatically, that your patient is not simply a broken collection of failed behaviours. It acknowledges that we all have, somewhere in our past, perhaps well covered or even deeply hidden, the kinds of experiences which can be dug up, dusted off, revitalised and brought to bear in the creation of the kind of future we want to have instead.

This is the hallmark of a solutions-centred approach. Starting with the end in mind, we can build a detailed, behaviourally based outcome that is stated in sensory-specific terms. We can ask about the things that really need to be there – the things that will really make a difference. And using the techniques described in this chapter, it does not matter whether a patient has had a particular resource for a day, an hour, a minute or just a few seconds. We can bring it to life again, revivifying it and making it as strong (if not stronger) than before. We can fan the flames of a flickering candle in the wind into a roaring flame. Then we can attach it exactly where we want, and in the process give our patients back the kind of self-mastery that they may have forgotten they possessed.

You can return again and again to this pivotal chapter as you continue to build up your resources in succeeding chapters ...

CHAPTER 7

Collapsing anchors

Introduction

Many patients have symptoms that only occur in a specific context or particular time frame and have not generalised out into the rest of their lives. Specific fears and phobias are top of the list. However, it is also possible to consider other conditions in the same way – for example, asthma, vertigo, recurrent vomiting, motion sickness, chemotherapy-induced nausea, insomnia, irritable bowel syndrome, nightmares and stammering, to name only a few.

In the 1950s, Joseph Wolpe became the first psychiatrist to use counter-conditioning techniques to treat phobias. Until that point, variations of psycho-analysis were the main therapies. By pairing deep muscle relaxation to the problem state, he offered a fairly swift (in those days) resolution of symptoms. Enterprising therapists since then have built on this by utilising other states, such as humour, laughter, sexual arousal and other emotive thoughts and imagery, to achieve similar results. The general model is to substitute positive emotional experiences for negative ones. It is still a much used tool in cognitive–behavioural therapy today.

NLP has gone another step further. Because both the problem state and any proposed resource(s) can be anchored kinaesthetically, this allows for their simultaneous triggering – the effect of which can have profound therapeutic results. And not only that, the specific anchors act as a set of precision tools, thus giving a degree of control over the process that was hitherto unheard of.

Many practitioners of NLP are apt to bypass this fairly simple technique in their quest to move rapidly on to other more complex approaches. However, my own experience is that collapsing anchors represents a very powerful tool in its own right – one that is well suited to the time-limited interventions that are required in medical practice. If done well it can have as much (or even more) impact as the techniques described in later chapters.

So would it be useful to have a simple, quick yet effective approach that is easily learned and utilised? The following cases will demonstrate its flexibility in a number of different situations. As you read through them, be alert for your own patients (or your own issues) which come to mind, and also other symptom complexes that might benefit from the same approach.

Violet's vertigo

Violet was a grandmother in her late fifties. For several years she had had episodic vertiginous attacks that had been put down to recurrent labyrinthitis. She would suddenly get very dizzy, vomit incessantly and end up in bed for several days. Usually she required a house call for an injection of prochlor-perazine and subsequent oral medication to last her the 10 days or so before resolution occurred. She had had three or sometimes four episodes a year for several years, and investigation had ruled out any serious pathology.

I happened to be the duty doctor on call for her latest episode, and duly attended her as she lay ashen-faced on her living-room couch. As I was drawing up the necessary injection, she said 'This *always* seems to happen to me before some important event I've been looking forward to. It's a blessed nuisance!' My ears immediately pricked up and I asked her to tell me more. 'Well, it's my niece's wedding in Ayrshire (200 miles away) this weekend, and I'll not be in a fit state to travel now. I get so fed up when this happens.'

As I asked her to recount the last few episodes of vertigo, it seemed that they all presaged weddings, celebrations or even holidays. The result of each one was that she had to cancel her trips. I explained for her in layman's terms the background to classical conditioning, and conjectured aloud whether this was the mechanism causing her present reaction. I did wonder whether there was any secondary gain to her symptoms, such as getting her out of something she did not want to do and simultaneously saving face. She seemed quite genuinely to believe that, given the opportunity, she would definitely want to go. I suggested that once this acute episode was over we could run the collapsing anchors process.

A couple of weeks later we met up at the health centre. I explained that we were going to search her memory banks for times when her proprioceptive system was firing on all cylinders and she was in dynamic balance. She went back a long way, all the way to childhood and early adolescence, where she unearthed two memories. The first was of riding a large-framed, bright red girl's bike which had been her pride and joy. The second was of climbing in the ruins of a wartime bombed-out building with her friends, dancing sure-footedly along the tops of narrow walls.

I usually like to get three resources (maybe I am superstitious!) and because she could only come up with two, I asked her what her favourite tree was – one that was solid, well rooted and strong. A large oak tree fitted the bill nicely, and she then spontaneously remembered climbing one in her youth. On this occasion, though, I had another plan.

Initially, in order to allow her to relax somewhat, I asked her to picture a favourite place where she was comfortable and felt at ease with herself. As she accessed a memory of curling up in a soft leather chair at home, I asked her to 'let yourself *go even deeper* into the feelings of ... *relaxing* ... letting them wash all over you ... with every breath ... embracing the *developing comfort* ... *sinking down* ... *easily* ... *drifting* ...'

One by one, as in Chapter 6 on building resources, we accessed the first two memories, anchoring one on each knuckle. We focused on the feelings of dynamic balance, turning easily, nimbly and sure-footedly on the wall, and how riding a bike successfully required one always to be on the verge of being out of balance. We accessed the third resource in a different way.

I asked her to vividly imagine the big, strong oak tree, and to picture its roots going deeply into the earth. No matter what the weather, from sunny windless days to winter gales and storms, it remained firmly secured to the earth. I said 'And as you see that oak tree over there ... imagine that *you can step inside* it ... become one with it ... feel its roots ... *your roots* ... going deep ... *deep down* ... keeping you stable ... no matter what happens ...' I anchored this to a third knuckle. This is a good example of building a resource state from an inanimate object, using the patient's own projected strengths. You can of course do exactly the same thing with people whom your patient views as mentors (*see* Chapter 14).

Having built the three positive resources, we were ready for the next step. I asked Violet to think about the worst episode of vertigo she had ever had, and to step inside that memory for a moment, reliving the experience and feeling the negative feelings of dizziness and nausea. As she did this, her face contorted, her skin became pallid and I reached over and anchored the state on the first knuckle of her *other* hand. It is really useful to use one hand for the positive resource states and the other for the negative ones. After this she stepped out of that memory and I spent a few moments getting her back into the relaxed state from which we had originally started.

Once she was back in a fairly neutral state, we were ready to move on. I said 'In a moment I'm going to touch all your knuckles at the same time. This can be a weird kind of experience and sometimes a bit confusing as *things change and rearrange* all by themselves. I'd like you to simply *go with the flow* as it happens, riding it out until we're completely done.' I triggered all of the anchors together, pressing more strongly on the positive ones as I continued 'letting all that dynamic balance ... sure-footedness ... sense of strong, deep roots ... *going exactly where they're needed* ... so it's as easy as riding a bike ...'.

As I pressed on each knuckle both individually and simultaneously I could see the play of the various emotions passing across her face, together with the colour shifts. Her breathing initially became a bit quicker and shallower, until after a minute or so she gave a big sigh, letting it all out as a smile spread across her face. I removed my finger from the negative-state anchor and held the others for 10 more seconds. As she opened her eyes I looked at her and said 'Now just imagine going into the future ... to a time that *would have been* like those past events ... and notice how *things are different now* ...' An even bigger grin spread across her face, and I said 'We're done!'

I didn't see Violet again for a long time afterwards – over a year, in fact. I was just coming back from a house-call and saw her pushing a buggy across the zebra crossing. I pulled in, parking illegally (!), and wound down my window. She beamed a grin at me in reply to my obvious question. She told me that she had had no episodes of vertigo in the past year, and had been to two weddings and a golden wedding anniversary (but no funerals!), all in the south of Scotland. She was delighted with the results.

Norman's nausea

Norman, aged 63 years, was an insulin-dependent diabetic who had disseminated prostate cancer. An honest, hard-working man with large calloused hands, he had come to terms with the fact that he was not going to get better. He was gaining excellent pain relief from his long-acting oral morphine. The only problem was his recurrent nausea, which was particularly troublesome first thing in the morning on rising. It played havoc with his diabetic control, and despite using various anti-emetics he was still symptomatic.

During one particular home visit I suggested that his nausea had become habitual due to a form of classical conditioning. Each time his feet hit the floor in the morning the nausea started. I explained about the possibilities of counter-conditioning, and he agreed to give it a go. I wanted him to access memories of times when he had successfully achieved something of great importance – times when he had felt on top of the world. A keen golfer in the years before cancer struck, he recalled a time when he had won the local 'medal' competition and stepped up to receive the cup, much against the odds. He relived all of the feelings in the telling of the tale, which he embellished suitably for my ears.

A second powerful memory that lived with him was the birth of his first grandchild. He could still picture the tiny tot's eyes looking at him shortly after birth, a most powerful connection that had a timeless here-and-now quality. The third memory was that of the Buckie Thistle football team in the 1960s, which had swept all before it. It was a strange coincidence that although I was not a local, my uncle had played for the team following a career as a professional footballer in the 1950s.

In exactly the same way as I had done with Violet, I induced a relaxing state as Norman lay on his couch in the living room, anchoring the three positive states and one negative state to the knuckles of both hands. I collapsed all four together, holding them until his breathing settled and his face had a symmetrical glow with deep red patches on both cheeks. Simplistic as it may seem, his morning nausea completely disappeared the very next day, and he required no further anti-emetic medication for the duration of his illness.

Based on this success and the positive feelings that he associated with it, we were able to do some other NLP interventions for localised pain control when the discomfort from his metastatic disease was not fully controlled by morphine and non-steroidal anti-inflammatories (*see* Chapter 17).

Debbie's dental phobia

Debbie, who was in her late thirties, really needed to go to the dentist, but could not get herself from the waiting-room into the dentist's chair. When I explored the situation further, it seemed that the main problem was her intense dislike of 'having lots of equipment inside my mouth'. Her actual fear of gagging brought on that very same response! She knew that she needed dental treatment, but was frightened she might 'choke to death' during the procedure. She realised that this was very irrational, yet at the same time found herself gripped with mounting anxiety at the very thought.

I asked her if there was anything that she could easily tolerate in her mouth for prolonged periods of time. Initially we spoke about food and drink, most of which she held in her mouth only for short periods prior to swallowing. Then a huge grin spread across her face. One of her 'pastimes' on holiday was filling her mouth with several ice cubes and slowly crunching them! We had found our resource state.

She allowed herself to relax more deeply by remembering her last beach holiday, enjoying the sun's rays, with not a care in the world. When she was suitably relaxed, and her face had become flaccid and symmetrical with slower breathing, I revivified a memory of drinking the Spanish wine cocktail 'Sangria', and anchored her ability to swallow this easily. Then she remembered the feeling of several very cold ice cubes in her mouth, and how the coldness also acted as a local anaesthetic agent. I went into more detail about just exactly how they felt inside her mouth, tongue and teeth, before anchoring it on a different knuckle. With these two states firmly anchored, I triggered the memory of the various intra-oral dental instruments, collapsing these all together, and then waited for integration to occur.

Once again there was a rise and fall in respiration followed by a peaceful sigh, indicating that integration had occurred. Still holding the positive anchors, I asked Debbie to imagine stepping into a future dental appointment and noticing the difference now. She has subsequently managed to have some major restorative dental work done, with several appointments lasting as long as an hour – even holding the plastic-tasting impression moulding material in her mouth without gagging!

Collapsing anchors process

Since we have already covered all of the steps in this process in the above examples, you will already have an intuitive feel for how it works. *You actually know more than you think you know!* The following exercise will simply make that understanding come more to the forefront of your conscious mind, allowing you to be more fully aware as you do it with patients. First, however, it is a good idea to find a willing partner so that you can practise on each other. This will give you a 'mind to muscle' type of experience that will markedly increase your degree of congruence when doing it 'live'.

Prior to doing the exercise, it is important to define just exactly what the problem state is. This process works best with *contextualised* problems – that is, reactions which occur in *specific* sets of circumstances, rather than generalised issues. If you can pinpoint the visual, auditory or kinaesthetic cues that trigger the negative state, this will increase your success rate. You must also decide beforehand which (and how many) positive resource states you are going to utilise, so that you can have them clearly in mind as you begin.

Exercise 7:   Collapsing anchors process

1   Having chosen your *resource states, elicit them* one by one and anchor them either to separate knuckles of one hand or on to a single stacked anchor. Ensure that you *get powerful representations* of each state, building the resources to peak intensity.
2   Next you can elicit a neutral state, allowing a clean break from step 1.
3   *Briefly step into the problem state*, accessing the negative feelings, and making sure that you get the visual, auditory or kinaesthetic trigger. *Anchor this* to a knuckle on the other hand.
4   Elicit the neutral state again, ensuring that all of the negative feelings have completely gone prior to the next step. *The patient must be dissociated from the negative state. This is very important!*

> 5   *Now collapse all of the anchors,* negative and positive together, *simultan-*
> *eously.* Press more firmly on the positive anchors as you say the words
> that suggest *integration is occurring now.* Watch as the breathing initially
> speeds up, and keep holding the anchors until it settles, often with a
> sigh. Then release the negative anchor first, holding the positive ones
> for 10 more seconds.
>
> 6   Now *think of a future time* which in the past would have triggered the
> old feelings, and notice what is *different now,* how things have *changed.*

The collapsing anchors process can be a very powerful intervention, and when
done well, it is as effective as many other more complex NLP techniques. There
are certain fundamental keys to ensuring that it works effectively.

1   The first is *always* to think context, context, context! You must get a specific
issue and draw a boundary around it, isolating the behavioural cues that
trigger the response. Failure to do this will give a wishy-washy result.

2   The problem state and the resources that you choose to utilise must be
clearly separated prior to integration, so that they do not cross-contaminate
each other. An effective break-state will dissociate them sufficiently so that
you can move cleanly on to the next step. If the patient seems to be stuck in
the negative state, ask them to stand up, move around and look up at the
ceiling. This change in physiology will quickly get them into a neutral state.

3   I generally like to ensure that the resource states are *far more powerful* than
the negative state. If they are of similar intensity, you are less likely to achieve
a good result. Build and stack some really great states (*see* Appendix 1) so
that your patient is glowing from the inside out and *you know* this will easily
overpower the negative state. Spontaneous states such as humour and
laughter that occur should always be anchored and utilised.

4   Sometimes it can be useful to utilise the *circle of excellence* process, with one
circle for the resources (favourite colour) and another circle (colourless)
several feet away for the problem context. This will help to give a more
effective dissociation, keeping the states separate. When you come to
collapse the anchors, the patient can place their colourful resource circle
inside the problem space circle. This is a useful alternative for those who are
more kinaesthetic.

Later in this chapter I shall give several more examples of the process in action
to stimulate your thoughts about the kinds of conditions with which you can
use this. In the meantime it would be useful to begin to think about how you
could fit each medical condition (both physical and psychological) that comes
in through the health-centre door into this framework.

How collapsing anchors works: connecting theory and practice

Collapsing anchors is a form of *systematic desensitisation*, the counter-conditioning process introduced by Wolpe in the 1950s. As it was originally conceptualised, because maladaptive responses (such as many symptoms) develop as a form of classical conditioning, substituting a competing response desensitises the original reaction. The classical approach is to develop a hierarchy of anxiety-provoking situations and to expose the patient incrementally, in their imagination, to each step of the ladder. The patient learns how to relax first, by being taught a progressive muscular relaxation technique. Successfully maintaining relaxation in the face of exposure to negative stimuli allows the patient to advance on to the next rung of the ladder. This may often take several sessions. Rather than employing gradual exposure, the collapsing anchors process does all of this in one step.

We could also view this process as a form of *extinction*. This occurs when a patient is encouraged to remain in a negatively charged situation, especially anxiety, without using operantly conditioned coping or avoidant responses. Extinction is used particularly in phobic reactions, and when the presumed negative consequences fail to occur, the anxiety diminishes markedly. Many practitioners who are trained in NLP believe that exposure to highly charged negative feelings simply conditions the response even more strongly. They are unaware that extinction by itself, through prolonged exposure, ensuring that the negative feeling peaks and *then* falls, actually has a high therapeutic success rate. In specialist hands, systematic desensitisation and exposure procedures are very successful and may have a durable lasting effect of up to 70% in certain phobias. The collapsing anchors version is a very useful variant for ordinary general medical practice, where there are more time constraints.

Reciprocal inhibition is the neurophysiological explanation for both of the above behavioural mechanisms. Intensely negative states, such as anxiety, are predominantly driven by sympathetic arousal in the autonomic nervous system. Relaxation, being a parasympathetically mediated state, is induced by progressive muscular relaxation, which may take between 4 and 30 hours to learn adequately. As it is the opposite physiological response, it means that anxiety cannot be generated so long as the muscular relaxation is maintained. In NLP we can make use of this by eliciting the patient's own deep relaxation memories first by revivification. However, parasympathetic states are not required to counter-condition all negative states, and indeed may have little or no effect on blood-product phobias, as we shall see shortly.

There are also *cognitive explanations* which augment the above behaviourally based mechanisms. With successful desensitisation procedures, the patient's *beliefs* about the event may change substantially. *Self-efficacy* and personal mastery are both strengthened by believing that future episodes can now be dealt with differently. This change in expectation allows for more objective and realistic thinking about the previously negatively perceived event. If we elicit the *submodality* structure of the event both prior to and after the collapsing anchors process, we shall see that it has also changed – often considerably so. Patients *literally* do see things differently because *cognitive restructuring* has taken place. NLP uses this as an extremely useful verification procedure to further deepen the conviction of lasting change.

Another potential mechanism for the therapeutic effect is that of covert *modelling*. The therapist is seen as someone who has the necessary skills to deal effectively with the presenting issue himself, and as such is a *coping* or even *mastery model*. The therapeutic process itself is modelled from successful therapists, and this gives it a considerable pedigree. The therapist's beliefs about the patient's ability to succeed may also have an effect, and are conveyed by a supporting and empathic relationship that can encourage risk taking in a safe environment. Of course, the patient is also involved in *self-modelling* of his or her own resource states, which makes for easier and more effective retrieval. This highly learnable skill can then be generatively applied in different future circumstances.

Looking at the collapsing anchors process from the perspective of *state-dependent memory and learning* together with *self-organising systems theory*, we can see again how change comes about. The negative anchor is a context-specific *systems attractor* around which current experience has been organised. Because this neural network is relatively independent, it functions autonomously to continue generating the problem state over and over again. The addition of the positive resources causes entrainment and admixing of two previously unbridged states, resulting in the formation of a new *stable attractor*. This alters the *attractor landscape* sufficiently to allow this new response to occur when the old cues are triggered.

The collapsing anchors process is the prototype for virtually all of the change mechanisms that we shall encounter in succeeding chapters. As such, rather than simply repeating much of the above, I shall highlight the most applicable part of the change model chapter by chapter.

Some more case examples

To allow you to begin to think about the other kinds of clinical situations with which you can use collapsing anchors, I shall give some more case examples that are pertinent to medical practice. These are only thumbnail sketches, and you can imagine the fleshed-out details by running the collapsing anchors steps in your mind as you read through them.

Barry's blood-product phobia

Barry, who was in his early forties, had a phobia of blood products and would literally faint at the sight of blood. He could not watch surgical procedures on television without feeling queasy and changing channel. He had recently visited a friend in hospital, but did not make it into the ward because he collapsed as he walked along the corridor. He was highly embarrassed to find himself on a casualty trolley!

Unfortunately, using relaxation makes this kind of situation worse, as it augments the fainting response. We used the circle of excellence process instead. In a bright yellow circle we anchored feelings of confidence, dynamic power and inner strength. I asked Barry to imagine lifting a heavy load, tensing all of his muscles to straining point as he did so. Then he took his yellow circle into the negative situation and, as he imagined being fully in it again, I exhorted him to keep his muscles tense, strained and strong. We repeated this twice more with different negative past scenarios, and within one short session his problem was resolved. This is very much in keeping with standard cognitive–behavioural approaches to blood-product phobias leading to a one-session cure.

Natalie's needle phobia

Natalie had had episodes of relapsing and remitting multiple sclerosis. Her neurology consultant had suggested daily self-injections of beta-interferon to see whether this would forestall further relapses. The only problem was that Natalie had a phobia of needles, which was made worse by the fact that she would have to self-administer the medication.

I induced a state of relaxation and elicited times when she had succeeded in a task despite thinking that she would fail, together with times when she had completed a task while ignoring personal discomfort (cleaning up her children's vomitus!). These, together with other examples of times of confidence and competency, were collapsed with remembered memories of her needle phobia, and future paced to her own self-administration. Although she did still initially have reservations, she has subsequently managed to use an auto-injector device on a daily basis.

Freda's flashbacks

Two weeks previously Freda had been involved in a road traffic accident. While turning at a junction she had been blind-sided by another car. She escaped with minor whiplash injuries, but continued to have distressing flashbacks of the crash itself which appeared out of the blue. Her confidence had been dented, and subsequently she had only been out in a car as a passenger. She appeared hyper-vigilant, was easily startled and complained of restlessness and poor sleep.

Again, having induced a state of relaxation, we revivified times in different contexts of confidence, competence, fun, laughter and determination to succeed. I asked her to think of the worst moment she had experienced in the crash, and then collapsed all of the anchors together. For a few moments she looked quite confused and appeared 'woozy'. Afterwards, when everything had settled down, she reported that when she thought of the accident it was 'as if it had happened to someone else' – major evidence of submodality shifts. She now felt comfortably distanced from the actual memories.

Kim's nightmares

Kim had a recurring nightmare of being in a burning house and being unable to escape. She invariably awoke drenched in sweat, with a strong physiological reaction. She had no history of an actual experience like this, and denied other precipitating stresses. The nightmares could occur three or four times a week, and had been going on for several months. Kim had heard from a friend that I had some 'weird techniques', and was keen to try anything that might help.

During deep relaxation, I elicited states of calm confidence, courage in the face of adversity, and a time when she had an uncontrolled fit of laughter while watching comedian Billy Connolly (one of my personal favourites)! We threw all of this into the 'burning inferno', mixing them together over a period of five minutes or so. The nightmares stopped, and to my certain knowledge nearly eight years later they have not returned.

Concluding

As you can see, the collapsing anchors process is very versatile and can be used in a variety of anxious and fearful situations, as well as with less intense everyday troublesome symptomatology. Sometimes, however, if the negative response is overwhelming, with major physiological reactions, it is best to use the phobia and trauma process described in Chapter 10. This ensures sufficient dissociation to allow the process to proceed successfully.

The most important part of a successful set-up is to ensure that the problem state is highly contextualised, occurring in a specific set of circumstances, with particular triggers. In this, the process is an example of *first-order change* where the benefits usually remain in the single context and are less likely to generalise out into other areas of life. It is a remedial type of process rather than being generative across contexts – *second-order change*. Occasionally, however, when a specific problem has caused a generalised and pervasive set of negative beliefs about oneself and one's capabilities, the solving of the issue can lead to a wave-like progression of cross-contextual positive change and enhanced self-efficacy.

Now that you have read about some of the types of medical conditions that you can use this with, I have a question for you. What if you were to note down the clinical case scenarios that enter your consulting room each day and formulate them in a way that fits the collapsing anchors paradigm? I don't know about you, but I am certainly interested in applying this type of thinking to conditions like asthma, allergies, skin problems, etc. What are your thoughts about this?

CHAPTER 8

Chaining anchors together

Introduction

Our patients often come to see us because they are stuck in a certain way and cannot seem to generate new options. It is as if the kind of thinking that goes on in those types of stuck states is repetitive and precludes movement towards solutions. Yet there are times – and we've all had them – when we seem to start off 'stuck', and then cycle through a series of different states that ends up with us being in the flow again. The kind of flow state where we are thinking easily and flexibly and once more heading in the direction of our goals and outcomes. In fact, we cycle through many states each day without consciously thinking about it other than having a vague sense of unease, followed by ease again. You probably know that feeling. So what is really going on at these times?

Think of a time when you have been temporarily *stuck*. What was happening then – the internal and external sights and sounds? What did it feel like bodily and what were you saying to yourself? What was it that got you moving again? Often after a period of time, a stuck state gives way to a sensation of building *impatience and frustration*. Just like when you have chosen the wrong queue in a bank – it's moving so slowly and you have another appointment for which you may be late. Remember that growing feeling?

When impatience and frustration build and reach a peak they often give way to a sense of *'enough is enough'*. If you have teenage kids you may know this state well! The arguments reach crescendo point, destroying your peace of mind, and you feel compelled to put an end to it once and for all. It is a strong kind of feeling, often accompanied by a firm voice and deliberate movements. Ever felt like that? What happens next?

Well, perhaps you get a sense of *determination* to do something different – the kind of feeling you get when you have decided to commit yourself to some action. As you think about it now, where in your body do you get that felt sense of being determined? In your chest? Your abdomen? Elsewhere? And is it a feeling that pulls you or pushes you forwards, towards taking the first steps in another direction? Before you know it, you are off, engrossed in something new, *in the flow again*, feeling good about yourself and what you are doing.

You have cycled through a chain of states, most likely without being consciously aware of exactly just what was happening. If you think about it, this is something that goes on many times a day, over and over again. We are *constantly* changing states. Yet sometimes, and especially for patients with problems, the stuck state and the behaviours that it encompasses do not spontaneously lead to resolution. They are simply repeated ad nauseum, spinning around yet getting nowhere. So what can we do instead?

Well, this chapter is all about deliberately setting up chains of powerful states that can propel you from specific behaviours you would prefer to stop doing into something that you would rather do instead. And although the examples we shall use are mainly about addictive behaviours, you will find that this is a versatile tool which can be used in many other circumstances, too, especially in conjunction with techniques from the other chapters. So keep in mind at least one question as you read on, and that is 'What other clinical issues could I use this pattern with?'

Kicking Suzy's smoking habit

Suzy, who was 27 years old, had smoked 20 to 30 cigarettes a day for a decade. With a new man in her life, and an urge to be fitter and healthier, as well as to use the money saved from cigarettes in other pleasurable ways, she was keen to kick the habit – permanently! There are a variety of different NLP approaches that you can use with addictions, especially smoking, and I have successfully used the techniques described in all of the other chapters in this book in this condition. However, what follows is a fairly quick, direct and simple approach that can be surprisingly successful without necessarily going into all the issues of secondary gain and other benefits.

Suzy's resolve to put off having a cigarette was greatest when she was by herself, but when she was with friends, especially when socialising at the pub, she found it harder to say no, and usually gave in readily. This was a context that we needed to pay special attention to. I decided to set up a chain of anchors which would fire off whenever she reached out for a cigarette, whether this was of her own choosing or offered by other smokers. First we discussed the kinds of states that we would need to elicit and for which we would need to find reference experiences.

We began with the end in mind, setting up an outcome to move towards. I asked Suzy to picture herself as a non-smoker. What would she look like, talk like, feel like, smell like and taste like, especially when her new man kissed her?

What would be her evidence for being fitter and healthier? What would she be doing with the money that she had saved? We continued in this vein, building up a three-dimensional life-size image to which she was really attracted, and her external physiology reflected this.

If you think about it, one way to stop someone doing something is to give them an aversive experience that forces them to move away from that behaviour. I asked Suzy about things that she could not stand, and which made her feel physically sick. She said that the sight and stale smell of a full to overflowing ashtray of stubbed-out cigarettes on a Sunday morning after the night before was something that could stop her smoking for several hours that day. She felt nauseated when thinking about it, especially when I asked her to make the noxious picture bigger and to bring it closer so that she could really smell and taste it!

Next we elicited a time when she was really determined to do something and she had done it. She had spent the previous year working and travelling in Canada, a time that she looked back on with many positive memories. She had planned to do this for some time previously, and although she did not have a job to go to prior to heading off, she had saved up for several months and had a single-minded focus on her goal. This single-mindedness would prove an excellent resource to use in the process.

I asked her to allow herself to sit comfortably and to recollect one of her most pleasant memories of Canada, which was of the Niagara Falls in summer. Revivifying the memory, the sights, sounds and feelings caused her to begin to drift into a relaxed state. One by one I elicited each of the states we had chosen and anchored them to separate knuckles. We actually started in the reverse order to that in which we would eventually fire them off. We built up the outcome image first, making it strongly compelling and attractive by pulling it closer, and giving it an all-round sparkle. We strengthened it by repeating the process again, emphasising the great feelings of success.

Following a break state of being in the Niagara memory again, we proceeded to get in touch with Suzy's feelings of absolute determination and focus, amplifying them as much as possible and anchoring them to the next knuckle along. Following another break state, I vividly described an overflowing ashtray of stubbed-out cigarettes and ash coming closer and closer to her nose and mouth. I asked her to imagine what it would be like if the contents spilled all over her face, so that she was inhaling the stale ash up her nostrils and tasting cigarette butts in her mouth. It was so noxious that I thought she was going to vomit! At that moment I anchored the toxic state to the next knuckle and gave her the much-needed relief of a break state.

We were almost ready to start the process, but we still required one more state, namely the trigger that set things off. I asked her to think about the feelings she experienced when she really craved a cigarette, and to put herself back into the times when she was in the pub with friends and felt that she could not refuse. She imagined herself reaching out for a cigarette, and I anchored the feeling to a knuckle on her other hand. It was time to start.

I pressed the anchor for needing a cigarette, asking her to 'really get in touch with those feelings of *wanting* it and *craving* it'. As the feelings began to peak, I fired off the noxious trigger, intensifying the feelings and imagining the bile rising in her throat – not a pleasant state! As the look of disgust began to plateau and recede, I said 'Now *step into* those feelings of *absolute determination and focus* ... noticing where they start in your body and how they *spread* (firing the next anchor) ... And as they *really build up* ... look at that image of you as a non-smoker ... and the closer you bring it *feel the feeling of being attracted ... to that you ... fitter ... healthier ... tasting* and *living* life to the full (firing the last anchor of the chain)'.

We used her Niagara memory as a break state once more, allowing her a spell of relaxing feelings before repeating the entire anchor chain again. We did this several times, ensuring each time that after running through each chain, we punctuated the process with relaxation. As well as the initial trigger, we imagined various different contexts (both alone and with friends) that would occur in the future. We covered all of the different scenarios that might cause Suzy to reach for a cigarette. And what was the end result? Well, she had no more cigarettes from that day on, and at a nine-month follow-up she remains a non-smoker.

Marie's weight loss

Marie, who was in her mid-thirties, was approximately two stone overweight. Although she ate reasonably healthily at mealtimes, her major penchant in between meals was for chocolate bars and crisps. A particular favourite was a Mars bar at bedtime! She felt that if she could have help with cutting out her snacks, then her weight would stabilise by itself. She was not keen about and did not feel the need for a major psychotherapeutic intervention, and when I explained the process of chaining anchors to her she wanted to give it a try.

Once again, beginning with the end in mind, we set up a sensory-specific outcome of how she would look, sound and feel after having shed two stone over the next three months or so. She acknowledged that this would mean buying some new clothes, as well as having the chance to wear others that were languishing in her wardrobe. We made certain that there were no major secondary-gain issues to take care of before proceeding. Ensuring that her new self-image was compelling and attractive, I anchored it to a knuckle.

Several years previously, Marie had had a nasty fall from a horse and had broken her collar-bone. Initially her confidence had been shaken, but she was *absolutely determined* to start riding again once the fracture had healed. And she did. I felt that this would be a particularly good resource to anchor, especially as it encompassed the determination to succeed despite a setback. Given the nature of the current challenge, it might prove to be very useful if her resolve temporarily failed her.

As for the noxious stimulus, that was really quite easy. She had a dog as a pet, which meant that she had to clear up its faeces from her back lawn. This was a task that made her stomach turn, and she generally put it off as long as possible. Revivifying the smell of rancid dog faeces was just what we needed, and I duly anchored this to another knuckle.

With the sight, smell and taste of chocolate and crisps separately anchored on her other hand, we were ready to start. Just as with Suzy, we began with a relaxing scene from a previous holiday and used this as a break state at the end of each cycle of chaining. From vividly imagining chocolate and crisps coming up to her mouth we connected the smell of rancid dog faeces, and as the noxious stimulus peaked we moved on to determination to succeed, followed by the compelling picture of her outcome. With deep relaxation interspersed we repeated the chain twice more to cement the connection further. I then asked Marie to simply imagine reaching out for chocolate and crisps, and the chain fired through spontaneously. We were finished.

And the final result? Well, the chaining anchors process was enough to stop her desire for chocolate and crisps. She actually joined the local gym, and after four months – slightly longer than her original goal – she achieved her two-stone weight loss.

Chaining anchors together: the process

What follows is a fairly standard method for chaining anchors together. As in all change work, it is important to begin with the well-formed outcomes process, obtaining a sensory-based description of what your patient really wants. Knowing the particular behaviour that they wish to desist from – the starting state – you can now decide which states to use to form your chain. In general, chains of four to five states in total length tend to work best. If there are more the process becomes unwieldy, and if there are too few the jumps between states are too large.

One thing to consider is that all states have a motivating direction – moving you towards or away from what you want. Consider states such as frustration or impatience. In fact, remember a particular time when you felt this way. What was it like? These states usually feel quite uncomfortable, and the underlying feeling is to get out of them as quickly as possible and move into something more comfortable. When used at the start of a chain they can provide the *push* to move you *away from* the undesired behaviour.

Now think of states such as determination or desire. What they have in common is an underlying feeling that moves you *towards* what you want. Used at the end of a chain, they can be utilised as the *pull* towards your outcome. This feeling of pushing away at the start of a chain and pulling towards at the end is sometimes called a *propulsion system*. It can have very powerful effects when it is set up correctly.

Once you have chosen the particular states that best suit your patient's needs, you can employ the format described in the following exercise.

Exercise 8:   Chaining anchors together

Ensure that you have first set up your outcome and chosen the states that you are going to use. In between each step choose a state such as relaxation to serve as a break state.

1   As you build your outcome, make certain that it is sufficiently attractive and compelling to really pull the patient towards it before anchoring it to a knuckle.
2   Build the various resource states that you have chosen into powerful anchors, attaching each one to a separate knuckle. You may want to repeat this to ensure the potency of each anchor. *Always break state between each elicitation.*
3   Anchor the problem state to a knuckle on the other hand. Obtain the visual, auditory and kinaesthetic cues that *trigger* the state.
4   Now fire off each step in the chain, starting with the problem state and finishing with the outcome state. Calibrate closely to the patient's responses, ensuring that each state reaches a peak before moving on to the next one.
5   Break state for a few moments by enjoying some relaxing feelings. Then repeat the chaining process again. You may wish to do this several times.
6   If you have followed the process correctly, then when you fire the trigger for the problem state you will see it automatically chain all the way through to the outcome without touching the other anchors.

One method that I often use is to condition the chain of the second, third and fourth states together *before* adding the problem-state trigger. By ensuring that the second and subsequent states run together very smoothly *first*, this can help to pull the patient rapidly through to the outcome state when you cue the problem trigger. In fact you can then attach several different problem triggers that occur in various contexts to the same chain, one after the other. Examples of different contexts for a smoker would include reaching for their own cigarette, being offered one by a friend, coffee break at work, socialising in the pub, etc.

The whole process can also be used in a very literal stepwise fashion. Just as in the *circle of excellence*, it is possible to lay out each state in its own separate location on the floor, one after the other in a straight line. You can use pieces of paper with the name of each state written on them. Once the states have been firmly anchored to each location, you can lead your patient from one to another, stepping into the next location as the previous state reaches a peak. Following a break state at the end of the chain sequence, you can repeat the process until it is sufficiently conditioned. This is often more useful for kinaesthetically oriented patients, who may include different postures and gestures for each state.

Chaining anchors together can work well in those situations where the secondary gain of the problem situation is minimal and the patient has no major sequential incongruities. If the patient appears congruent with regard to their decision to make the change, and you are relatively certain that they have no other parts waiting in the wings to sabotage the process, then it is worthwhile using it as a first step. If there is a more major degree of secondary gain, *six-step reframing* is a better process to use (*see* Chapter 13). If there are incongruities, *parts integration* processes give better long-term results (*see* Chapter 16).

In a patient who is overweight, this method can be useful if they only have one or two stone to lose. However, for those who are morbidly obese, with much more weight to be shed, there are often multiple factors to take into account (sequential incongruities, past traumas, etc.), and this simple process will almost certainly fail if it is used by itself (*see* Chapter 17 for details of multifactorial approaches that you can use in this and similar conditions).

Chaining anchors has also been used to manage conditions such as anxiety and anger, alcohol abuse and sexually deviant behaviours, utilising their triggering cues to direct the patient to a more useful contextual response. However, my personal experience is that other techniques which deal more adequately with secondary-gain issues and past initiating events give more ecological overall results. Nevertheless, chaining anchors can be used following resolution of these issues and, like the swish pattern (*see* Chapter 9), it can be the final nail to lock home the solution.

How chaining anchors works: connecting theory to practice

Chaining anchors is built very much on *classical and operant conditioning* methodologies. Each individual step of the chain is typical of classical conditioning, where we set up a stimulus–response cue. We also make use of the so-called *aversion–relief response*. This is when the increasing feeling of comfort that naturally occurs when a noxious stimulus is removed is connected to the direction in which we want to go instead. The aversive states act as *negative reinforcers*, while the moving-towards states are the *positive reinforcers.*

Change also occurs at a cognitive level, with the occurrence of *cognitive restructuring* together with *skills training*. We can think of the linked chain as being a new cognitive strategy that takes the place of the old 'problem' strategy. Thus we establish a different set of pictures, sounds and feelings, which by repetition installs the new strategy as a streamlined skill that operates below the conscious threshold. In the outside world, successful completion of the strategy allows all of the various *self-efficacy* factors to come into play, acting as a self-reinforcing loop.

In *self-organising systems* terms, each of the steps is a specific *attractor* that controls the firing of its own neuronal networks. Repeated firing of the attractor sequence leads to rapid propagation of the linked neuronal impulses which, strengthened through Hebb's law, leads to the automatic formation of a new pathway. The stimulus that formally led to being stuck in the problem attractor basin now takes a different route through the attractor landscape.

Concluding

As you can see – and perhaps have already experienced for yourself if you have done the above exercises with a colleague – the chaining anchors process can be a versatile tool in its own right, as well as in combination with the various techniques that you have yet to encounter. It is important to remember that state chaining occurs automatically in everyday life in any case. Just think of the state you are in after a morning of difficult consultations when you have run well over time, and the relief that occurs following a cup of coffee. After a short time your muzzy head begins to clear, you start thinking straight again and you become galvanised with an energy surge that takes you through your next set of engagements (or maybe not!). All that we are doing when we are using the process formally is choosing carefully the states we want to link together so that they run together automatically when we really need them.

There are many other areas that you may like to think of where the principles of chaining might be fruitfully used. Any situation where you want your patient to stop doing one thing and start doing another is a candidate for this approach. You can even use parts of it conversationally to build a covert visual anchor for a noxious stimulus on the one hand and really great feelings on the other hand. You can use them as a propulsion system, attaching a move away from response to health-harming behaviours and a move towards response to health-affirming ones. Of course, I shall leave the utilisation of this type of application up to your own personal ethics!

CHAPTER 9

Basic submodality patterns

Introduction

Did you ever wish that your patients could get a new perspective on a troubling issue? What about yourself? Have you ever had a problem that loomed large and forbidding in your life – encompassing and enveloping you in feelings that you did not want to have – and yet you could not get away from it? And as you look back on it now as a resolved issue, with the benefit of hindsight, do you have a sense that it had all been grotesquely blown out of proportion? Perhaps now you are picturing it from an entirely different viewpoint.

And when you do look at what *was* an issue from your past, do you still have some negative feelings associated with that event? Or have they subsided in the mists of time so that you now have an air of equanimity? As many people will testify, time heals, memories fade and what was once perhaps acutely painful is consigned to the scrapbook of yesteryear – maybe even accompanied by a rueful smile. But why wait for days, weeks, months or years to pass? What if there was a way to view currently disturbing events – whether they are actually of the here and now or continuous reruns of unresolved past memories – in a new light, rapidly transforming any accompanying feelings? Would you be interested in this? One of the patterns we shall be exploring in this chapter, namely dissociation of affect by changing visual submodalities, will literally reframe these situations in an instant.

On the other hand, perhaps you or your patient have a recurring annoying habit, such as nail biting or something similar, that gnaws away at you time and time again, despite your best intentions. The kind of habit that you will yourself *not* to continue – yet it happens anyway. It is as if when you notice that you are consciously doing it, it is far too late and it has already happened. The triggers have occurred outside your everyday awareness. And you may have noticed that the more attention you give the habit, the harder you try to catch yourself before it starts and make an increased effort to try to stop it – all of this leads in only one direction – more of the habit!

Trying hard in this way invariably leads to failure. Most people, when questioned closely about the problem, are usually picturing the habit occurring in their mind's eye and attempting to alter the picture *as it is happening.* This is too late! We need to back up to the beginning, to the very triggers that cue the unwanted behaviour, and reassociate them to the direction in which we want to go instead. You may be asking if this is possible – and not only that, but whether this can lead to rapid lasting change. In the second half of this chapter we shall explore the *swish pattern,* one of the earliest submodality patterns to be developed by Richard Bandler in the early to mid-1980s. You will find that its principles can be used in a variety of change formats.

There is an old saying about changing habits that I shall return to shortly. First, however, I shall give some examples of everyday clinical issues that have been helped by dissociation of affect.

Sandra's suicide

Sandra had had an unfortunate encounter. The previous week one of her neighbours, a young man in his twenties, had hung himself from a tree that she could see from her kitchen window. Although she had not actually seen him hanging there, she was in attendance when the police mortuary van had arrived to take the body away. As it was wheeled out on a trolley covered by a white cloth, his right arm had rather grotesquely slid out and dangled awkwardly as he bounced rather unceremoniously to the back of the van. This image and the way in which she subsequently imagined he would have looked swinging from the tree had haunted her each night since, preventing her from sleeping.

I asked her about the structure of the troubling images – not the content *per se,* but simply the visual submodalities of the experience. The images were big, bright, colourful and close. It was as if she was there in real time, zoomed right into the small details which replayed over and over again, like a never-ending movie loop, generating a feeling of revulsion.

Taking each of the images in turn, I asked her to do several things in quick succession. 'First I want you to imagine *stepping back* from the image ... and as you see it with an increasing sense of distancing yourself from it ... allow it to get *smaller* ... drain out all of the colour so that it's *black and white* ... and shrink it down to a *still-framed photograph* ... the size of a *postage stamp* ... *way over there* ... And just take a moment ... as you're *comfortable here with me* ... to look at it way over there ... and know that it's *over now* ... and you've *dealt effectively with* something that had troubled you back then ... And you can *preserve anything you've learned* from that event ... *consciously and otherwise* ... and know that you can *use this automatically* in the future ... whenever you need to.'

In the space of a 10-minute consultation we had completed a very simple process that had markedly changed her feelings for the better. Of course, the question that everyone asks at this point is 'How long will this last?' Well, I saw Sandra for review two weeks later, when she told me that from that night on the images had no longer troubled her. Around six months later I was doing a routine contraceptive check and she confirmed, with a smile, that she had not thought of the event for a long time.

Rhonda's RTA

Road traffic accidents are a fairly common occurrence in my neck of the woods, and occasionally it is not simply the physical injuries that may have untoward consequences. There can be psychological issues, too. Although I may have to use collapsing anchors or the phobia cure for more problematic cases, often a simple visual submodality pattern can quickly do the trick.

Rhonda, a teenager, had come off the road at a particularly bad series of bends and had hit a tree, writing off her father's car. Thankfully she walked away without any physical injuries. However, over and over in her mind, like a never-ending loop, she replayed the images of the tree rushing towards her and the sickening jolt as she hit it square on. Two weeks later and her sleep was poor, she was off her food and wondered if I could do anything for her.

I explained to Rhonda that we were going to watch a video rerun of the event again, this time from *before* she had lost control of the car, all the way through the accident until *after* she was safe again. She was to imagine that an observer had taken a *black-and-white* video recording of the whole incident from quite a distance away. She might have to peer to get a sense that she could see herself in the car and watch what had happened to her from this different perspective.

We ran the video through twice, and by the second time she was pointing out things that she had missed previously, such as the excessive speed, failing to slow down when she was coming into the bend, and also the fact that that particular area was notorious for crashes. Her demeanour as she did this had changed markedly. She was speaking in a 'matter-of-fact voice' and was looking far more comfortable in herself. I asked her to imagine the worst part of the whole experience, and to make sure that she had drained out all of the colour and turned it into a small postage stamp-sized memory. She now knew exactly what she would do differently in the future. She had learned her lesson. Her last words were 'Don't tell my dad just how fast I was going, will you!'

These two cases, which are drawn from many similar ones, show how effective it can be to change one's visual perspectives of an event for the better. The next section will give you a format to use with your own patients.

Dissociating affect from memories

The following pattern can be used for any previous life experience. You can disconnect from any unresourceful negative feelings that are involved and see the event in a new light. You can learn any new information that arises from attending to a different perspective and incorporate this into the future so that you now have an updated response if the same circumstances reoccur. This pattern works best for events of medium or low intensity. If you are dealing with a severe trauma or phobia, use the NLP phobia cure described in Chapter 10.

Exercise 9:   Changing perspectives

The following steps are from the viewpoint of the practitioner addressing the patient.

1   Choose a negative experience that still troubles you today. As you *remember it*, imagine that you are seeing that younger you *over there*, as if on a movie screen in your mind's eye.

2   If you are bothered by a single image, *imagine draining out all of the colour* from the image, *turning it into black and white* and shrinking it way down so that it is like a small postage stamp in the distance. Stay here *comfortably* with me, as you see that image way over there.

3   If you are bothered by many images or a recurring movie of an event, imagine that someone has taken a *black-and-white video* of that younger you. Now, in the movie theatre of your mind, imagine a small screen *over there* at a distance. Run the movie again, way over there, all the way through from beginning to end, as you sit here *comfortably* with me, watching what had happened to that younger you.

4   Ensure that, as you *complete the process*, any negative feelings have subsided and you are *now much more comfortable* with the event. If not, cycle through it again, making it smaller, more distanced, adding another perspective such as 'looking down at it as if from a mountain top', etc.

5   When your patient has observed this experience from a completely different perspective, ask 'Is there anything new that *you have learned* and can incorporate into your future?' Help your patient to *verbalise any new thoughts* about the event which they can put to good use both now and later.

6   Imagine that you are now in the future, at a time when an event similar to the past event might occur. This time notice *how you are dealing with it differently*, putting your new thoughts and learning to good effect.

This is a fairly simple process and can be used both formally, as shown above, or informally in casual conversation for any number of troubling memories. It is a very useful first-step procedure, as by itself it can resolve many simple issues quite easily. Of course, if your patient is still in the throes of negative emotions despite this, you can utilise their ongoing response as important feedback that another NLP process is required. Here is an example of how you might set up the situation in casual conversation:

> *'That wasn't a particularly nice experience you* **had** *back then. As you tell me about it, imagine that someone* **had** *followed you around with a video camera that only uses* **black-and-white film**. *Pretend that we're* **watching it from the outside**, *and describe what had happened to* **that you** *back then.'*

In this way you can learn to use the kind of language that helps patients to dissociate from strong feelings, recoding their memories in more useful ways and allowing them to change perspective more easily.

In the next section I shall introduce you, again via case histories, to the swish pattern, one of the earliest submodality patterns to be originated by Richard Bandler.

Norma's nails

For as long as she could remember, Norma had bitten her nails down to the quick. She recognised that some aspects of this habit – which she had tried hard to kick – were related to anxiety. She certainly chewed more when she was tense. Yet there were other times when, for no apparent reason, her hand had mysteriously made its way to her mouth without her conscious knowledge. She desperately wanted long shiny nails – their current look did not fit with the kind of person she considered herself to be.

She was a bit sheepish when she came to ask for help, recognising that although the habit troubled her greatly, it really could not be regarded as a major medical problem. She was quite surprised when I said we could probably do something about it in the next 10 minutes. She had thought I would have to dig deep into 'her murky past' in a kind of psychoanalytical probe for an archaeological find.

I said 'In your mind's eye, imagine that you're getting that feeling of needing to bite your nails, and see the picture you're making as if you're inside it, seeing through your own eyes what's happening now'. She described her picture as a bright, colourful associated image of her hand coming up to her mouth. The closer it came, the more she had the urge to bite. I asked her to lay that image aside for a moment.

'Now I'd like you to make a picture of the "you" for whom nail biting is no longer an issue. The "you" who's solved that problem. You may not know exactly how you've done this – just picture her over there, her nails looking great, and immersed in all the good qualities and attributes that you know you possess.' I encouraged her to make a big, bright, colourful, three-dimensional picture of a Norma as she wanted her to be, ensuring that it was an attractive and compelling vision that really drew her towards it. I waited until it was clear from her physiology that she was glowing from the inside out, and then I asked her to lay the picture aside.

I explained to her what we were going to do next. 'Norma, I want you, in a moment, to go back inside the first picture, seeing your hand coming up to your mouth, and feeling the urge to bite. Then I'd like you to very quickly drain out all of the colour, making it black and white as you zoom it away into the distance, so that "that Norma" becomes a tiny spot on the horizon. At exactly the same time I'd like you to see the Norma for whom this is no longer an issue start off as a small black-and-white spot in the distance and then zoom up to you large as life and in full colour.' I used my hands to show her just how quickly this could happen, making a 'swishing' noise as they crossed over.

I got her to do this five times, with each swish getting faster, so that the last one was almost a blur. In between each attempt she cleared her mental screen by simply imagining a blank sheet of paper. This ensured that she 'swished' in the same direction each time. After a final pause I asked her to think of her original cue picture of her hand coming up to her mouth. All she could see in-stead was the big, bright, colourful picture of the Norma she wanted to become. I suggested that she should try to bite her nails now and see what happened. A strange look came over her face as her hand remained in her lap. She said 'It's odd – like I don't need to do it any more'. And she didn't!

For a while after learning this pattern I practised the technique on any nail biters I could find. I must have successfully swished 20 to 30 people using both similar and different variations of the pattern (*see* below), which really helped me to get to grips with the process. In cases of nail biting there is often very little secondary gain to deal with, which makes it ideal for generating your confidence in the technique.

Craig's cigarettes

Craig, who was in his late twenties, generally smoked 10 to 15 cigarettes a day. He had cut down and almost stopped several times, yet found it difficult to say 'no' if he was offered a cigarette when out socially with friends. This inevit-ably got him started on the downward spiral back to his usual daily number. He wanted to stop, and he wanted to have a social life, too! He reckoned that he had good self-control when he was alone, but this evaporated in company. I saw him at a time when I was just mastering the swish pattern and was using it on anything that moved!

Since one of the main triggering cues was the offer of a cigarette from another person's packet, we used this as the first image. Craig pictured in his mind's eye an open cigarette packet advancing towards him as he heard the words 'Fancy a cig?' He could feel himself divided into two minds, and the beginnings of relief as he started to reach out for one. I asked him to lay that image aside.

Next we developed his desired self-image. This was a dissociated picture of the Craig who was no longer a smoker. I asked him to ensure that his image contained his best qualities and showed him as leaner and fitter, and with a healthier heart and lungs. We made the image as attractive as possible, yet his demeanour told me that something was not quite right – he had a look of slight consternation. He said 'Although I really like what I see, I'm concerned that that Craig would come across as being a bit obnoxious, pious even, and actually lose the friends he's got!'

We certainly did not want a Craig who would aggressively reject his friends' well-meaning offers or, worse still, preach to them about the evils of cigarettes. So I asked him 'What would it be like if you could see a Craig who could deal respectfully with his friends and the choices that they had made for themselves *and* at the same time was respectful of his *own* choices and his *own* long-term health and well-being?' His face immediately softened and his head nodded as he said 'That looks *much* better!'

I was now satisfied that his self-image picture could be used as an appropriate cue for the swish. Just as with Norma, I asked him to shrink down his original associated cue picture, zooming it out to a spot on the distant horizon, while at the same time rapidly bringing his dissociated desired picture up close, large and bright. However, even after several attempts the original cue picture still surfaced, driving his desire to accept the offered cigarette. This distance-based swish was not working, so I tried a variation on the theme.

'Craig, this time, as you see the first cue picture in your mind's eye, look at the bottom right-hand corner and see a small black-and-white "smudge" containing the desired state picture. Now as I say "Swiiiiiissshhhh", shrink the original cue picture into the right-hand corner smudge, and simultaneously explode the desired state into a huge, brightly coloured, compellingly attractive picture.' After the first attempt he broke into a large grin, and although I knew that the other four attempts were probably superfluous, we went through them anyway.

Craig later told me that this intervention had worked well in the social situations for which we had designed it. He had retained his friends and maintained his composure when he was initially pressurised to accept a cigarette. Surprisingly for him, though, he had actually experienced some difficulties with the desire to smoke when he was by himself. Intuitively he had run the swish pattern again, this time substituting the original cue picture with one of his desiring hand reaching for a cigarette of its own volition. He kept the desired state picture the same as the original intervention, and was delighted when it worked perfectly.

Although I used the swish pattern a lot in my early NLP days, I found that many smokers had more complicated addictive issues which needed some of the other types of interventions that you will encounter elsewhere in this book. However, because the swish pattern is a relatively quick intervention, it can be used as a 10-minute first-line approach, keeping the 'bigger gun' techniques to use as a follow-on if necessary.

Patsy's pregnancy

Several years ago we had a small maternity unit attached to our local community hospital, and we would be on hand during the second stage of labour, or earlier in the proceedings, for any maternal or paediatric complications that required assistance. Patsy was admitted in reasonably advanced labour with contractions occurring every three minutes. The midwives were reluctant to give her opiate analgesia, as they felt that delivery was reasonably imminent. Fortunately I already knew Patsy from a previous encounter when we had used the swish pattern to successfully cure her nail-biting habit.

In between contractions I suggested that we could utilise the same pattern to reduce her labour pains. The first cue picture involved looking at her distended abdomen through her own eyes (associated) as the contraction started. The desired state picture was how she would look (dissociated) if she felt an increasing sense of comfort and ease. We customised it a little more than in the standard swish by having *that Patsy* standing apart from the situation as if *she* were looking at *another Patsy* who was going through the contraction some distance away. The purpose of these manoeuvrings was to induce a *double-dissociation* effect to further reduce any discomfort (*see* the phobia cure in Chapter 10 for further explanation).

We practised the swish pattern in between the next set of contractions, and because of Patsy's previous experience with the process, she learned how to do it very swiftly. Using an actual contraction as the real-world trigger, I led her once again through the swish. This time, as the dissociated desired-state picture came up, I kept it there, talking to her in a hypnotic voice tone to further maintain and prolong the dissociative experience. I said 'And you can watch *that Patsy* ...

over there ... with an increasing sense of *comfort* ... with every breath you take ... noticing her watching that *other* Patsy ... *way in the distance* ... like a tiny speck ... *safe and secure here* ... looking at her *over there* ... until you're ready to come back ... *now* ... as the contraction subsides ...'.

Within the space of a couple of contractions the whole process became automatic, so that she simply seemed to drift away in her thoughts. Yet between times she was fully lucid and able to chat away to the midwifery staff and her husband, who had belatedly appeared. Not long afterwards, she delivered a healthy baby girl, Louise, and in the newspaper birth announcements she commented 'arrived with a *swish*'.

If you are interested in using NLP for aspects of pain control, you will find more information and applications in Chapter 17.

The swish pattern

Originally conceptualised by Richard Bandler, the swish pattern has been around since the mid-1980s. It can be utilised in a variety of circumstances, and for those who are particularly interested in the nuances of the pattern, Steve and Connirae Andreas have thoroughly investigated the important aspects of what makes it work in different circumstances (*see* Bibliography).

Exercise 10:   The swish pattern

1   Think of a *recurring behaviour or habit* that you would like to change. Clearly *identify the context* in which it occurs. You may want to see, hear and feel again what is happening in this situation.

2   As you *imagine that you are just about to perform the unwanted behaviour*, identify what it is you are seeing that triggers it. Ensure that this is an *associated* picture, seen from the perspective of your own eyes. Once you have it, set this cue picture aside.

3   Now *create a resourceful*, dissociated self-image of the *you* who no longer has this behaviour or habit. How would you look, sound and feel if you had already resolved this issue? What particular qualities would you be exhibiting? Ensure that this outcome picture is both *attractive* and *compelling* – something you are really *drawn towards*.

4   Now *go back to the original cue picture* and, as you do so, simultaneously see the resourceful picture as a small dot on the distant horizon, with no detail yet visible.

5   Now perform the swish! Make the *original cue picture* go black and white and zoom out into *a small dot in the distance*. Simultaneously, allow the *resourceful image to expand rapidly into a big, bright, close, colourful image that fills the whole screen of your mind*.

6   As soon as you have done the swish, do a '*break state*' by blanking out your mental screen or opening your eyes. *Repeat the swish* at least five times, breaking state in between each one. Do each swish *as quickly as possible!*

7   After a moment or two's distraction to allow the change to settle in, *try to get the original cue picture back*. If you cannot, or if it fades and is unstable in some way, or you immediately *get the outcome picture instead*, then you have finished.

The above exercise is one of the standard ways to use the swish technique, which utilises the submodalities of association and dissociation together with distance and colour/black and white to effect change. Other pairs of submodalities, such as size and brightness, still frames and movies, can be used to exchange the two images. You can test your patient first to see which submodalities are actually their own personal drivers for the experience, and use them instead as a *designer* swish. I personally have found that using the options of distance and brightness seems to work best.

There are several tips which you can follow to make the swish more effective. A few are listed below.

1   Always have the problem picture as an associated state and the solution picture dissociated.

2   Back up and get the earliest trigger possible to use as the start of the swish. This trigger is usually in the external world (a sight, sound, touch, smell or taste), although it may be in the internal world of your patient's mind.

3   Ensure that the solution image is about the *kind* of person they want to become, rather than a specific behaviour. Detail the qualities, skills, attitudes, values and beliefs they would want to have.

4   Make sure that the solution image is not in a specific context (i.e. that it is uncontextualised). This ensures that the new self-image will generalise across more contexts as a generative change.

5   Use a different voice tone and physiology when you are talking about both problem and solution pictures. This will anchor them to your voice and give a strong non-verbal cue when you are carrying out the process.

6   You can enhance the non-verbal cues even more by using your hands to gesture as you demonstrate the process.

7   Always test! Usually the patient can no longer access the problem picture –
     all they see is the outcome picture, or that the submodalities of the problem
     picture have changed significantly.

As well as using the swish for problems, you can also use it to take anything you
do well and make it even better. In this case, the cue picture is of you performing
the skill as you do now. The outcome picture is of that same you having made a
quantum leap in skills improvement. You can utilise this in any area of life.

The swish can also be performed using auditory and kinaesthetic submodalities,
although many people find this a little more complicated. Steve and Connirae
Andreas have discussed this at length in *Change Your Mind and Keep the Change*
(*see* Bibliography).

I generally tend to use the swish pattern when the issues and behaviours
involved have little in the way of secondary gain for the patient and the problem
can be well contextualised. Personally I do not use it for 'heavy-duty' problems
that are cross-contextual, or in areas where there is a major degree of simultaneous or sequential incongruity (e.g. life-disrupting addictions). However, once
these problems have been dealt with by the other techniques you will read
about in subsequent chapters, you can use the swish to 'nail shut' the changes
that have been made and to provide a strong directional future pace.

Submodality patterns: connecting theory and practice

One of the main actions of submodality processes, especially the swish pattern,
is on the initial stimulus, which leads to an entirely different response. This in
turn causes a totally different set of consequences to occur instead of the original
behaviour. It breaks the *classically conditioned* reaction, substituting a completely
new response when the same trigger is reapplied. If you get the earliest trigger
possible, then you will completely bypass the problem behaviour – a neurological
short-circuit. There are also elements of *operant conditioning* akin to a rapid
two-step chaining of anchors – directly from the original stimulus to the outcome state. This then becomes its own positive reinforcer of the new directionalised link.

This bypassing of the original problem response results in *cognitive restructuring*,
whereby a new set of thought processes automatically comes into play. It is like
installing a new cognitive strategy – the original is now unobtainable. In the
case of using the swish to improve on an existing performance, this is essentially
the application of *skills training*. Metaphorically we are saying to our brains 'not
this ... but that instead'.

The desired-state picture that is used in the swish is a major application of *self-efficacy* theory – building a detailed image of possibility, capability and deservedness. At the unconscious processing level this acts as a strong *systems attractor*, powerfully aligning and directionalising current resources toward future change. In this way the triggers of the previously learned *state-dependent* behaviour propel the patient toward a new set of behavioural responses.

Concluding

In this chapter we have considered two of the basic submodality patterns, namely dissociation of affect and the swish. In the right circumstances both can lead to the rapid resolution of a presenting issue with a literally changed perspective, as well as allowing the patient to actually *do something different*. Rather than waiting for time to heal and for events to fade into the past, we can take charge of our own perceptions and *make those changes now*.

Whatever happened to that old saying 'Old habits die hard'? This kind of thinking is the product of a mentality which says that change, if it happens at all, is a long-term and arduous process without guarantees. Yet that kind of thinking is simply that – a kind of thinking, not the literal truth! Rather than trying to change the old saying directly, simply identify your mental triggers for it and then lay them aside briefly.

Now consider this. What if you were becoming the kind of person who, even if you didn't know exactly how, was developing the kinds of qualities that could automatically lead you in the direction of believing that 'change is *easy* – and I'm learning the steps, now'? What if you were already making a big, bright, colourful self-image of the *you* who was consciously and unconsciously assimilating all of the skills in this book as you continued to read on? And lastly (before the next chapter, at any rate) what if you fired those original 'old-saying' triggers, heard a swishing noise in your ears that increased in volume and intensity, and found instead that 'Old habits ... *change easily*'!

CHAPTER 10

Phobias and traumatic memories

Introduction

Up until now, the kinds of techniques and processes that we have been learning about have been really useful for applying to memories, behaviours and contexts that have had only a mild to moderate negative emotional charge. If we were to use a scaling rating, where the number 1 represented the least traumatic and 10 the most traumatic memory that your patient was dealing with, then in general the previous techniques are useful for ratings of 5 or under. So how do we deal with those situations that are rated between 5 and 10 (or above!)? And what kinds of situations are we alluding to?

Although we dealt with some simple phobias with the collapsing anchors process, you may often find that the traumatic response is so huge that it engulfs any positive resource states with which you attempt to resolve it. In the case of a phobia, you can calibrate to this quite easily. The very mention or thought of the situation may give rise to an overwhelming physiological reaction. Of course, other situations, such as post-traumatic stress disorder (PTSD), sexual abuse, major accidents or trauma, emotional abuse, etc., can all give rise to a similar reaction. You may well be asking yourself 'What is really going on here? What is the representational system and submodality structure of this response?'

In NLP terms, these memories are stored as *synaesthesias*. This occurs when two representational systems are inextricably linked together so that you cannot have one present without immediately and simultaneously accessing the other. In most phobias and traumatic memories a visual/kinaesthetic (V/K) synaesthesia is the most common form – where a remembered picture or movie evokes the response. However, it is possible to have auditory/kinaesthetic (A/K) and even kinaesthetic/kinaesthetic (K/K) synaesthesias. An A/K synaesthesia occurs when a particular sound or voice triggers the phobic-type state. A K/K synaesthesia occurs when a sensory stimulus, such as a particular kind of touch, triggers an overwhelming negative reaction. Of course, those of you who are becoming even more astute will recognise that strongly positive synaesthesias can also occur. I shall leave further examples to your imagination!

The good news about all of these types of negative synaesthesias is that there is an NLP process, the *phobia cure*, which can quickly disconnect the previously formed link, leading to rapid resolution of even the most traumatic of issues. Given that the most common synaesthesia is a V/K linkage, this is often called the V/K dissociation process, although the procedure can easily be adapted for the other types, too.

Just as a reminder, Richard Bandler modelled the early prototypes of the process when he encountered some people whose phobias had resolved spontaneously. They each seemed to report a variation on the theme 'It's like it had happened to someone else in the past'. They could picture themselves *over there* as they felt comfortable talking about the event here and now. They had disconnected the strong, overwhelming negative feelings. And what is more, encountering the same event in the future generally elicited only neutral feelings of the 'ho-hum' variety.

As you continue reading the next section, you can keep in mind those of your patients who might also benefit from this process. You might even consider whether you, too, have carried certain memories of events in less than useful ways that could easily be updated using this technique. Occasionally, simply reading about similar circumstances can cause spontaneous, often unlooked-for changes to occur automatically!

Stella's spider phobia

Stella, a young woman in her twenties, had a long-standing phobia of spiders. Curiously, the smaller they were, the more she reacted. Interestingly, spider phobias are the number-one fear in the UK! Yet for most people, encounters with spiders are few and far between, so the tendency is to simply live with the phobia in the knowledge that only a tiny proportion of life is affected. However, Stella was different. Her phobia of spiders had become almost an obsession that markedly affected her behaviour in everyday life – whether a spider was in view or not!

Things were generally at their worst in summer, although her pattern of behaviour continued throughout the year. She kept all of her windows shut and double-checked this in summer, no matter how hot it became inside. She could never let herself go to sleep with an open bedroom window. Each night her husband had to check the bathroom – just in case! Things had come to a head when her brother was due to be married in England during a spell of glorious weather. Her husband had to close all of the hotel-room windows and check out every inch of the bedroom and bathroom before she came in.

Now it was clear that there was an element of obsessive-compulsive behaviour in Stella's actions, rather than just a simple phobia, yet when she tearfully came for help I decided that the standard phobia cure would be my first-line intervention. One of the most important things you can do before attempting the process is to ensure that you have anchored some powerful resource states to use as a 'bail-out' anchor in case things go awry and your patient gets caught up in the phobic state in front of your eyes. I had already calibrated to Stella's initial reaction when I produced a matchbox and told her there was a spider inside it – and then proceeded to show her the empty box! Now we searched her history to find out which resources would be useful in the upcoming process.

I was absolutely fascinated to find two amazing resources which I resolved to use. The first was when Stella had actually ridden on a crocodile when on holiday in Australia! The second was when, during her travels in India, she had been photographed with a snake around her neck. She had clearly enjoyed both experiences and had been fearless during each episode. Her husband had flatly refused to do either! This was as clear an indication as I had ever had that people can have fantastic resources which they are unable to bring to bear on a state-dependent memory, which can fire off autonomously and take control of their life. The first step was to revivify both states and anchor these on her knuckles. This was our 'bail-out' anchor in case things got tough.

When we were ready to begin, I said 'In your mind's eye, I'd like you to imagine you're in a cinema, sitting in a comfortable chair, watching a blank movie screen over there'. She closed her eyes as she did so, and for a moment or two I simply added some words about her ability to develop a deepening sense of comfort and relaxation as we went on with the process. I continued 'Now I'm going to ask you to do something that might seem a little odd. I'd like you to imagine that you're floating backwards out of that you in the cinema ... floating all the way back to the projectionist booth ... and when you *arrive there* you can feel even more safe and secure as you *watch that Stella* down there in the cinema watching the blank screen. As soon as *you've done that ... fully and completely* ... you can give me a nod to let me know *you're there now.'* We had completed the first part of the process and I squeezed her knuckle to anchor this dissociation. The bail-out anchors were ready and waiting – just in case.

'Now, staying safely and securely in the projectionist booth, I'd like you to identify the first time, or the most intense episode of your "spider response". As you do that, you can imagine it's stored in an old movie newsreel ... black-and-white film ... gathering dust in the archives.' She actually uncovered the very first episode she could remember, which was as a seven-year-old child, when her older brother had put a spider down her nightdress while she was reading in bed – a typical 'fun' thing for a big brother to do!

'Stella, you know that there was a time before that event occurred when you were totally safe ... (head nods) ... I'd like you to put a black-and-white still-frame photo of that young Stella up on the screen ... (nods) ... and you know that after the event had occurred, when it was all over, there was a time when you felt OK ... I'd like you to put up another black-and-white photo of *that* young Stella on the screen.' In this way we created a 'safety sandwich', so that when we came to run the movie we could frame it between those two times of safety and prevent it continuing as an endless loop.

'Now *staying here safely* in the projectionist booth ... feeling all these good feelings (squeeze resource anchors) ... you can watch *that Stella* down there in the cinema as *she* watches that *younger Stella* on the screen go through that event again ... all the way through to the end ... *in black and white* ... until she's safe again.' During this part of the process it is important to calibrate carefully and notice whether your patient is slipping back into the phobic experience. You can keep firing both the dissociation and the resource anchors to prevent this happening. By distancing the movie screen, so that it appears smaller and even further away, you can maintain the dissociation from any negative feelings.

'Once she's past the end and safe again, I'd like you to *freeze the frame* ... (nods) ... then I'd like you to *float down* into that Stella who's watching in the cinema ... (nods) ... and from there ... *step inside* the still-frame picture ... give that young Stella a big hug ... and tell her she's safe now ... as you pull her right inside yourself ... *integrating* with her fully and completely again.' During this part of the process, having reviewed the situation from a new perspective, we must then integrate the 'watching self' with the 'participating self' to realign the experience fully. In the early days of the V/K dissociation process this was where the therapy finished, with some additional future pacing. However, in order to make the process even more robust, Richard Bandler added another section.

'Stella, now that *you're inside the movie* I'd like you to turn on all the colours ... then very quickly feel yourself being pulled back through the memory ... all the pictures going rapidly in reverse ... all the sounds ... all the words in reverse, too ... getting faster and faster until you "pop" out of the beginning again ...' Her eyes fluttered rapidly as she completed this phase, letting me know with a nod of her head that she had finished. Moving back through a memory in this way totally scrambles the submodalities of the experience, stripping away any remnants of the phobic response from its triggering cues. This stage can be repeated several times if necessary until the emotional response has been completely neutralised.

The final stage of the process was to embed the changes that she had made into the future. 'Stella, I'd now like you to picture yourself at a time and a place in the future, and notice your response to spiders now.' I simultaneously fired off her resource anchors and she laughed, saying 'Oh my God, I'm riding around my living-room on the back of a crocodile with a snake round my neck, chasing away spiders of all shapes and sizes. And what a mess the crocodile's making on the carpet!' We took her new self-image into three further future contexts as we finished off.

I saw Stella by chance in the waiting-room two weeks later, when she confirmed that she had hardly given the spiders a thought, and her husband had stopped checking bathrooms and bedrooms. Later that summer they both had a carefree weekend visiting her brother and his new wife.

Margaret's motor-bike

Margaret had been a keen biker until she had been involved in a collision at a crossroads. The driver of a car had failed to notice her, and had turned right on to a main carriageway and struck her broadside on, causing her to somersault and land several yards away. She had extensive soft tissue injuries to her shoulder and upper back, and was lucky to escape without any fractures. Since that incident, some nine months previously, she had neither ridden on her motorbike nor driven her car. With two young children to look after, her inability to use private transport was becoming more and more of a nuisance. Knowing of my interest in NLP, she came to see what could be done about the problem.

Whenever she thought of the accident she felt as if she was reliving the whole episode again from the 'inside out', in full Technicolor. She was tense and winced several times during the telling of her tale, rubbing her left shoulder, which was still painful with restricted movement from her injuries. She was keen to try anything that could get her back on the road again.

We ran the standard phobia process from beginning to end, in a similar way to that described above for Stella. Margaret found it a really odd yet very calming experience to watch herself for the first time from 'outside in'. She recalled many other details from the incident that had been 'forgotten', which gave her a more complete picture of the event and an inner sense of comfort that it was now 'finally over'. Interestingly, when we had finished she rubbed her left shoulder, surprised that the ache had gone and it felt 'much freer and more flexible'. Indeed, from that day on not only was she able to get back on her motorbike *and* drive a car without any further mental trauma, but also she found that she rapidly regained full mobility of her previously stiff shoulder.

Margaret's recovery from her physical symptoms would not have surprised NLP trainers Tim Hallbom and Suzi Smith. They believe that if the memory of a physical trauma is stored as an associated memory, then the remembering of the event triggers the same micromuscular movements as the original trauma. For this reason many people repeatedly 'relive' their accidents, and carry around with them chronic muscular tension that can lead to prolonged healing times and even chronic pain syndromes. These authors anecdotally report obtaining good results using the phobia process together with re-imprinting of the original event (*see* Chapter 15 for details of re-imprinting). Perhaps this is an area that would repay further study.

At this juncture I shall describe the various steps of the process before going on to discuss its use in two other cases.

The phobia/trauma cure method

This process is mainly used for those kinds of overwhelmingly negative emotional response that require some degree of V/K dissociation in order to dissolve the synaesthesia. Although it was originally used for simple phobias in cases where collapsing anchors was ineffective, it can be utilised for any severe emotional or physical trauma.

If you think about it, phobias are the doyen of one-trial learning – a significant, often lifelong (unless treated) automatic response occurs with one exposure! The fear is anchored very strongly to the originating stimulus, whether that is an insect, another type of animal, a person or a situation. The anxious feelings that are generated become so intense that the situational cues trigger an avoidance response – it must be escaped from at all costs! Of course, psychologists would like to use the same structure to engender overwhelmingly powerful *positive* emotional responses to enable one-trial learning in the field of education. What a joy education would be then!

What follows here is the standard phobia cure model as it is taught on most NLP practitioner courses. It is best to use this format with another person to guide you through the process. It is not recommended that you should attempt to use this on yourself! I have presupposed that you have already established rapport, calibrated to the patient's phobic physiology and excluded and/or dealt with any secondary gain issues.

Exercise 11:   The phobia/trauma process

1   First, and most importantly, *establish some powerful resource anchors* that you can use throughout the process, especially if your patient inadvertently accesses the phobic state. This is called a *'bail-out' anchor*.

2   Establish the first dissociation by asking the patient to imagine sitting comfortably in a cinema, watching a small screen 'over there' that runs only black-and-white movies from the past.

3   Establish the *second dissociation* by asking the patient to imagine floating backwards out of their body up to the safety of the projectionist booth. You can *anchor this* with a touch and a different voice tone. You can also fire the resource-state anchor when they are there, so that they can feel comfortable 'watching that you (name) down in the cinema as he or she prepares to learn something new'.

4   In the projectionist booth, select the reel of film from the past that contains the *earliest/most intense example* of the phobia/trauma. Ensure that this runs from when they were safe *before* the incident occurred, through the event until *after* they were safe again (safety sandwich).

5   Maintaining the double dissociation, *run the movie in black and white* all the way through to the end. Watch your patient closely to prevent them from reaccessing the phobic feelings. If they do this, use the resource anchor and run the movie again, altering the submodalities to give more distance, fuzziness of the picture, or anything else that further minimises the response. *Freeze frame the final image* when they are safe again. Ask them what they have learned from this new perspective.

6   *Now reassociate* all of the previous dissociations. Ask the patient to float down into their watching self in the cinema, fully reconnecting, and then step into the screen itself and *fully integrate with their younger self*. This is an important part of the process to ensure free access to all resources and learnings.

7   Staying inside the movie, fully associated, *run the movie quickly backwards* in full colour. Make sure that all of the actions, words and sounds are going in reverse. The patient may have the feeling that they are being rapidly pulled back through it until they literally 'pop' out before the beginning. You can repeat this step two or more times to *fully diminish any residual emotional charge*.

8   Once you are certain that the negative feelings have either completely gone or are markedly reduced, ask the patient to *imagine the same situation occurring in different contexts in the future*. Use their resource anchors as you *ask them what is different in their experience now*.

This pattern is one of the most powerful in the NLP toolkit. You can adapt its principles to fit many different contexts and problems. For example, rather than using the 'cinema' analogy, you can facilitate dissociation in a number of ways. One patient imagined that she was sitting comfortably in her living-room – a context that she knew well and was 'at home' with – watching her television set. The second dissociation was achieved by imagining that she had floated out of the window and was outside the house looking in at herself sitting on the chair watching events as they unfolded on the television screen.

Maintaining dissociation during this process is probably the most important element in making it work. You can facilitate this more expertly by using your voice pitch and locus adroitly. When you address the 'you sitting in the cinema', direct your voice to the person and speak at normal pitch. When you are addressing the 'you in the projectionist booth', turn your head and direct your voice up and behind them, speaking in a slightly higher pitch. When you are addressing the 'younger you on screen', turn your head away from them to the front, speaking in a slightly lower pitch. If the patient happens to keep their eyes open during the procedure, you can also gesture appropriately. You can easily practise doing this by rehearsing the process with an empty chair.

For simple phobias, ecology is not usually an issue. However, after more major traumas, especially post-traumatic stress disorder and sexual abuse, many other life contexts may have been adversely affected. After such an event it is easy to form limiting beliefs that may further constrain the expression of certain behaviours with specific people or in particular places. Some patients may require many extra resources and skills to deal with relationships and social situations in a new way. If there has been a prolonged period of incapacity, they may have to completely rethink their life's course.

We shall now consider two more cases which illustrate other clinical situations that can benefit from this approach. You can watch out for minor adaptations of the technique that more easily facilitate each encounter.

Sharon's sexual abuse

Sharon was in her early thirties. Between the ages of nine and 15 years she had been sexually abused by a friend of the family. The abuse ranged from touching and petting to full sexual intercourse. Like many who have been abused, she had felt deeply guilty that it had all been her fault, and had kept it secret from everyone apart from her husband. Her frequent nightmares and thrashing about in bed had forced her to tell him a little about what had happened to her, although he didn't know the worst of it.

I knew nothing about it myself until she came to the health centre one day very upset. Several weeks previously a policewoman had arrived unexpectedly at her door. She told her that the perpetrator of the abuse had been accused by another woman who had suffered in the same way, and that in the course of the investigations Sharon had also been named. Preparations were being made for Court, and she was requested to be a witness for the prosecution.

Initially she told no one else about this, and over the next few weeks she was deluged with flashbacks to her younger years. They could occur at any time, but especially when she was doing domestic chores such as ironing. She said 'One minute I'm in the here and now and the next it's like I'm back there again, aged nine or twelve or whatever, reliving it all, with no way out.' Her nightmares increased and her sleep was even more disturbed. During our initial consultation I explained about the phobia/trauma technique, and we set up a longer appointment to run the process.

We started off by following the protocol, and I made sure that I had created sufficient dissociation *and* that I had a powerful 'bail-out' anchor. Rather than go through each individual event, I created a safety sandwich that started just before the age of nine, prior to the abuse, and finished just after the age of 15, when the abuse had stopped. I asked Sharon to run the movie of all those years from beginning to end. It did not matter if the events were at all blurred, perhaps hard to see and in the distance – only that we counted off the years until 'that little girl had become a young woman and was safe again'.

I asked Sharon to step into the end of the movie and to give that young Sharon a big hug. 'Please let her know that you're from her future, to let her fully understand that she never needs to go through any of that ever again. I'd like you to tell her that she did the very best she could under the most difficult of circumstances that anyone could face. And not only that – tell her she's the reason that you survived and are here today, a living, full-grown, adult woman. Once you're sure she understands all that completely, I'd like the two of you to integrate fully, as one whole person, and take everything you've learned here today out into the kind of future you deserve to have.'

That one session effected an 80 to 90% improvement in her condition. Interestingly, she did have a setback after a prolonged police interview in which she had to give a detailed statement about all that had happened to her. This forced her back into the position of reliving some of the events from the 'inside out', and gave her some more sleepless nights. We had a repeat session and dealt with the more troubling memories. However, having gone through the phobia process again, she found that some of the other memories were really hard to get into, and she struggled to remember the kind of detail that had previously haunted her – so much so that the veracity of sections of her earlier police statement was questioned!

The worst thing about the Court procedure was the recurrent cancelling of the case at the last minute. This happened several times – once within a day of the proceedings starting. It really made me wonder about the whole process of giving evidence and how it could be improved from the victim's point of view. Some 18 months later the abuser was sent to prison for eight years, and Sharon could finally get on with her life.

Barbara's baby encounter

Barbara, who had been a social worker for nearly 15 years, found it very difficult to deal with a particular situation that arose when she was on call for emergencies. A little baby, the product of a concealed delivery outwith hospital, was found dead in a house, wrapped in a polythene bag. The images haunted her and prevented her going to work. Her employers arranged for counselling, but the psychodynamic approach – which involved performing a ritual with a doll – seemed to increase rather than alleviate her symptoms. A very practical and straightforward woman, she could not understand why she was unable to deal with the situation.

When I described the phobia/trauma process to her, she was very unconvinced about how it would help. She could not imagine being in a cinema, and as soon as she closed her eyes she said she could see nothing at all. I decided there and then to use a variant of the process which I had read about in an article by NLP trainers Richard Bolstad and Margot Hamblett.

I placed two chairs one behind the other, facing the front wall of my room. As Barbara sat in the front chair, I asked her to simply project out her memory of that particular day's events on to the wall. I said 'You know when you left home that morning to go to work, *before* it all happened, you were feeling relatively comfortable, right? And when you arrived back home *after* all the trials and tribulations of the day, Sam (her husband) was there to give you a hug. Now just pretend that you can see both of those times out there on the wall'. She nodded, and I knew that we had just set up our safety sandwich.

Then I asked her to get up and move to the seat directly behind. 'Now from here, Barbara, I'd like you to pretend that you're looking over *that Barbara's* shoulder in front of you. I know she's not really there, yet just imagine what she would look like from behind if she were.' Once I was certain that we had this second dissociation in place, I led her through the traumatic memory itself. 'It doesn't matter whether *you really see it clearly in black and white ... from beginning to end ... over there on the wall ...* or not. Just pretend that you do.' Using a question-and-answer format, over *that Barbara's* shoulder, I talked her through the sequence of events which had occurred that day until the details were literally plastered all over the wall.

I asked her to sit for a moment in the first chair looking at the Barbara *over there* on the wall, and said 'You might think that this has been a really *"off the wall"* experience so far, and to *complete it*, you can simply imagine *reconnecting* all aspects of *yourself together*, so that what's *all past now* can be the foundation for a new *look to the future*'. And with that having been said, we had successfully completed the process.

What we did here was to use spatial anchors to mark out the different states and keep them separate. The chairs were situated so as to ensure a different visual perspective from each position. Much as before, I used my language and gestures to maintain the dissociation as Barbara participated in an eyes-open procedure. Paradoxically, I have noticed that patients may develop an even more deeply dissociated state when doing the process in this way, rather than with their eyes closed. It is certainly worth your while experimenting with this approach.

How the phobia cure works: connecting theory to practice

The phobia cure is an example of the more general category of interventions known as *systematic desensitisation* (*see* Chapter 2 on models of learning and changing and Chapter 7 on collapsing anchors). This is a form of *counter-conditioning* whereby a competing state such as relaxation is paired with the anxiety-provoking situation. In the classical methodology of Wolpe, the patient is gradually introduced in his or her imagination to a hierarchy of increasingly anxiety-provoking imagery. The key of course is to remain in the relaxed state throughout. At the very least the phobia cure utilises two competing states to counter-condition the original event, namely the relaxing effect of dissociation together with application of the resource anchors. In my experience this combination allows the complete viewing in one session of very traumatic memories with little or no provocation of anxiety.

It is also possible that the phobia cure could work by means of *operant conditioning*. This is where more prolonged continued exposure to the feared stimulus *without* the usual consequences causes *extinction* of the response. This is a key feature of cognitive–behavioural therapy exposure techniques, such as imaginal and 'real-life' *flooding* and *implosion*. However, the tendency with these techniques is to actually *increase* the fear or anxiety first, keeping the exposure going until the response has peaked, faded and been replaced with relative ease. They are therefore sometimes called *anxiety-induction* therapies, and many patients find them very uncomfortable although effective. However, most patients who encounter the phobia cure experience anxiety *reduction* from the start of the process. The rarely used NLP technique of *compulsion blow-out* works in a similar manner to flooding and implosion techniques.

A major element of *cognitive restructuring* takes place in the phobia cure, as the feared stimulus is literally 'seen' differently. Processing previously vivid visual imagery, by turning it into black and white and then running it backwards, randomly scrambles and disconnects all of the triggering cues, reassociating them to a neutral response. This restructuring has a profound effect on the patient's *self-efficacy*, markedly strengthening their belief that they can now cope with future *in vivo* exposure. In addition to this, it installs a different strategy of future response by imaginal rehearsal – a form of *cognitive skills training*.

As a *state-dependent* memory, the negative emotion can be used to track back to the original trauma. Whether you actually deal with the earliest memory of the response is not that important. So long as you utilise the memory of an event that was of high intensity, the resolution will generalise to all other memories in the chain. The *attractor basin* of the phobic reaction is narrow and deep. This means that falling into it is relatively uncommon, yet when this happens the response may be overwhelming in its intensity. Rather than simply creating another attractor to move towards instead, the phobia process systematically dismantles the existing one, leaving the landscape smooth and flat.

Having read this section, you might find it useful to review the function of the amygdala in fear-based conditioned responses (*see* Chapter 4). It may be that the phobia cure allows elements of the non-conscious memory store to be reprocessed via the hippocampus and then moved into long-term memory as a resolved event.

Concluding

Phobias are an exquisite example of one-trial learning, yet once you appreciate their structure – how they exist as a synaesthesia – it becomes relatively easy to take them apart and neutralise the response. The phobia process can be applied to any clinical situation in which the patient has an overwhelming fear- or anxiety-based response, including rape and post-traumatic stress disorder of any origin. The procedure itself is based on a raft of well-supported cognitive–behavioural interventions, and is a particularly good example of systematic desensitisation in action. The major benefit is that your patient is very likely either to have a one-session 'cure' of their problem or at least to experience a substantial reduction in symptomatology.

You may already have in mind some patients who might benefit from this approach. However, before you launch yourself on them with gay abandon, you must ensure that they *do* want to go through the process and that you have excluded or taken care of any secondary-gain issues prior to your intervention. In Chapter 19 on 'the dark side of the force', I give some salutary examples of the potential pitfalls of failing to consider these aspects. Nevertheless, this is one of the most powerful NLP techniques, and it is a most valuable addition to your therapeutic toolbox.

CHAPTER 11

The counter-example process

Introduction

What is it that is always at the cutting edge of scientific advancement? What is it that scientists are actually looking for? What is the one thing that can blow a scientific theorem out of the water? The answer is a counter-example. Scientific theorems represent our best current thinking and explanation about the world at large. Like our beliefs, they are broad, acceptable generalisations that help us to navigate the various contexts of our life. And again like our beliefs, they can be changed and updated by a single counter-example that disproves the theorem. An effective counter-example may be the single most powerful catalyst for change.

Generalisations are usually examples of what NLP calls *universal quantifiers*. These include words like *all, every, always, never*, etc. Whenever someone complains that something *always* occurs in a particular context – an invariable response – then the provision of one effective counter-example may often be enough to permanently change that response, or at least to make it as permanent as the problem used to be! And it matters not a whit whether the problem has been there for only a short period, or whether there is a seemingly infinite number of examples of proof extending back as far as can be remembered.

Perhaps you have had this kind of experience yourself. Maybe you can think back to one of those times when there was something you knew that you could not do. Something that your own personal history told you that you could not accomplish. Then one day, for some reason – possibly even without knowing why – you spontaneously succeeded for the first time. Now your brain may still have coded this as a 'lucky fluke', which is one way to deal with the cognitive dissonance that arises with success. Yet no matter how you initially code it, this counter-example may well prove to be the turning point that allows you to re-enter that context both with increased choice and confident of a different outcome.

Robert Dilts first modelled the counter-example process when he was researching allergies, which he regarded as a *phobia* of the immune system – creating a response that was grossly out of proportion to the initial stimulus.

A response that could be triggered not only by being in the presence of an allergen, but also in some people simply by *thinking* about it in a certain way. In his experimentation, Dilts looked for those times when the expected allergic response failed to occur – that is, a powerful contextual counter-example. If he failed to find evidence of that in the patient's personal history, he searched for something that was sufficiently like the allergen, but for which they had a normal, non-allergic response. Anchoring this normal response state, he then brought it to bear on the allergen in a controlled way, and in many cases eliminated the allergic reaction.

In this chapter, then, we shall explore how the counter-example process can be used not only in the field of allergies, but also in other non-related areas. You will find it a versatile tool for a variety of circumstances.

Katrina's cats

Katrina, who was in her fifties, had had a 'lifelong' allergy to cats. She found that being in the presence of a cat brought on symptoms of itchy, watering eyes, sneezing and a widespread urticarial reaction. Many of these symptoms were controlled by antihistamine medication which she used on an intermittent basis. Most of the time she simply avoided the situation as best she could, 'popping a pill' when appropriate. However, this coming summer she was due to spend two weeks at her daughter's house in Hertfordshire, and her daughter had two cats! Much as she wanted to go, she was also experiencing trepidation at the thought of what this prolonged exposure might do to her. She had already had to take a course of oral steroids for a severe reaction on one previous occasion. Fortunately she had never had an anaphylactic response.

When she first consulted about the impending problem, my initial thought was to explore any issues of secondary gain that the symptom might have for her. I was especially curious about the relationship she had with her daughter, and whether her condition might 'fortuitously' prevent her summer visit, by acting as a ready-made excuse in lieu of inability to say 'no' for more deeply held reasons. This kind of area needs to be explored very sensitively! Having explored it thoroughly, it was clear that Katrina had had symptoms on and off from early childhood, obviously preceding her daughter's birth. It did cross my mind that her daughter might derive some secondary gain from having the cats in the first place, although living about 500 miles away did provide her with a great deal of protection from spur-of-the-moment parental visits!

I asked Katrina to imagine being in the presence of a cat, so that I could calibrate to her physiology, eye-accessing cues and symptomatic response. She sneezed twice, her eyes reddened and her face went pale. I had seen enough of a response to know that I could check after the process to identify what had changed. I explained to her that her immune system had 'made a mistake' and was reacting out of all proportion to the stimulus. I told her that our job today was to retrain her immune system to provide an appropriate, more neutral response. I calibrated her non-verbal communication carefully to ensure that this pre-frame had been accepted. I also made sure that I checked what her life would be like without the allergy. Exploring the positive and negative consequences in this way fully respected the ecology of the situation. We were ready to begin in earnest.

The most important part of the process is to find an appropriate counter-example. The ideal kind of example is an occasion when the patient has previously been in the presence of the allergen but *did not* experience the allergic response. Unfortunately, this had never happened to Katrina. We then searched for a convincing counter-example that was similar enough to cats to use instead. I asked her which animals she could easily be in the presence of and remain completely well. We excluded horses straight away – they were simply too big, even though she had ridden many times over the years. Dogs were a possibility, but from her initial response I did not think they would fit the bill. Then we found our counter-example – a guinea pig! This was of a similar size to a cat and could be held and petted on her knee with no ill effect. Given that she nodded vigorously in response to this idea, I decided to proceed.

I said 'Katrina, I'd like you to think back in your mind's eye to a particular time, a particular place, when you were comfortably in the presence of a guinea pig. And as you *go be there now*, I'd like you to *see* what you're seeing, *hear* what you're hearing and *feel* all those feelings as if it's happening *here ... right now*. And you can know that your immune system is responding appropriately ... normally ... the immune cells getting about their routine, day-to-day business ... feeling this (set touch anchor on knuckle) natural connection'. By anchoring this state I had captured the essence of her normal physiological response to the counter-example.

Now that we had our resource state available, it was time to move on to the next stage, which was to create a safe place of dissociation, much like the phobia cure process. 'Katrina, I'd like you to imagine a wall-to-wall Plexiglass shield in front of you ... the kind of shield that can fully protect you from the feelings on the other side ... yet at the same time allow you to see clearly what's happening over there.' I waited until she had nodded her head before proceeding. 'And on the other side of the Plexiglass, I'd like you to see another Katrina ... a Katrina who's about to learn something new ...'

Once I was certain that we had established the necessary degree of dissociation, I continued 'As you look at that Katrina, beam across to her this new resource ... this new immune response ... and see her light up from the inside out ... knowing that *things can be different now'*. I fired off the anchor on her knuckle and kept it active throughout the rest of the process. Now it was time to gradually introduce the allergen.

'Katrina, I'd like you to *keep watching* that Katrina over there ... her face, her skin colour, her breathing ... and ensure that throughout this process she remains in this really good state. Gradually ... from a distance ... let her see a cat approaching ... and only let it approach closer at the rate and speed at which you see her *maintain and even intensify* this resourceful state ... (pressing the anchor even more). Watch her closely and see how her breathing is normal ... her skin colour is normal ... her eyes are normal ... her nose feels normal ...' I calibrated closely, ensuring that the anchored response was strong as I encouraged her to see *that Katrina* with the cat on her lap, as she stroked its fur and heard it purring with delight.

'Now imagine that five minutes have passed and Katrina's looking fine ... then 10 minutes ... half an hour ... an hour ... two hours ... half a day ... a full day ...' I future paced her newly acquired normal response over the next 24 hours, ensuring that the old response did not get a chance to recur. When I was satisfied, I said 'Let the Plexiglass shield dissolve ... and welcome Katrina who's learned something of great value to you ... pulling her back inside you ... fully connecting ... spreading this new response through every cell in your body'. I completely reassociated her to the here and now as I continued to hold the resource anchor.

·'Katrina ... you can now imagine being on your summer holiday ... at your daughter's house ... for two whole weeks ... and notice how things are different now ... with your new response ... the cats around you ... you're continuing well ... and everything's fine ...' We future paced her response throughout the two weeks and beyond, ensuring that the old reaction failed to surface.

Later that summer she reported back that everything had indeed gone well. She had had an initial tingling feeling in her nose which had settled with one antihistamine tablet – she required no more. Although she had a 100% success rate, I have found that on average the success rate is around 50%. The less secondary gain there is and the more identical the counter-example, the more successful the process will be.

Pete's pollen allergy

Pete, a married man in his early thirties, had a recurrent summer problem with hay-fever symptoms. He usually required antihistamines, nasal sprays and eye drops, and he had occasionally been given intramuscular steroids. He had heard about the success of another patient of mine with NLP techniques, and was keen to have a go himself.

Because an almost identical counter-example is the best resource to use, we racked our brains to think of one. Pete could not remember any time when he had not had a response to pollen. A keen runner, he had to confine his summer runs to coastline paths. Anything inland, especially near fields of oilseed rape, brought him to an eye-watering standstill. Our initial difficulty was that we could not think of anything that was like pollen – floating invisibly in the air. However, a 'chance' remark about how different it was in winter, running through pine forests and smelling the distinct aroma in the air, gave us our resource.

We set up the process in exactly the same way as I have described for Katrina. I associated Pete back into one of his favourite pine-forest runs. I completely revivified the experience, amplifying the sounds, smells and tastes as he heard his feet padding softly through the pine needle-laden tracks. Focusing on his breathing, he concentrated on his normal immune response to the smell of pine in the air, which I duly anchored. We ran through the rest of the process holding this anchor throughout.

We did this four years ago, and Pete had what he termed an 80 to 90% response rate. On days with a very high pollen count he takes an occasional oral antihistamine, and he no longer requires the other medication. Generally, however, with more non-specific allergens (such as pollen) it is more difficult to find an acceptable counter-example, which is probably why my success rate is no higher than 50%!

The counter-example process

Initially modelled by Robert Dilts for allergy resolution, the principles of the counter-example process can be utilised in a wide variety of circumstances. In fact, any problem for which you can conceptualise having a counter-example is a candidate for its use. One way of mastering the various NLP patterns is to focus exclusively on one of them for a period of time, and to see every presenting issue through that pattern's lens. In this way, rather than merely exhibiting *the* particular technique for *the* specific problem, you will more quickly realise the deeper fundamentals of the principles of effective change. The various steps for you to begin using this process successfully are described below.

Exercise 12: The counter-example process

1 First, it is important to *flush out any areas of secondary gain* that might need to be addressed. What will the consequences be after the problem is resolved? How will life be different? What else may change?

2 *Calibrate to the allergic response.* Ask 'What happens when you are in the presence of the allergen?' Notice the patient's eye-accessing and projection cues together with physiological changes.

3 *Find an appropriate counter-example* to use as a resource. If you can find an instance when the expected reaction did not occur, then use it. If not, search for a counter-example that is sufficiently like the example. It is best if the patient spontaneously comes up with their own choice.

4 *Reassociate the patient fully to the counter-example.* Step them back into that experience and revivify it completely, emphasising their normal immune reaction in these circumstances. At the peak of the state, *anchor it to a knuckle.* Keep this state active throughout the rest of the process.

5 Now *create an effective dissociation* by imagining a wall-to-wall and floor-to-ceiling Plexiglass shield. If necessary you can use the additional steps in the phobia process. Get the patient to 'see that other you, over there, on the far side of the screen, with this new and updated immune response'.

6 Keeping the dissociation in place and *firing the resource anchor, gradually introduce the allergen.* Calibrate carefully to ensure that they do not slip back into the allergic state. Get them to 'watch that other you over there, paying special attention to their breathing, posture and other reactions ... until they can successfully be in the presence of the allergen ... having this new immune response instead'.

7 When you *notice the physiological shift* that lets you know their responses have now been updated, dissolve the Plexiglass shield and *fully integrate the new responses inside them.* Keep holding the resource anchor as you do this.

8 Finally, *take them out into the future* when they may meet the allergen that used to cause the allergic response, and *notice how things are different now.*

It is not usually possible to do an on-the-spot 'live' test to check that the response has changed. However, you can ask the patient to 'try hard' to get the old allergic reaction back, and calibrate to check that their physiology and accessing cues are different from those at the start of the procedure. If their state switches to that of the resource, then you have a good indication that change has occurred. Although it is possible to use this process with life-threatening, anaphylactic-inducing allergens, it is very important to ensure that the patient takes all of their usual precautions, including medication, etc., when they are next in the situation. They must remain cautious and vigilant.

There are certain important points to bear in mind that allow the process to go more smoothly and successfully.

1   Always address any issues of secondary gain that arise before or during the procedure. The extent of your success may well depend on flushing them out adequately and dealing with them appropriately.
2   Regardless of your thoughts about what the patient chooses as a counter-example, if they really believe that it matches the example, then use it! Their unconscious processes may well be helping you out here. However, you can still clarify the important similarities in detail. This will help to build the resource state.
3   Before you introduce the allergen, build up the patient's self-image 'over there' to be the 'you' with a completely normally functioning immune system, and fully resourceful in the way that they want to be. Add other resources, too, if you feel that this will help.
4   Always have the allergen approach gradually, and only come closer as quickly as the patient maintains the physiology of the resource state. If either they or their internal self-image 'over there' falls back into the old response, then you must do two things. First, increase the dissociation by distancing, turning the image into black and white, etc. Secondly, make the resource state stronger, either by intensifying it or by adding other resources (both general and specific) to help to stabilise it.
5   Spend some time on the integration step, ensuring that the new knowledge is fully available to each and every cell of the patient's body. They might like to imagine this information coursing through their bloodstream, reaching every part of their body in a way that allows them to respond far more effectively.

If you bear all of the above in mind, you will increase the chances of a successful outcome. As I mentioned previously, the more specific the allergen and the better matched the counter-example, the more successful is the result. Cases involving non-specific allergens and those for which it is challenging to obtain a believable example do much less well. I usually confine my use of the process to those with significant and specific allergies who are highly motivated to make the change. I make sure that they are not suffering acutely from the condition when we do the intervention, but even then the overall success rate is in the region of 50%.

What follows next is an adaptation of the process for a swallowing problem.

Terri's tablets

Terri, aged 16 years, suffered from dysmenorrhoea. Each month she had painful prolonged periods, and sometimes she had to take time off school. She had a complete inability to swallow tablets, which meant that it was difficult for her to take standard analgesics for pain relief. She coughed and gagged when trying to take a simple paracetamol tablet, becoming sick in the process. She dreaded the last few days of every month. The target outcome for our session was for her to be able to swallow tablets easily whenever she wanted to.

During preliminary questioning I asked Terri to picture herself in her mind's eye the last time she attempted to take a tablet. As she described the submodalities of the picture, it seemed that she looked very small compared with the tablet, which looked huge. No wonder she thought that she would choke! I suspected that she must have had some kind of negative imprinting experience when she was much younger. However, instead of exploring this, I simply asked her to 'make that Terri over there much bigger and adult life-size, while at the same time shrinking the tablet down to make it small'. She had an immediate physiological shift, and looked much happier.

Next I made sure that there were no secondary-gain issues. I wanted to be certain that if we removed the barrier to taking tablets, she would not be going around 'popping pills' indiscriminately. I was reassured by both her verbal and non-verbal responses and decided to continue with the process.

We initially searched for a counter-example with little success. Then I asked her 'What is your favourite thing to eat, so much so that you really enjoy it, and it slides over and down into your stomach with ease?' She surprised me with her reply: 'Red Leicester cheese sandwiches!' So I asked her to vividly imagine eating a Red Leicester cheese sandwich, focusing on the feeling as it slid easily over her throat and down her gullet to end up satisfyingly in her stomach. I amplified the feeling and anchored it to her knuckle. We were ready for the next stage.

Setting up the dissociation, she saw *that Terri over there* with the Red Leicester response. Then we gradually brought up an analgesic tablet, watching as *she* easily swallowed it with a glass of water. I really amplified the Red Leicester anchor as we repeated the swallowing over and over again with increasing comfort and ease. I made sure that by the time we had finished this step, Terri was glowing with satisfaction and triumph!

Then we future paced her success to the next three menstrual cycles, finishing off the session on a high note. She phoned me excitedly the next day to say that she had just had to experiment that evening to make sure that it really worked – and it had! Now some of you may be wondering why I did not just use some NLP technique to reduce her period pain or some other such intervention. Well, I focused on the particular outcome that Terri herself wanted, not my outcome for her. Interestingly, however, she reported that her dysmenorrhoea 'spontaneously' settled of its own accord shortly thereafter.

How the counter-example process works: connecting theory to practice

Many allergies can be thought of as examples of *classical conditioning*. Although there is no doubt that an actual physiological reaction involving the release of adrenaline and histamine takes place when in contact with an allergen, the same response can take place without the allergen's physical presence. For example, one of the earliest documented allergies to roses showed that the response could occur when the subject was exposed unknowingly to a paper rose that was *believed* to be real. Intensely imagining being in the presence of an allergen can also mediate the response. Thus it may well be that psychological factors can intensify the response, in much the same way as occurs with a phobia.

This then suggests that an element of *state-dependent learning* can account for the persistence and reactivation of the reaction. Thus by using a counter-example as a form of *counter-conditioning* we can reduce or even eliminate it. This seems to be the principal way in which the counter-example process works – by substituting one set of physiological responses for another. This does make some sense, as a severe allergic reaction is usually accompanied by a sympathetic arousal state that recursively increases in intensity. In theory at least, countering this state with a parasympathetic relaxing state instead may be an important mechanism for change.

Expectation can play a large part in determining whether or not a future reaction takes place. If you have already suffered a reaction in a certain context, then the thought of going back into this context may prime the physiological response. Successfully future pacing a normal encounter increases *self-efficacy* at the level of belief not only that change can occur, but also that 'I' am in control. The locus of control shifts from external (being a 'victim') to internal (having personal choice). This is more likely to be an important additional mechanism in situations such as Terri's case, where the intervention works more at the *cognitive* level by *restructuring*.

Concluding

Using the counter-example process with allergies is a very specific example of a much more generally applicable change pattern. Virtually any problem with which a patient presents can be formulated in terms of examples and counter-examples. It is probably best to experiment with the pattern in situations where the issue is confined to a single context, rather than being pervasive across contexts. Yet, as with Terri, successful unicontextual change may spread cross-contextually in a generative fashion.

Allergies are a very good place to start to learn the technique. They are generally very clear-cut, with specific, identifiable triggers. Success is usually easy to measure, and patients with troublesome reactions are truly delighted when the process works well. The experience that you gather in this area will stand you in good stead when you are conceptualising different presenting problems in the same way. As very little active research has been performed on NLP interventions thus far, allergies may be one area where it is possible to set up a validated scientific intervention. Those of you who are more research-minded may like to take this topic up with your local immunologist – but only after you have elicited a counter-example to traditional thinking on allergies!

CHAPTER 12

Resolving grief

Introduction

How many patients do you have who have experienced bereavement and have still not fully come to terms with it, months if not years after the event? And I'm not just speaking about the classical abnormal grief reaction with deep depression more than six months later. What about those patients who simply continue in a sort of 'quiet mourning', generally managing reasonably well in the rest of their life, yet still shedding tears and feeling a sense of empty loss many years on? Have you ever experienced a bereavement reaction yourself? They do not necessarily occur just with the death of a relative or very close friend. They can happen with the death of a pet, the loss of a prized possession of sentimental value, the 'empty-nest syndrome' when children grow up and leave home, or even the loss of a job or the run-down to retirement.

Since 'loss' is something that we all go through at one stage or another in our life's transitions, would it be useful to have a process that allowed our patients – and ourselves – to let go and move on in an appropriate way? What if there was a method by which you could, in one session, turn grief into the kind of gratitude for a life lived that frees up previously bound energies for sustaining future endeavours? Would you be interested? In the late 1980s and early 1990s, Steve and Connirae Andreas modelled and developed a process that did just that. So what exactly did they do?

They compared those people who had resolved their grief and could look back with joy and gratitude while moving on into their future with those who looked back with sadness and felt stuck and unresolved, dragging themselves more wearily through each succeeding day of loss. What they found was that the submodality structure of resolved grief was quite different to that of grief which was unresolved. Not only were there differences in internal feelings, words and sounds, but also both the type and location of the 'picture' of their loved one had changed markedly. It was as if the brain had a code, a configuration of submodalities, to let us know the difference between what *was* resolved and what was not. Steve and Connirae Andreas formulated a process that successfully led those who were still grieving into the peacefulness of resolution – a process that we shall explore thoroughly and master in this chapter.

Martha's mother

Martha was an unmarried lady in her early fifties. She had both lived with and looked after her mother for many years prior to her death some five years previously. She had had recurrent low mood since then, and had been prescribed treatment with antidepressants. Although her mood was never low enough to require psychiatric referral, as she said herself, 'life isn't exactly a bed of roses'. Even now she could not talk about her mother without tears coming to her eyes. I explained a little about the grief resolution process and asked her if this was something that she would like to experience for herself. She agreed to give it a go.

I said 'When you picture your mother in your mind's eye now, I'm going to ask you some questions which might seem a bit strange. Just go with the first answer that comes to mind'. I asked the various visual submodality questions (*see* Appendix 2) and found that she pictured her mother off to her right-hand side, beyond arm's reach, as a dim, almost translucent picture. It was like a still-frame photograph, with no movement or sound at all. The tears came again, and she said that she had an empty feeling in her chest, just like a deep, dark void. I asked her to lay that all to one side for a moment, and waited until she had regained her composure.

'Now, Martha, the next thing I want to do is find out how you picture someone who's been in your life in the past but you haven't seen them for a long time. It could be someone like an old school friend you haven't thought about in years, or a relative on the other side of the country or even the world. Someone who, as they come to mind right now, fills you with a nice warm feeling of presence. In a sense, they've been "lost" to you for a while, yet when you think about them, you can't help feeling as if they're here now.'

She remembered a friend from a long time ago, Deborah, whom she had been at school with, and who had moved away in her early twenties. 'She was such fun ... I can see her now with her two pigtails ... jumping around ... making us all laugh.' Calibrating to Martha's state, I could see that she was fully engaged in the memory. She was smiling, the sides of her eyes were creased and her cheeks were pink. This was going to be a good resource to use! I checked out the visual submodalities. Deborah had appeared on her left-hand side, within arm's reach, in full colour, with movement and sound, too. We were ready to go through the process of mapping across one to the other.

I said 'Martha, as you go back to that picture of your mother, I'd like you to move it now, all the way across in your mind's eye to the same position as Deborah'. I mimed with my hands, taking her mother's picture from her right side and placing it quickly over to her left, close by. 'And as you *do that* ... see your mother *there now* ... bright, colourful, close, within arm's reach, with full movement and sound ... a spontaneously happy memory from the past.' You could see the physiological shift taking place almost immediately. She sighed and shuddered, and then broke into a smile.

'Now Martha, it doesn't matter if you do this next bit with your *eyes* open or *shut now* ... beginning to *relax more deeply*. And just behind where you see your mother now ... in her new place ... you can imagine ... like a pack of cards ... a whole series of pictures ... each with one of her particular qualities ... her attributes ... a special, happy event or memory ... and you don't need to see them all clearly ... just get the sense that they're there ... perhaps the corner of each card peeking out ... one behind the other.' She closed her eyes and a relaxed look came over her face.

I continued 'And keeping your mother in her new ... and rightful place ... I'd like you to imagine taking the rest of the cards ... spreading them into where you picture your future ... some in the foreground ... some in the middle ... and others further out ... in the distance. And just notice them now ... as they begin to sparkle ... and turn into stars that light the way ahead ... so that you know ... no matter where you go ... no matter what you do ... that you can have a comforting sense of her presence ... left with you always ... as you live your life ...'

Two weeks after this session Martha reported that she had awoken the next morning following the session, after a deep sleep, feeling at ease with herself 'for the first time in ages'. That was around eight years ago, and since then she has not had any depressive symptoms or required medication. It never ceases to amaze me how, following this process, most people report that they feel better within 24 hours. As I say to them, 'crazy but true'!

Anna's uncle

Anna was one of the very first patients with whom I tried this process. Her favourite uncle had died two months previously. She had found him lying on the floor, his face grotesquely skewed from his terminal stroke, in a pool of urine and faeces. She knew that she had to clear the house of all his belongings, but could not face doing the task. Every time she thought about it she would see his sightless eyes staring up at her as he lay on the bright red carpet. She even avoided driving on the street in which he had lived, and her sleep was disturbed and unrestful.

The image that she kept seeing in her mind's eye was a potential barrier to using the grief pattern successfully. It loomed up at her whenever she thought of him. Before continuing, we needed to do something else first. I said 'Anna, I'd like you to take that picture, drain out all of the colour, and as it becomes a black-and-white snapshot, push it way over there into the distance'. Once we had successfully changed the submodalities that had made the image vivid and intruding, she felt more resourceful.

'Now, Anna, what was it you really valued about your relationship with your uncle? What were the particular qualities, the times and the events that made this special for you?' It was important for Anna to focus on the positive aspects of the relationship that had been lost, rather than the final event itself. In fact, the process will really only work well when you ensure that this step is completed. If you fail to do this, it is likely only to result in more misery! Anna replied: 'Well, he was kind, caring, and always said something to make me laugh'. I asked her to make a representation of her uncle with these qualities. She smiled as she described her projected picture at arm's length in front of her.

We used this representation of her uncle as we went through the process in a similar way to that described above for Martha. She had a relative, a close cousin, who had emigrated to Canada 10 years previously, and we used this as the template to map across her experience of loss. Her submodalities were of a full-coloured movie at 45 degrees to her left. I knew that the session was successfully completed when I spoke about her uncle again and this time she looked spontaneously over to her left and broke into a wide smile. There were some tears, but they were now tears of reunion rather than of loss.

Anna phoned me the next day to say that she had spent the best part of the morning cleaning out her uncle's house, and she had felt fine. The next week she sent her mother (her uncle's sister) to see me, and we used the same process to resolve her grief.

Angie's angst

Angie's grandmother had died a year previously after a long and harrowing illness, and in her final weeks was looked after in our local community hospital. At the age of 22 years, this was the first death that Angie had witnessed at first hand. During the last year she had lost her usual sparkle and energy, and everyday tasks seemed like major chores. She had not initially consulted specifically about grief, just about her 'tired all the time' symptoms. As she was not a regular patient of mine, and this was the first time I had seen her, I had not known about her grandmother. When I asked about recent family bereavements she burst into tears, with racking sobs.

I gently explained that I had a process which would help her, and we set up another appointment.

Angie had been really quite traumatised by her grandmother's death, particularly the manner of her passing. Etched on her brain were vivid pictures and sounds of the whole event, especially the last few hours, when the rattle of retained secretions seemed to go on and on. The terminal episode had been like an epileptic fit – quite grotesque. This memory was imprinted on her to such an extent that it blocked out any of the good times they had had prior to the illness.

This particular memory had become like a phobia – a strong visual/kinaesthetic synaesthesia. Therefore, prior to using the resolving grief pattern, we used the phobia cure. In exactly the same way as described in Chapter 10, we ran the whole of the movie of the terminal event in double dissociation, disconnecting the negative synaesthesia and reassociating Angie to a much more resourceful 'Angie'. Once this was out of the way, the rest of the process proceeded smoothly.

If you are going to approach grief resolution in this way, it is important that you use the phobia process only on the 'traumatic' elements of the terminal process (e.g. road traffic accident, etc.). To use it on prior 'good' memories would strip them of all their positive feelings, thus *intensifying* the grief. In a sense, grief *is* the dissociation from the ability to feel connected to the positive past experiences in the present moment.

We shall now move on to the step-by-step details of the process itself.

The grief resolution process

Steve and Connirae Andreas have done much to elucidate both the structure of grief and its resourceful resolution. I first read about the process in *Heart of the Mind*, and adapted it to suit my way of working as described below. It is important to honour the positive intention of grief, which is the wish to be reunited in some way with the deceased. Because many people believe that to stop grieving is in some way to dishonour the dead, you can reframe these types of objections before starting the process. This is known as pre-framing.

I usually suggest that rather than letting go and forgetting about the person who has gone, this process is more about reconnecting them in a wholesome way and honouring what the relationship meant to them, carrying that forward into the future. Sometimes it is useful to state a variation of the following: 'If you were to die, would you want your relatives to keep grieving, being unable to carry on with their lives? Or would you tell them to remember all the good times as they move on in life?' It is unusual for someone not to see the logic in that statement. Surprisingly, however, one or two have not seen it! It turned out that they still retained some anger and resentment which needed to be dealt with first. For those who are still uncertain, I let them know that if they do not like the changes, we can put it back the way it was (I've never had to do this).

Exercise 13:   The grief resolution process

1   Ask the patient to *think of the situation of grief* and loss (it could be an object or a job, as well as a person). If this is a very traumatic event you may have to do a submodality shift or the phobia cure first. Ensure that the patient is thinking about the positive value and the good things about what has been lost. *Identify the submodalities* of this picture (often beyond arm's reach, dissociated, dark, dull or transparent). Notice *especially the location* – this is the main submodality driver.

2   Now ask the patient to *think of a situation of 'loss' that their brain codes in a pleasant and joyful way*. This may be someone they have not seen for a long time – at school, college or university, a friend, relative, etc. It may be someone who is already dead, but they still feel connected to all the good feelings. Identify the submodalities of this experience (usually closer, colourful, with movement, sound, etc.). Pay special attention to the *location* of this image.

3   Ask if they have *any objections* to seeing the person who has gone (from step 1) in this new light, connected to them in a resourceful way. Pay attention to any objections that come up, and *reframe them* before moving to the next step.

4   Now comes the 'mapping-across process'. *Change the submodalities of the experience of loss into those of connection.* Usually location is the main driver – you can imagine physically holding their picture of 'loss' in your hand and transferring it to the location of 'connection'. You will probably *notice an immediate physiological shift*. Calibrate to ensure that the change has occurred prior to the next step.

5   Thinking of *all the positive qualities*, attributes, past happy events and memories of this relationship, ask the patient to imagine that these are all represented in some way *on a pack of cards*, each card representing a different quality. They don't have to see them clearly – just notice the edges of the cards situated behind this new image of connection.

6   Now, keeping the new image of connection safely in place, ask the patient to imagine these cards *streaming out into the future* – their future. And as they begin to settle in the foreground, the middle distance and out into the far future, let them turn into sparkling stars of light. And as the patient walks out into this new future they can *enjoy the continuing sense of connection* – spreading out to encompass others whom they know, and those whom they have yet to meet.

This process is an example of *submodality mapping*, where you identify the critical differences between two experiences and map one on to the other. This can be used in a variety of different ways (e.g. confusion to certainty, doubt to belief, problem to opportunity, failure to success, etc.). However, before making the changes it is important to address any objections that hold valuable information about ecology.

You can adapt the above process very easily to deal with loss of objects of sentimental value, job loss, moving house, etc. When resolving any type of grief, there are certain things you can do to ensure that the process goes smoothly.

1   Always pre-frame! Let them know that they are *not* forgetting the person, but simply reconnecting in a more enhancing way. Deal with residual anger and resentment before going any further.
2   If the images of loss are traumatic, use another submodality pattern or the phobia cure first. You want the patient to have an image of the loss of what was most valued in the person, relationship or object.
3   The fundamental driver of the process is the submodality of location. Simply changing the location is often enough to allow the other submodalities to spontaneously change as well.
4   Be very aware of any responses that may be objections. You must reframe them before moving on to the next step.
5   If they do not have an experience that is coded as 'pleasant loss', then ask about how they represent someone who is currently in their life to whom they feel connected but who is not in the room at present. Use the sub-modalities of this representation for the mapping across.
6   If you use step 5 above, ensure that the patient recognises that, unlike the person currently in their life, the deceased person is still gone and will not be physically present and contactable in the same way.

Let us continue with another example – this time a job loss.

Eric on the scrapheap

Eric, in his early fifties, had been made redundant from his engineering job a year previously. He had felt tired and lethargic, with a complete lack of motivation, lamenting that he was now on the scrapheap of life. His whole identity had been bound up in his job, and he now felt an aching sense of loss at the thought that he would never work again. He felt ill at ease, and was unable to settle on the mundane tasks that faced him at home.

He had two pictures in his mind. The first was a distant still photo of his last day at work. He saw this on his left side. The second was a closer, yet stark picture of him actually sitting on a scrapheap off to his right. I asked him what he had valued in his job, and he replied 'A feeling of doing something important and making a difference. A sense of being part of a team, and the security of a good wage'.

I asked him about times in the past when he had experienced loss, yet had moved on purposefully into the future. We explored various options and came up with one which I thought would work well. When he had been employed in England many years previously he had lived in a cottage near the Lake District. He had changed jobs 10 years ago and moved back up to his current residence in Scotland to a new job. The release of equity from the desirable cottage had given him substantial funds to buy outright a much larger property in the north. He had a colourful, panoramic mental picture of the cottage and its surroundings, projected down and off to his left, about five feet away.

I decided that I would use *both* the picture of his last day at work and that of him sitting on the scrapheap in the grief resolution process. I intuitively felt that this might give him a deeper sense of connecting the past, the present and the future together, allowing his resources an unrestricted flow. He released a big sigh when he turned each of them into a colourful, panoramic picture down and off to the left. Then, when creating the 'pack of cards', I asked him to think of all the qualities he had back then, especially doing something important, being part of a team, making a difference and the sense of security engendered. We added in the various skills he had manifested when dealing with other people, particularly communication and rapport, together with his ability to get the job done and produce a first-rate product.

'Now, Eric, I'd like you to take all of those qualities ... and the others of which you're not yet consciously aware ... and scatter them into your future ... and not only in the immediate few weeks ahead ... .but also spreading out over the many months and years to come ... knowing that as you look back into the past that was ... you can feel a developing sense of reconnecting with the very best of you ... passing through the present ... and on into the kind of future possibilities that are yet to come ...'

Although he was initially sceptical, he noticed an increased feeling of ease within himself – the frustration and boredom quickly disappeared. A few weeks later he enrolled on a computer training course at the local college. One thing led to another, and he now has a part-time job with the local enterprise trust, helping to give advice to new business start-ups.

How the grief resolution process works: connecting theory to practice

Grief is of course a learned behaviour, and can be thought of in *state-dependent* terms. When you look at the various world cultures and see how their reactions to loss vary from abject misery and prolonged mourning to happiness, acceptance and celebration, then it is clear that the same event can be given many different meanings. Therefore your own reaction will depend not only on the country in which you were born, but also on your experience moulded by parental influence, and your developing religious and spiritual beliefs.

At its most fundamental, the structure of grief can be thought of as a dissociation process. There is a profound state of disconnection, which creates feelings of emptiness and loss. However, resolved grief is a reconnection with all that was and is wholesome, good and resourceful about the relationship. This is an associated state, with access in the here and now to nourishing past memories which give continued future sustenance. There are several ways to think about how the process works.

The submodality shifts of mapping across are a way of visually collapsing anchors. This is a type of *counter-conditioning* process in which two states – one negative and the other positive – are simultaneously brought to bear on each other. This is often accompanied by easily seen physiological shifts, sometimes of major proportion. The seeding of changes into the future acts via *operant conditioning*, providing a stimulus to move towards. Of course, each of these events could be recast as different types of systems *attractors*, with a subsequent profound shift in the attractor landscape.

There is also a large element of *cognitive restructuring*, with a major and often instantaneous shift in visual imagery processing. This is accompanied by a simultaneous modification of self-talk and beliefs *about* the deceased, which further embeds the changes. The future pacing of values, qualities and attitudes is a strategy installation typical of modified *skills training* and rehearsal, thereby enhancing *self-efficacy*. When the session is facilitated by someone who has gone through the process him- or herself and has a deeper unconscious imprinting of the pattern, this too can have a powerful *modelling* effect.

Concluding

Grief and loss are major elements of our day-to-day encounters in medical practice. By widening the scope of loss to involve life transitions of all kinds we become equipped with a very potent tool for change. There is an immense amount of psychological and physical energy bound up in unresolved grief, which can lead to a heavy stagnancy and sense of being stuck that prevents contemplation of the future, let alone action. The grief resolution process can be thought of as freeing up, reconnecting and recycling these energies, allowing them to be channelled in a worthwhile direction. It is often quite amazing how liberating this can be.

Remember that people's beliefs about loss and grieving may be substantially different from yours. Yet it does no one any good if they continue to carry around a debilitating burden. It will repay you many times over to practise your pre-frames so that you can help your patients to honour what is past as you assist them in moving on. I have even used the process to help people to recontact their unfulfilled dreams of yesteryear, so that the qualities and attitudes which they espoused then could be resurrected in a new and more fulfilling project. As we conclude this chapter, I suggest that you find some of your own unresolved losses to experiment with and further ground you in the technique. As you step back now and look at the mapping-across process from a wider perspective, you may find it valuable to think about the other types of personal and clinical experiences with which you can use it.

CHAPTER 13

Six-step reframing

Introduction

Have you ever had a particular kind of problem that seemed to dog you for a while and you couldn't get away from it? Perhaps it was one of those kinds of issues for which you developed 'tunnel vision' – everywhere you looked it was all you could see, looming large. Maybe you told yourself over and over again that there must be a solution, yet the answer was elusive, a poorly heard whisper on the breeze that strained your ears. Perhaps you felt that things would never get better. Yet one day, somehow, maybe even simply out of the blue, your perspective suddenly shifted and you could see the big picture, the ephemeral whisper became a clear, resonant answer, and you found yourself able to move on again.

So what was it that happened at that moment? What was it that changed and led to resolution? If we imagine metaphorically that our problem was originally set in what appeared to be a rigid frame, then the solution occurs when the frame changes. It may be that we do literally see things differently – like the visual submodality shifts that we have explored previously. Or we hear an inner voice from a deeper part of ourselves that announces the positive intention underlying the problem – an 'aha' moment. This is what NLP calls *reframing*, and changing perspective in this way is typical of many of the change processes in this book.

However, in this chapter we are going to explore a particular type of reframing called the *six-step reframe*. The pattern was originally elucidated by NLP co-founder John Grinder while he was teaching a seminar at a psychiatric institute in Vancouver, a quarter of a century ago. Like many discoveries, it arose from the fortuitous co-operation by both conscious and unconscious processes which laid the foundation for the subsequent development of New Code NLP (*see Whispering in the Wind* by Bostic St Clair and Grinder).

The crux of the pattern was the recognition that behind every problematic behaviour lay a positive intention for the patient – one of the key presuppositions of NLP today. By holding the positive intention constant, the more creative problem-solving aspects of the patient's mind could generate many alternative behaviours that fulfilled the original intention. From a position of being 'stuck' with only one problem-generating choice, the solution gave a series of new choices – not only expanding the frame but also allowing movement in a different direction.

This six-step process can be used both as a formal procedure and also informally in conversation to facilitate change in those with troublesome symptoms and behaviours. Working with this perspective in mind can be a very liberating experience – for patient and practitioner alike.

Mandy's migraines

Mandy, aged 42 years, had been a chronic intermittent migraine sufferer from her early teenage years. Occasionally she had clear spells for several months, and then the migraines returned with a vengeance, wreaking havoc on her work and social life. She had tried various preventative medications, although she generally opted for more acute 'on-the-spot' relief. Very occasionally she required an intramuscular injection of anti-emetic and painkiller. After a series of particularly trying headaches she sought me out to ask about alternative help.

As we chatted I initially asked her about any recurring precipitating factors. Apart from occasional premenstrual exacerbations, she denied any major life stresses. She was single – and enjoyably so! Her family consisted of two cats and a dog, on which she doted. There were no specific food or drink triggers. She worked as a personal assistant in an oil company, and was meticulous and well organised in her job.

Her migraines usually began as a mild throbbing around her left temple and eye, developing fairly rapidly into lightning-like stabs with waves of nausea and disturbed vision. I asked her to remember her last episode, which had occurred mid-afternoon at work the previous week. I said 'I'd like you to imagine being back in that experience again so that you can begin to feel a little of those feelings again'. Getting the patient back into the problem context is the precursor to accessing the state-bound information that is contained within the symptom.

Mandy nodded, and I continued 'And it would be useful to have the deeper aspects of your mind set up some involuntary signals for *yes* and *no* which can help us to get to the kind of information that can assist us in resolving this. As you're aware of those feelings in the side of your head, I'm going to ask your mind to increase the intensity of the feelings to represent a *yes* response'. An almost startled look came across her face as she gasped 'It's doing it all by itself!' I asked for the intensity to fall towards zero as a signal for *no*, and she duly complied.

Setting up communication with unconscious processes in this way is a pre-requisite for successful change. With Mandy we focused on the feeling response, yet other patients may get unconscious communication in the form of pictures, sounds, words, smells or tastes. Because the kinaesthetic system is mostly out of conscious awareness in the Western world, I tend to favour this modality for unconscious communication, as there is much less chance of conscious interference.

Next I wanted to find out the positive intention of the migraine symptom. I explained that behaviours and symptoms which we regard as problematic keep on being expressed because a 'deeper' part of us has important information to provide about the situation. I asked 'As you turn your attention inwards, ask that part of you, if it has a positive intention for you underlying the symptom, to signal with the *yes* response'. As she got the 'yes' answer, I continued 'And ask that part if it would communicate its intention to you in a way that you can understand consciously, by words, pictures, sounds or feelings'. Mandy got a 'yes' response together with the sense that the message she was receiving was about slowing down, taking her time and being less obsessive, particularly at work.

I asked her to thank that part of her for this valuable information, and decided to see whether we could chunk up to a higher-level, more encompassing response. 'If you got all of those things, *what would that do for you* that was even more important?' This is an especially vital question to ask if any of the original intentions were perceived as negative responses. She replied 'Balance and harmony in my life'. We discussed how odd it seemed that on one level she had a symptom that often debilitated her, while on another level its intention was almost the exact opposite! She explained 'As I think about it in this light, I can see that many if not most of my migraines come on when I'm trying to do too much, especially at work, burning the candle at both ends. Maybe it's a signal that I need to do something different'.

The next step was to create some new alternative behaviours that could satisfy the positive intention in more healthy ways. 'Mandy, we all at various times in our lives have used our skills and resources to *solve problems* and come up with *creative solutions* ... whether that's solving the crossword, coming up with *new ideas* for decorating the kitchen or something similar. As you *get in touch now* with those *automatically* creative and problem-solving aspects of yourself ... you can ask your *deeper mind* to provide you with three new and alternative behaviours that fulfil the positive intention of *having more balance and harmony* in your life and work ... behaviours that are *as good if not better* than the original behaviour. And your deeper mind can let us know by using the "yes" signal that it has accomplished this task ... whether you are consciously aware of the new behaviours or not.'

Sometimes patients will get a clear and full picture of the specific new behaviours that they are going to use – in glowing Technicolor. More often they may gain a general sense of the *type* of behaviour without knowing exactly how it will occur in the previously problematic situation. Occasionally they get a clear *yes* signal that new behaviours have been chosen, yet they have absolutely no conscious clue of how things will change.

Mandy was fairly clear about her newly generated options. 'Firstly, I'm going to go to yoga classes. I've been meaning to for ages, but never got round to it. Now I will! Secondly, I'm going to go for a 15- to 20-minute walk every day at lunchtime. Usually I get back to work too early and just get stuck in. Now, even if it rains, I'm going to take my full break. Thirdly, I'm going to stop taking so much work home with me at night – only rush jobs.'

I could see that the first two choices were ecological and under her control, but I had some concerns about the third one. We discussed the issues involved, namely her boss's demands, her desire to do a good job and be on top of her tasks, and her new-found commitment to balance and harmony. Eventually she found a form of words that respected both her needs and those of her boss, while preserving her employment! I asked her to check again that her deeper mind would agree to try out these new behaviours, perhaps for a month or so in the first instance. She got an answering *yes*. If she had received a *no* response instead, we would have checked which specific new behaviour did not fit and either updated it in some way or asked for a new one in its place which would fulfil the positive intention more completely.

Finally, we performed an ecology check. I asked Mandy to 'go inside again and ask your deeper mind if there are any other aspects of yourself that may object to carrying out the new behaviours ... and if there are they can signal with the *yes* response ... and if not ... with the *no* response'. All was quiet, and we had completed the process. Of course, if there had been any objections we would have gone back to the second step of the procedure and identified the positive intention that lay behind the objection. With that new information we could then cycle through the rest of the steps again.

The six-step reframe is a model for ecological change. Over a very short time frame Mandy's migraine headaches disappeared almost completely. When she did get twinges it was almost a kind of 'warning signal' that she was beginning to do the kinds of things that would lead her to being out of 'balance and harmony'. Most of these episodes occurred in relation to work schedules and deadlines. The upshot was that the impending headaches became the stimulus to further develop her assertion and negotiation skills. She actually ended up negotiating a higher salary for less work!

Steve's smoking

The six-step reframe is another powerful way to help smokers to become non-smokers. In many cases the positive intentions behind smoking are concerned with relaxation, time for self, peer group inclusion, an aid to thinking clearly, creating distance to prevent others getting too close (they might get burned), creating a smokescreen, etc. Many people find that when they are feeling stressed out, smoking a cigarette can help them to calm down rapidly and gain a perspective on the situation. The two or three deep inhalations that often occur at the start of smoking a cigarette activate the diaphragmatic muscles, which in turn stimulate parasympathetic nerve activity, leading to a feeling of relaxation.

For Steve, relaxation was the main key, followed by social inclusion in his peer group. He had found that he felt himself to be 'part of the crowd' if he had a cigarette in his hand in the pub. We used the feeling that he got in his throat when he needed a cigarette to act as the signal for 'yes' (increase) and 'no' (decrease). Using 'relaxation and inclusion' as the positive intentions, we went through the process step by step.

Steve's new behaviours were fairly simple. They included taking a deep diaphragmatic breath and letting it out slowly, planning more regular time-outs at work, and smiling as he spoke to his friends in the pub, to engender more of a feeling of connection. These may not have been behaviours that you, I or other patients might have chosen, yet Steve's deeper mind gave an unequivocal *yes* to putting these into action, and he stopped smoking without experiencing any withdrawal effects.

Nowadays, nicotine replacement treatment is available on prescription, and this has markedly increased the number of people making plans to 'give it a try'. In these situations you can use the six-step reframe in a casual conversational manner in an ordinary consultation to aid the patient. Questions such as the following are very useful:

- *'How committed are you to stopping smoking now?'*
- *'Is there anything that would prevent you from stopping smoking now?'*
- *'What are the kinds of situations in which you must have a cigarette?'*
- *'Which is the most enjoyable cigarette of the day?'*
- *'What are the important things that smoking does for you?'*
- *'What are the current benefits of smoking?'*
- *'How will you get those benefits in other ways when you stop smoking?'*
- *'What will you be doing differently once you have stopped?'*
- *'If things get tough and the desire for a cigarette increases, what will you do instead?'*
- *'What will you do with the money you've saved as a result of stopping?'*
- *'In what ways will you be healthier?'*

- *'If you happen to momentarily lose your resolve and have a cigarette, how will you get yourself back on track again?'*
- *'If you imagine that three months have passed and you have successfully stopped, how would you feel looking back on that success now?'*

I am not suggesting that you ask all of these questions! I am simply proposing that you use one or two of them to fine-tune your patient's approach and deal with potential areas of difficulty ahead of time. If you refine your calibration skills, you will easily be able to notice your patient's out-of-awareness *yes* and *no* responses that occur unconsciously. This will help you to gauge which questions to use.

Barbara's bingeing

The six-step reframe is a very powerful tool, and can be used with the patient being completely consciously unaware of the unconscious processes and choices that are being made. John Grinder believes that using NLP in this way – content-free therapy – is the most ethical way for any therapist to work. Working exclusively in this way prevents the therapist from imposing his or her own solutions on the situation.

Barbara was able to control her appetite until just after she had put the kids to bed. Then, despite her good intentions, she would literally 'stuff her face' with any food that was available. Putting the kids to bed was the signal that her responsibilities to others were temporarily over and that the time between then and her own bedtime was exclusively for her. Her weight had ballooned up, and she was desperate to get back in control.

I stepped her back into what it felt like just after she had put the kids to bed. She described an empty, gnawing ache in her solar plexus which we amplified and used as the *yes* and *no* signal. When I asked if there was a deeper positive intention behind her eating behaviour, she got the *yes* response. However, she got a clear *no* when asked if this part of her could communicate its intention consciously. We knew that her deeper mind was communicating with us and, remaining respectful of its purpose in keeping this information from her, we continued with the other steps.

Utilising her problem-solving aspects and creative functions, she generated three new behaviours to use instead of bingeing. However, once again she had no idea what these were at a conscious level. She got a clear *yes* signal that the step was complete, yet was wholly unaware of what she would do differently. Her deeper mind was in full agreement with implementing these new choices in the future, and there were no other objections! She had completed the whole process at an unconscious level.

To this day she still has no clue about what she is doing differently. All she knows is that she stopped bingeing, her weight gradually decreased over a period of a few months to a comfortable level, and she now feels more content in herself. This is an excellent rebuttal of the traditional view that 'insight' is required for successful change.

Six-step reframing: the process

The six-step reframing process can be used for any habit, behaviour or even physical symptom that seems to defy your attempts to change it. It is a particularly good choice for problems such as smoking, weight control and other symptoms that persist because of secondary gain. The fact that these habits or behaviours have all failed to change despite many attempts is a sign that they are all sustained out of your conscious awareness. It is an indicator of unconscious positive intention – the habit or behaviour, even if you dislike it intensely, is getting something of great importance for you. You will not be able to move on until this positive intention is incorporated within the solution.

Although the process seems to work best with unwanted habits, it can also be useful for problems involving sequential incongruence (e.g. bulimia) and physical symptoms (e.g. chronic pain syndromes). I would encourage you to think of all presentations in medical practice along these lines. It can sometimes be very surprising how the finding of a meaningful positive intention for a symptom can cause profound change – for both you and your patient. Practise the following steps on a variety of clinical issues.

Exercise 14:   Six-step reframing

1   *Identify the problem behaviour* and establish the context in which it occurs. Often patients 'can't stop doing x' ... or seem 'unable to start doing y'.
2   *Establish 'yes' and 'no' signals.* Often this is best achieved by imagining being in the context and attending to whatever spontaneously arises when asking 'Will the part responsible for this behaviour please give me a signal now?' Although communication can be in any modality (VAKOG), I usually prefer kinaesthetic responses because they are less easily consciously manipulated. Ask the part to *increase the intensity of the response for a 'yes'* and decrease it for a 'no'.

---

3   *Find out the positive intention.* Ask whether the part knows the positive intention behind the behaviour and if it is willing to communicate this consciously. If you get a 'yes', then verbalise the answer. If you get a 'no', assume a positive intention anyway and carry on. If the initial intention is expressed in the negative, then chunk up until you get a positive (e.g. 'I want to stop worrying' chunks up to 'I want to feel more relaxed').

4   *Generate alternative behaviours.* Get your patient in touch with their inner problem-solving and creative aspects and functions. Ask for three new behaviours that are as good if not better in achieving the positive intention. Once these have been generated, their deeper mind can give the 'yes' signal. They do not have to know what these choices are consciously. The process works just as well – often better – when they remain unconscious.

5   *Check that their deeper mind will take full responsibility* for ensuring that it will use these three new behaviours in the future instead of the original one, by getting the 'yes' signal. If they are consciously aware of what the behaviours are, they can imagine doing them in the future to make sure that they fit. If there are any objections at this stage, you can go back to step 4 to creatively modify any of the new choices.

6   *Final ecology check.* We want to ensure that any new behavioural choices are congruent with the patient's overall functioning. Occasionally, new choices can conflict with behaviours generated by other parts. Ask if any other aspect or part of them has any objections to these new choices, and pay attention to 'yes' and 'no' signals. If there are objections to a particular behaviour, you can generate a new one to replace it in step 4. You may want instead to find out the positive intention of the objecting part (step 3) and cycle through the reframing process again.

You can get into the habit of thinking about reframing by asking the following question – inside your mind or directly – of every patient who passes through your door. 'What is the positive intention of this symptom for this patient?' The very question itself helps you to generate a much deeper level of rapport as you are getting in tune with their underlying positive intentions. In fact, instead of merely trying simply to get rid of symptoms, you can start to regard them as providers of valuable information – symptom as friend rather than enemy!

Of course, the current behaviour is only one of a whole series of choices that can fulfil that positive intention. For example, if the patient smokes for relaxation then many, many different behaviours can give that outcome – including smoking itself. However, what happens in the process is that smoking is relegated to being simply *another* choice within a multitude, rather than the only available one. Six-step reframing underlines the fact that *NLP adds choices* in every situation – it takes nothing away from the patient.

There are certain things that you can do to ensure that six-step reframing goes as smoothly as possible.

1   It is always a good idea to specify the context for change in some detail. If you are too vague, this will be reflected in your results.
2   Always make sure that the unconscious *yes* and *no* signals cannot be manufactured consciously. If your patient can manufacture them at will then they are not reliable indicators of unconscious processes. They may even provide false information that prevents ecological change. Involuntary signals give the best results.
3   Never try to change the patient's underlying positive intention. Accept whatever response you get and work with it. If the initial intention appears to be negative, chunk up as many times as you need to get it phrased in the positive.
4   When asking for creative and problem-solving resources in step 4 you can revivify appropriate memories of creativity, etc., build up the states and anchor them on a knuckle. You can fire off the anchor when asking their deeper mind to generate the new behavioural choices.
5   During the ecology check you may occasionally get a very marked objection that is difficult to reframe. This is usually a sign of a deeply dissociated aspect that functions as a sequential incongruity. You can use this as a signal to apply the *visual squash* model instead (parts negotiation) (*see* Chapter 16).

Once you have mastered the above you can add some finer nuances. It is possible to set anchors on separate knuckles for the problem-state feeling and the positive intention as well as the creative resources. You can fire off the positive intention and creative resources together to help to generate the three new behaviours. Once this has been achieved, both of these anchors can be collapsed into the feeling for the problem state, which then becomes the trigger for the new behaviours. Of course, the originator of the process, John Grinder, might describe this as overly complicated, and suggest that one should simply trust the unconscious processes fully instead!

Six-step reframing is one of the few NLP approaches that do not need the prior delineation and setting of a detailed outcome – only a problem context. There is therefore much less opportunity for conscious mind interference. After all, it is usually this interference which has prevented adequate resolution in the first place! For this reason, Grinder prefers to conduct the whole process at a completely unconscious level. In fact, the patient may only find out which new behaviour they have employed after successfully coming through the problem context in a different way. This is a demonstration of the kind of generative change that typifies this pattern.

How six-step reframing works: connecting theory to practice

The principal mechanism of action for six-step reframing is *cognitive restructuring*. The pivotal point is step 3, with the uncovering of positive intention. This puts the problem behaviour within a completely different frame, and rapidly changes the patient's perspective. Their beliefs about the situation appear to be instantly updated, and this allows the introduction of a *skills training* response with the trial and rehearsal of several new future behaviours. Of course, the very act of either envisaging in detail or at least having a general sense of expectation that the future is going to be different can have a strong effect on *self-efficacy*.

We could also view this as a form of *conditioning and counter-conditioning*. The original problem is a *state-dependent* phenomenon which automatically triggers without conscious awareness in the troublesome context. Uncovering the positive intention causes a major state change, like an 'aha' experience, which collapses anchors with the original negative state. The newly selected behaviours are also state-dependent phenomena that are now triggered by the old contextual cues. Done well, the solution becomes as automatic as the problem used to be, with no conscious thinking required to behave differently in the old context. Of course, each success becomes its own positive reinforcer through recursion.

Concluding

As you think about all that we have covered in this chapter, some of you will feel that you can simply go ahead and apply six-step reframing in your daily practice. However, others might be just a little reticent. Perhaps you need to ask yourself what it is that could prevent you from easily utilising this process in the future. The main benefit of staying as we are is usually the sense of comfort and security that doing things in the same old way often brings. And of course, the trick in both learning *and* doing something new is to ensure that you can bring at least some of that comfort and security with you as you do so.

So how can you begin to incorporate this as you go about your daily practice? Well, you could simply break this down into small chunks. In some consultations you could ask your patient what benefit, if any, their current symptoms may be providing them with at a deeper level. In others, you might think of one or two reframes yourself and wonder out loud whether any of them fit while you calibrate to the patient's unconscious *yes* and *no* responses – they are always there if you know where to look! You could try the whole process out with patients who have chronic symptoms (especially psychosomatic ones) and with whom you already know you have developed a great deal of rapport and trust over the years. This could be framed as follows.

> '*I've been learning some new approaches that might be helpful to your situation. Although I'm still at the early stages, it might be to our mutual benefit to try out something new. It may be that this could help to improve your symptoms. You'll certainly be helping me to learn more about helping others in similar situations. Shall we give it a go?*' (And there's nothing to stop you using a crib sheet!)

Of course, the other ways to make sure that the skills are 'in the muscle' are to practise with one or more of your colleagues, friends, family, etc., or even go on a short training course. As you think about it now, what would it be like if you were three months along the road, looking back on having used this process successfully several times already? There are a huge number of clinical conditions on which you could try it out, ranging from mainly psychological conditions, through psychosomatic to mainly physical disorders. You might find as you check in with yourself that there really are no further objections to your going straight ahead and doing it now!

CHAPTER 14

Relationships through the looking glass

Introduction

Have you ever had a personal difficulty with a friend, colleague, patient or even a close relation, such as a family member or spouse? One of those times when you had very differing opinions and could not see eye to eye – you were on different sides of the fence. How did it feel to be in that situation? What thoughts were going through your mind and just how did you view the other person? When we are at odds with someone in this way it can affect how we deal with them every time we meet them. It is as if we set up a template in our minds of how they are likely to behave, and of course, the next encounter usually goes the way of that self-fulfilling prophecy!

So, given that there have been times in the past when this happened to you and you were later able to resolve the issue satisfactorily, just how did you do that? For some people it is as if they have a sudden insight into the other person's point of view. A bit like the old Indian saying, 'Walk a mile in the other person's moccasins'. Once you understood their perspective, and saw where they were coming from, even if you still did not agree with them the new knowledge led you towards a solution.

For others, it is as if they simply got to that point of exasperation, or even beyond it, when they did not know what to do any more. Perhaps that feeling prompted you to review the various encounters again, dispassionately, like a 'fly-on-the-wall' observer. Of course, this is exactly what mediation and conciliation services suggest. As a neutral onlooker you can see more clearly information that was previously obscured – information that can have a major effect in ensuring successful future encounters.

So what is the process that just went on there? What was it that you did in your mind's eye? It is certainly a truism that not everyone shares our view of the world – there are many different points of view. Yet NLP co-founder John Grinder presupposes that there are three perspectives which are pivotal in coming to an overall understanding of a situation. Each of the perspectives has its own truth, but each is partial and limited. Together they allow the first steps in acting with greater wisdom and integrity.

The *first position* is your own view and perspective as seen through your own eyes. You act from your sense of what is important to you in the situation and what is in keeping with your deeper values. You are assertive in your behaviours and make your needs known. However, if you only acted from this position without recourse to the others, you might come across as insensitive, or even arrogant and overbearing.

The *second position* is like stepping into the other person's shoes and imagining reality as experienced from their perspective. Of course, this is the fundamental position for building empathy and rapport. You gain a clearer understanding of their emotional state and intellectual knowledge. However, spending a disproportionate amount of time here can cause you to neglect your own needs, leading to misery, burnout and even loss of self-esteem.

The *third position* – sometimes called the meta-position – is a detached perspective, a bit like taking a step back outside the situation, viewing yourself and the other person from some way off. This allows you to re-examine a difficult situation from a distance, with much less emotion, gleaning valuable information about what to do differently. However, spending too much time here can make you appear austere and unapproachable.

These three *perceptual positions* are fundamental to using NLP effectively. Using each position sequentially, Robert Dilts conceptualised a process that he called the *meta-mirror* for helping to sort out difficult relationships. In the rest of this chapter we shall explore just how to put this process into action to gain favourable outcomes both for our patients and for ourselves.

Mattie and mum

Mattie was in her late teens. She had completed two terms at university studying languages, and her ultimate aim was to travel the world. However, things were not going according to plan. Her mother phoned me to ask if I could help. It seemed that Mattie had become increasingly isolated and depressed, coming home from Aberdeen most weekends and getting anxious almost to the point of panic on Sunday evenings when she had to return. She had seen the doctor at the student health services, who had recommended medication which she did not want to take. Her mother had arranged for her to see a psychologist privately, but despite several sessions she had made little progress. Mum wanted help now! However, to her initial consternation, I said that I would prefer to see Mattie by herself.

Mattie was a little withdrawn at the beginning, but with much prompting she told me of her feelings about university and her dread of going back each Sunday night. It became clear that, if we were to use diagnostic terms, she was suffering from 'separation anxiety' – she was homesick. Her symptoms improved when she was home at weekends and got worse each Sunday afternoon. She phoned home every day for an hour or so, and had not gone out to do much socialising from her room in the halls of residence. It became clear that her mother was a major influence in her life, so I thought that the meta-mirror would be a good place to start. I framed this intervention as 'wanting to gather more information about her relationship with her mother'.

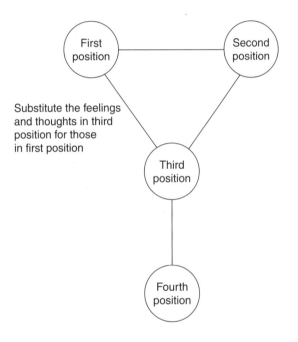

Figure 14.1:   Perceptual positions for meta-mirror.

I laid out four pieces of paper on the consulting-room floor to represent the positions that we would use during the process. I then asked Mattie to think about a typical interaction she had with her mother prior to going back to university on a Sunday. Stepping into first position I asked her to pay attention to her thoughts and feelings as she looked at her mother 'over there in your mind's eye'. First of all I asked her to describe just how her mother looked – her posture, gestures and voice tone. 'She looks angry, her cheeks are flushed, her eyes are glinting, her finger is pointing directly at me and her voice sounds harsh and loud.'

Next I wanted to know how she felt inside. 'I've got a sick feeling in my stomach, coming in waves, and I feel very trembly. I don't think I can do what she's asking. The angrier she gets the worse I feel.' Rather than go into any deep and meaningful conversation to explain what she was feeling, I asked her to focus on the process and the submodalities of her kinaesthetic experience. 'The sick feeling is like a pulse and it spreads from my solar plexus up into my chest and throat. It feels very heavy.' Having obtained this valuable information, I asked her to step out of first position and shake off all of those feelings.

Next I walked her round to the opposite side, imagining that she was now behind her mother and looking over her shoulder at 'that Mattie over there'. Wanting her to move into second position, I continued 'Knowing what you know both consciously and unconsciously about your mother over the years of living with her, I'd like you to step forward and imagine you've become her completely. Pretend that you can see through her eyes, hear through her ears and feel what she's feeling as she's looking at Mattie. As you do that, imagine you're the same body shape as her, with the same posture, gestures, voice tone and mannerisms'.

I asked her from this position to look over at 'that Mattie' and describe what she saw. 'She looks tense and pale – her lips are grey. She has tears in her eyes and she's looking down at the floor.' I wanted to find out 'as mum' just what feelings she had inside. 'I feel very angry, with a burning feeling in my chest that moves up towards my face.' I thanked her and asked her to step out of second position and shake off the feelings.

We now moved round to third position, which was equidistant between first and second positions, like the apex of a triangle. I asked her to imagine that she was observing the situation dispassionately as a 'fly on the wall'. I said 'As you look at them both over there, I want you to think about *who* is triggering *what* in this situation. And also *how* do they reinforce one another's behaviours? What can you learn from this viewpoint? You don't need to answer out loud. Simply think about it'. She looked very contemplatively from one to the other for a few moments.

Staying in *third position*, I asked her to turn her attention to the Mattie in first position. I asked her 'How is *that* Mattie coping with the situation? How do you feel about that and what advice would you give *her?*' She thought for several seconds, and then said 'I feel quite angry as I look at her. I feel frustrated that she's behaving that way. I want to give her a good shake and tell her to get on with it!' She stepped out of third position and shook off her feelings.

I took her to a *fourth position* from which she could see the other three positions from a completely disconnected point of view (simply another meta-position). To make sure that this was happening, I suggested that she let any residual emotion drain back to the position in which it really belonged. From this impartial view it was clear that the Mattie in third position was treating herself (in first position) in exactly the same way as her mother was doing – a mirror image! This was a revelation to her. She was caught between a rock and a hard place – and some of it was entirely of her own doing.

From fourth position I asked her to mentally swap round the images and emotions of first and third positions. We were creating a *new* first position which was now composed of the frustration and anger she had felt in third position. When she had done this she stepped out again.

I moved her over towards the newly transformed first position. 'Now, Mattie, I'd like you to step into this revised and updated first position, taking this new way of thinking and feeling with you. And as you do so, look across at your mother over there. What's changed now? What's different? How does she look now? How do you feel acting in this new way?'

'Well, Mum looks really surprised – shocked even! She's stopped speaking and her hand has fallen to her side. I feel really quite strong and I have a fiery feeling in my chest. It's not unpleasant – in fact it feels very powerful indeed!' When returning to this revised first position it is important to make the patient very aware of any changes that have occurred, to the extent of amplifying them so that they become a positive resource. Now I wanted Mattie to see this from her mother's second-position perspective.

I continued 'Mattie, I'd like you to step into second position now and notice the changes from your mother's point of view as she looks at *that* Mattie over there. What's different? How has she changed?'

Mattie replied 'Well, as Mum I feel quite shocked initially. My "baby" looks so grown up now. She's standing tall, pointing her finger and has a determined look on her face. I wouldn't like to get in her way!' This was obviously a complete contrast to her initial observations a little time earlier. Again it is important to ground the changes by making the patient aware of all the nuances of difference and amplifying them appropriately. You are literally creating a map of a new self-image.

To finish off, I brought Mattie back to her updated first position and let her think about how different the future would be if she brought all of this back with her to university. I said 'And you don't have to think of every single context that you could take these new resources into just now ... you can simply let the deeper aspects of your mind organise things in a way that best fits for you and your changed circumstances'.

The meta-mirror process was the key to allowing Mattie to go back to university the next term. Prior to that we had a follow-up session in which I used many of the anchoring techniques that you have already learned so far to further embed the changes and allow her to feel really good in previously challenging situations. She is now in her third year of university, and had a great time during a two-month elective studies period in Africa.

Joe's lung cancer

Relationships do not just occur between two people. We also relate to our own symptoms in a variety of ways. The meta-mirror and variations of it can be fruitfully used to explore how we relate in especially difficult circumstances, such as terminal care. Although there are many anecdotal claims of spontaneous remission following mind–body interventions, my own experience is that these interventions usually tend to bring a more 'accepting' state of mind – accepting in the sense of an increased peacefulness and calmness in the face of dealing with whatever the future holds. Although we shall deal next with Joe's relationship to his symptoms, the meta-mirror process can also be used in these difficult terminal care circumstances to facilitate the healing of previously fractured personal relationships.

Joe had been diagnosed with inoperable lung cancer several months earlier. His breathlessness at rest was exacerbated by his major anxieties about his tumour's progression and his thoughts of impending death. On several home visits I had chatted to him about mind–body interventions. He had been interested enough to borrow one of my books on the subject, and more recently asked for some help with his anxieties. At this stage he had difficulty moving around, so we did the meta-mirror process in his mind's eye.

From first position he told me of his anxious feelings about death and the 'nothingness beyond'. He pictured his tumour as a grey-black mass with slimy tentacles that were choking the life out of him. His anxiety was a tight constricting feeling that he felt in his upper chest and throat.

Initially he was reluctant to go into second position with the tumour, recoiling at the thought. I reminded him that the tumour was like a very estranged part of himself, composed of one of his cell lines that had run amok. It might have important information that could be of assistance to him. He took a deep breath, closed his eyes and imagined stepping inside. After a moment or two his breathing subsided and he became aware of a sensation in his abdomen that he described as a very powerful feeling of 'survival'. He said 'This part really wants to live'.

In third position he observed both himself and his tumour from a distance. He could see that the tumour's need to survive was inextricably linked to his feelings of choking to death. I asked him to turn his attention to his first-position self. He remarked how frightened and strained he looked. He felt a welling up of a sense of inner strength, and said 'I really want to live, too!'

In fourth position it was as if he had entered a deep open-eyed trance. His face was symmetrical, his breathing slowed and his eyes were unblinking. He switched first and third positions around and then floated into his *revised and renewed* first position with feelings of inner strength. He noticed that the tumour looked smaller, the slime had dried and many of the tentacles that had been choking him had shrivelled up. He felt a warm glow in his belly.

He then entered second position, feeling immediately that the tumour had shrunk considerably. When he looked across at *that* Joe over there, he noticed his breathing was easier, with his chest expanded and a wry smile on his face. It was as if the tumour now had a sense of watchful wariness.

On returning to his updated first position with all of the information that he had gathered along the way, he felt very tired and sleepy. I suggested that he should simply allow himself to drift off while the deeper parts of his mind put all the new knowledge to use in the days, weeks and months ahead.

There was no happy ending in the sense of a 'miracle remission'. Joe lived for a further three months before dying peacefully in his sleep. However, during that time his anxiety lifted, his breathing remained settled and he had sufficient energy not only to cope with but also to enjoy his many visitors. He calmly planned his funeral arrangements, and he maintained a sense of tranquillity up to the time of his passing.

The meta-mirror is only one of many techniques that you can use in this kind of situation. I have also found that *parts negotiation* (*see* Chapter 16), *six-step reframing* (*see* Chapter 13) and the various anchoring approaches have been very useful for a variety of terminal care symptoms. This is certainly an area that will repay further in-depth study.

The meta-mirror process

The meta-mirror process is an excellent way of sorting out difficult or entangled relationships, whether they be with other people or with parts of ourselves. In these relationships we often end up treating ourselves in exactly the same way as the other person does. Not only do we feel beaten up by them, but also our own 'inner self' – what NLP calls meta-position – beats us up, too. We are caught between a rock and a hard place.

I learned about the following process from UK trainer Ian McDermott, who based it on Robert Dilts' original conceptualisation. It blends very nicely with other NLP interventions, with which it is easily combined. The steps are as shown overleaf.

According to John Grinder, experiencing and utilising the three basic perceptual positions is fundamental to both mastering and using NLP technology with wisdom and ecology. Dilts' conceptualisation of the meta-mirror is only one of many ways to address relationship issues – albeit a most useful one. Each of the perceptual positions carries with it a different perspective together with a

Exercise 15:   The meta-mirror process

1 Step into first position

Imagine the other person across from you in your mind's eye. Notice how they stand, sit, walk, talk, breathe, move, etc. *Look* at their eyes, their direction of gaze, the tilt of their head, and whether they are looking towards or away from you. Notice their posture and gestures. *Listen* to their voice. Is it fast, slow, loud, soft, deep or shrill? Which words are emphasised? What are you thinking and feeling in this relationship? What makes it difficult? How do you feel and where in your body do you have that feeling?

Now step out, go neutral and shake it all off!

2 Second position

Step into the shoes of the other person. Try them on for size and fit. Use *their* posture and *their* gestures. Become them as completely as you can. Look across at that 'you' over there in first position. How does that 'you' walk, talk, sit, stand, breathe, move, etc? Go through all of the other questions as in step 1, and end by naming the feeling and where you feel it in your body (as them).

Now step out, go neutral and shake it all off!

3 Third position

Step into third position and view the relationship dispassionately. Who is triggering what in this situation? How do they reinforce one another? Now turn your attention to the first position 'you'. How is he or she coping with the situation? How do you ... here ... respond to that you ... there? What advice would you give that 'you'? What should that 'you' do more of? What should they do less of?

4 Fourth position

Step into a fourth position, *disconnected from the other three*. Allow any residual emotions to go back to the positions where they belong. Think about how the 'third-position you' is relating to the 'first-position you'. What is the predominant reaction/state/feeling of third position?

Now *mentally switch* your first-position and third-position reactions spatially. Quickly replace one with the other.

5 Return to first position

This time, *take the new way of thinking and feeling* from third position into this, a *revised and updated first position*. Experience the new feelings as you look across at the other person in second position. What has changed now? What is different? How do they look, sound, breathe, move, etc. (revisit the original questions if you wish)? How are you resourceful now? How does this allow you to act differently?

Now step out, break state and shake the feelings off.

6 Revisit second position

Step into second position once again, experiencing the 'other' person. See how the 'new you' in first position has changed. Revisit the original questions if you wish. How is the relationship different now?

7 Come home

Return to the updated first position in the here and now, and contemplate what will be different in the future.

specific set of information. None of the three main positions by itself provides the whole 'truth' of a situation (and of course fourth position is simply a variant of third position – with a wider perspective). However, synthesising the fruits of all three together can allow the spontaneous resolution of many challenging relationships – with both self and other!

The revelation which most people have is finding that their 'inner self' (meta-position) is treating them in exactly the same way as the other person – a mirror image. When looked at in another way, you can see that the original first and second positions are not in rapport – their states, postures, gestures and voice characteristics are all quite different. Substituting third position for first position allows rapport to be re-established with the other person – the states now match! This allows for a much more productive interchange of ideas and information.

Although I have described the process in its entirety as a single intervention, it is quite possible to use only specific parts in casual conversation during an ordinary consultation. Most people will understand the concept of 'taking a fly-on-the-wall view' or 'stepping into someone's shoes'. Used adeptly, it can open up a most useful perspective on a difficult situation. As usual there are some important pointers that can help the process to go more smoothly and effectively.

1   Always ensure that you step cleanly into and out of each position, allowing a 'break state' between the steps. Contamination of one position by another will give confusing information and fail to achieve the 'sorting out' that is required prior to re-integration. We already have all of the information from each position in our neurology – unfortunately most of the time it is in a bemused morass!

2   When in first position, build up as detailed a picture of the other person as possible. Elucidate all of the visual, auditory and kinaesthetic submodalities. Do the same when in second position looking over at first position. When you revisit each position later, this will let you know with precision what has actually changed, giving a strong feeling of conviction that things really will be different.

3   There will be a predominant feeling associated with each position. This is representative of the state you are accessing at that time. Pay careful attention to the kinaesthetics of that state, mapping it out in more detail if you wish. Again this gives a strong conviction of change to the patient when revisiting first position – the original internal state will have been replaced by a new resourceful state. If it has not been replaced, then you know that you have more work to do!

4   In each position you can ask questions at each of Dilts' logical levels in order to obtain more useful information. Is the challenge that you are facing about your environment or behaviours – what you are doing? Is it more at the level of your skills, competencies and capabilities? Is it to do with your beliefs, values and attitudes? Is it about who you are – your identity or your current role?

5   However, you can use a quick yet very effective version of the meta-mirror simply by focusing on the feelings that are engendered in each position. Each state is a container for the expression of specific behaviours, skill-sets, beliefs and values. Changing the state will change everything else – out of conscious awareness, of course.

6   You may find when you revisit first position that change has not yet occurred. You can take whatever the current situation now offers through the whole process again, returning in depth to steps 3 and 4, which are particularly important. If you wish, you can add whatever resources are required to further strengthen first position through anchoring and circle-of-excellence techniques.

Many of the relationship issues that abound in medical practice at present are gathered under the heading of 'co-dependency'. This is when the intertwined behaviours of both parties are fundamental to preventing change. When looked at from the meta-mirror perspective, two main factors stand out. First, there is a type of 'polarity rapport' between the two individuals. Instead of operating out of relatively similar states when in rapport, the opposite happens. If one is aggressive, the other is submissive; if one is distant and aloof, the other is overly caring, etc. Of course, these transactions happen episodically and sequentially, and are typified by the statement 'I can't live *with* him and I can't live *without* him!'

Secondly, at the times of the 'difficult' encounters both parties are acting from an isolated first position that fails to incorporate useful information from the other two positions. This information is present in their neurology, but appears to be inaccessible *at the time when they need it most.* It would be trite of me to say that simply exhibiting the meta-mirror will magically solve these issues. However, my experience is that it opens up a far greater degree of choice with regard to behaving differently *in the moment.* Of course, this is only one way of looking in a very simplified form at a very complex situation. Experiment and see what happens!

Mastering perceptual positions is fundamental to practising excellent change work. I encourage you to take this way of thinking with you into as many different contexts as you can currently perceive – and especially those you cannot yet perceive!

How the meta-mirror works: connecting theory to practice

One way to consider perceptual positions is as *state-dependent* information systems. Some people (but not many) are able to access all three positions easily at will. It is as if they have semi-permeable neurological boundaries that permit the free flow and interchange of information which allows the most appropriate response moment by moment and situation by situation. However, most of us tend to favour mainly one way of operating, without easy recourse to the others save by dint of 'hard thinking'. In times of stress we respond automatically from our fixed perspective.

Each state is an *attractor basin* that allows the emergence of certain beliefs, values and behaviours. In first position 'I' am important, and my needs must be met. In the extreme, 'I' will display whatever behaviour is required to fulfil those beliefs. In second position 'your' needs are more important than mine. In the extreme I will behave in whatever way is required for 'you' to get your outcome met. In third position 'our' needs in combination are important. 'We' must do whatever is necessary for both outcomes to be fulfilled. However, in the extreme we may endlessly analyse all of the options and paralyse ourselves by inaction.

Of course each of these positions and its extreme has a different set of attached cognitions and emotions. The third (and fourth) position perspective provides a physical and mental space for *cognitive restructuring* to take place. The beliefs of the first and second positions are evaluated, and their synthesis gives rise to the updated cognitions of the revised first position. Restructuring also takes place at a representational and motor level. There are spontaneous submodality shifts, the recognition of which helps to cement the changes. Posture, gestures, breathing and patterns of movement can all automatically shift as an expression of the reconfigured states.

The internal representation that we have of individuals in our lives is something that we carry with us wherever we go. Usually we are operating out of the summation of past memories which feeds forward into each future meeting. By changing and updating this summary representation, we open up the possibility and even the expectation of dealing with the future differently. Changing in the here and now brings with it a strong sense of *self-efficacy* for the next encounter. We now have access to the necessary skill-sets.

If you calibrate carefully you will notice major physiological shifts accompanying the significant realignment of resources. In effect we are collapsing the anchors of first and third position together – a form of *counter-conditioning*. In fact, each of the marked-out positions can be seen as a spatial anchor for a set of resources. Cycling through the positions will update each one significantly with the infusion of different states similar to *parts negotiation* (*see* Chapter 16). Following this, a successful encounter with the other person will act as its own reinforcer for future success – *operant conditioning*.

Concluding

The three main perceptual positions are fundamental to effective and ecological change in NLP. They are the organisers of and containers for all of the other change processes that you will read about in this book. One or more of these positions is implicit in each of the main techniques – for example, third position is implicit in successful application of the phobia cure (*see* Chapter 10). However, they come to the fore in relationship issues. They are capable of handling large chunks of information, much of it unconscious, and resequencing it in a more useful way.

You can use the various elements of the meta-mirror in every aspect of life. If we focus on consultations, you can see how it can improve your information-gathering and therapeutic skills. Going into second position with your patient is the basis for developing rapport and even deep trust over time. You can obtain much seemingly intuitive information about just how this particular person structures their world – almost to the point of 'mind reading'. However, you must always remember to check out these insights for continuing veracity!

Third position, where you imagine seeing both the patient and yourself 'over there', gives valuable information about just which point you have reached and what direction to choose next. It is an essential checkpoint for giving structure to the consultation, which you can do in the form of meta-comments – 'this is what we've done so far, and this is the next step'. This is also a useful position to adopt at times during teaching, especially when demonstrating change work to a group.

However, you must always take any information obtained in this way back to first position. This is the position in which you have most easy access to all of your current resources – you are in the moment and flowing! Failure to do this will leave you feeling strangely at odds with yourself, interfering in a self-conscious way with behaviours that are normally automatic. Ensuring that you have fully 'stepped into yourself' will remove any obstacles to your acting out of your best intentions.

As well as the above, I would encourage you to start thinking about how patients relate to their symptoms. Common in the western world is the attitude that we must get rid of all troublesome symptoms – both physical and psychological. However, what we resist often persists, and sometimes the harder we try to get rid of a problem, the more trouble it gives us. Exploring the information that lies behind a symptom (*see also* Chapter 13 on six-step reframing) can yield valuable clues about what to do next. Although occasionally this can be curative in its own right, you will usually find that changing the relationship in this way allows a far greater sense of an inner locus of control, and an easier trip along the pathway to health and wellness.

CHAPTER 15

Using time for a change

Introduction

I introduced you to the NLP concept of timelines way back in Chapter 3. If you did the accompanying exercise, you will already have found out how you personally organise time. If you have not yet done so, do the exercise now. It will pay dividends as this chapter unfolds.

Throughout our lives we have all gone through good times and bad – often rejoicing in very pleasant experiences, and sometimes being engulfed in the pain of unpleasant ones. We store all of these memories in particular ways on our timelines. Occasionally the way in which we store a particular memory actually causes us problems in the here and now. In a sense, Freud was right – the roots of many problems do lie in the past. The difficulty that Freud had was that he needed to inch his way back in time by a laborious free association technique to uncover the repressed memories that drove the current problem. His other difficulty was the belief that this uncovering, together with 'insight', would alter the situation for the better. Sadly this is not the case.

NLP recognised that it is not the content of the actual memory (repressed or not) which causes the problem, but *how* the memory is coded by the brain. This is a *process* distinction which Freud and his colleagues did not have. Stored in a particular way, the past memory can act as a template on which present experience is matched and compared. If there is a 'fit', then the problem recurs. The task of the NLP practitioner is to change the *structure* of the memory in some way so that the problem is resolved.

Until the advent of timelines, most practitioners had to take many examples of the problem from the past, changing each one as an isolated event and hoping that these cumulative changes would generalise into the rest of their patient's life. The discovery of timelines changed all that. Our personalities are tightly bound up in the way we think about time. To a large degree our enduring personality traits are the product of all our past experiences and our future expectations. We know who we are today by what we have done in the past.

Timeline techniques can cause major shifts in how we think about ourselves and how we behave. And these key changes can take place in as little as one brief session – a far cry from Freud.

Steve and Connirae Andreas were among the first NLP trainers to investigate both the way in which people stored time mentally and how changing the submodalities of the timeline itself could effect lasting change. Richard Bandler came up with a technique called the 'decision destroyer', whereby taking resources back into the past *before* the problem had even started resulted in rapid change. Robert Dilts externalised the timeline and had people walking up and down it. His technique of 'reimprinting' can cause profound, in-depth transformation.

In this chapter we shall utilise both internal 'visual timelines' and external 'kinaesthetic timelines' to demonstrate powerful effective change. This will provide a most potent set of tools for your therapeutic toolbox.

Alan's asthma

Alan, aged 29 years, had had asthma for as long as he could remember. Although it was well enough controlled on bronchodilators and inhaled steroids, he wanted to explore any mind–body approaches that could help him to reduce or even stop his medication. He had never had a life-threatening asthmatic episode, but had occasionally required oral steroids and brief use of a nebuliser over the years. Being an asthmatic just did not fit with how he saw himself. He wanted to try out hypnotic regression techniques to see whether he could unearth the cause of his problem. Because he was keen to investigate alternative approaches, I suggested that we could use timelines to explore the issue and perhaps give him a new measure of control over his symptoms.

Before starting any therapeutic technique, I asked him about his asthma and the kinds of situations that caused him problems. It became clear that although he had the usual exacerbations with upper respiratory tract infections, there was also an emotional component. Working as an executive in the oil industry, he often had to deal with high-pressure situations. In particularly stressful moments, especially before major business meetings, he would find himself getting chest tightness and reaching for his inhaler. He described these as 'life-and-death decision' situations. Although no one's life was actually on the line, his words were to be strangely prophetic.

As he was right-handed, Alan's timeline was arranged in a fairly standard way, with the past diagonally over his left shoulder and the future diagonally off to the right. I asked him to think about one of those business meetings that had made his chest tight. He identified a particularly troublesome one about two months previously – the one that had prompted him to take things further today. I said 'Alan, I'd like you to imagine floating upwards, out of your body, so that you can look down and see your timeline ... past, present and future ... stretched out below you. And as you get used to seeing it in that way, I'd like you to begin now to float back to that time ... just before that particular meeting ...'

I waited until he signalled by nodding that he had arrived at that point, seeing himself down below in the memory. 'Alan, I'd like you to float down into that memory so that you can get in touch with some of those feelings again ... just enough to know what they feel like ... in your chest.' I wanted him to experience as much of the feelings as I required to anchor the state without precipitating an asthmatic attack. His breathing increased slightly and his face went a little pale as I anchored the state to a knuckle. I brought him back out of the memory again, floating high above his timeline once more, and as he returned physiologically to a more neutral state we continued with the next step.

'Now, Alan ... as you keep floating above all that ... I'd like you to take a *little bit* of this (touching the anchor) ... and take it all the way back in time ... all the way back to where it really belongs ... .floating back along your timeline ... until you get to the event that started it all off.' Known as a *trans-derivational search*, I wanted him to ride on that particular familiar feeling back to his earliest memory of its original occurrence. I continued 'And you may get glimpses of images ... snatches of sounds ... other feelings ... that may not initially make much sense to you ... yet soon ... very soon ... things will clear ... and when you get a feel for where and when it is that ... *you've arrived* ... you can let me know (head nods)'.

I asked him to come all the way back to the here and now, and looking back into the past from the safety of the present moment, to describe what had happened back then. 'Well, it was me, looking like I was about four or five years old – a thin scrawny-looking kid. I was at the beach and I'd been playing at the breakwater and got knocked off by a big wave and dragged under. I couldn't breathe and I panicked, inhaling salty water. My father pulled me out leg first. I was gasping for air, then vomited in the sand. It looks funny now, but back then I can tell you it seemed like a real *life-and-death situation!*'

It was clear from his comments just how that event – what we might call a negative imprinting experience – had played a part in triggering his asthmatic episodes. Every time he went into a 'life-and-death' business situation, he experienced the same tight panicky feelings in his chest and needed to use his inhaler. It was a very powerful demonstration of a state-dependent memory cueing his current symptoms. What we needed to do now was to bring some new resources into that past situation so that we could change the way in which he remembered the event – into a more productive and positive imprint.

I asked Alan just what kind of resource he would have needed back then to navigate the event in a more productive way. He replied 'Well, it seems odd to say this, but it's as if I would have needed to know beforehand that, even though the situation was potentially traumatic, everything was going to turn out fine. I would have needed to have been a five-year-old mind reader!' We turned a few ideas over in our minds, thinking about potentially hair-raising experiences that were ultimately really quite safe. Then he hit on it: 'It's like one of those scary adventure-park rides I was on two years ago – the Screaming Banshee – a huge vertical drop followed by a wild roller-coaster. You know that you'll get butterflies in your belly and sweaty palms beforehand, but that ultimately it's safe – you'll come out of the other end intact.'

I took him back along his timeline to that particular ride. Focusing on the knowledge that he knew he was *going to survive*, he relived the memory again as I set an anchor on another knuckle. We now had the resource we needed to reimprint the earlier memory. I said 'From where you are with me in the here and now, I'd like you to beam that resource all the way back along your timeline to that young Alan. Ensure that it's fully in place and he has complete access to it, standing on the breakwater *before* the traumatic event occurred (fire anchor). You could beam it as a colourful light ... a stream of sound ... an energetic feeling ... and you'll get a signal from him ... perhaps a smile ... maybe a nod ... that he's received it all ...'

When it was clear that five-year-old Alan was re-resourced, I said 'Now from here ... looking at him from a distance ... watch how he goes through that event again ... this time with the new resource ... and see the difference it makes to the outcome'. It is important to run through the event with the new resource in a dissociated way first to make sure that it really does turn out better. If it is not quite right, you can continue to add different resources until you get the best fit. Alan was satisfied that the run-through seemed fine. 'He's not distressed any more ... in fact he's laughing loudly and playing with his dad as if nothing had really happened!'

Once you are certain that you like the result, it is time to associate into the event and generalise the changes throughout the timeline. I said 'Alan, I'd like you to float all the way back in time and *step into* that five-year-old "you" ... this time with the benefit of knowing that *the new resource is there* ... ready and waiting ... and as you feel it building up inside (press anchor) ... you can imagine going quickly through that event again ... noticing at one level *how different it feels* ... and at another how you can continue past it ... growing up through your timeline ... all the way up to the present day. And it doesn't matter whether you know consciously ... or not ... that *all of the other events between then and now are changing and rearranging themselves as a result* ... updating with the new resource ... as it spreads throughout the times of your life ...'

When Alan had 'grown up' through his timeline to the present moment, I continued to future pace the changes. 'And from the here and now ... you can look out into the future and watch ... as that Alan continues his journey into the days ... and weeks ... and months ahead ... even further ... and notice how *he's dealing with things differently now* ... how events that used to trouble him are being dealt with in another way ... *your own way* ... and see how good it feels ... to know that kind of future awaits you ...'

In the months which followed that single session, Alan was able to deal with high-pressure meetings far more easily and without the need to resort to his inhaler. He still kept it with him for the few times when a high pollen count triggered an occasional wheeze, yet on the whole he was vastly improved. Now this is not to say that all asthmatics can be treated this easily. Yet this approach is very useful, particularly when emotional factors play a significant role, and even when the problem appears to be 'all physical'. Some people, in the trans-derivational search, have reported being back at birth with the umbilical cord wrapped around their neck. Whether that really happened or not is in a sense immaterial. Changing whatever memory perception seems to be driving current experience can provide many unexpected benefits.

Angry Andy

In the above scenario the reimprinting involved only the one individual – young Alan. Often, however, there are other significant characters involved in the original imprinting experience. Because they are so intertwined in the problem's beginnings it is very useful to include them in the reimprinting process. Robert Dilts' refinements of the basic procedure have given us a versatile tool which can be used in a variety of circumstances. In essence, he uses elements of the *meta-mirror* (*see* Chapter 14) to reconfigure the imprinting memory so that it becomes a resourceful experience instead. We shall see how this works with Andy.

Andy, in his forties, was generally an angry man a great deal of the time. Separated from his wife and two children, and unhappy with his current partner, he often took his pent-up anger and frustration out on his employees. After literally blowing his top he would immediately feel remorseful, and then become angry with himself for his stupidity – a vicious circle indeed. Recognising that he needed to do something different, he had received hours of counselling, and although he understood himself a little better he still could not control his angry outbursts.

I took Andy back to a recent outburst which had occurred over a very trivial matter. Initially he was a little bemused that all I wanted him to do was to focus on the angry tight feelings in his chest – he wanted to talk *about* his experience, whereas I was more concerned with the *process* of anchoring the state as a prelude to a trans-derivational search. Finally he understood, and we traced the feelings back in time. Initially we stopped off en route in his teenage years, to various violent escapades when he had been a 'hard man' in his native Glasgow. I simply kept asking him to trust his mind to take him back to the earliest event and, lo and behold, a memory of when he was six years old surfaced. He was crying and cowering in a corner while his father angrily punished him for a misdemeanour.

Interestingly, Andy was behaving today in the same way that his father had done in the past. As he put it, 'It's just like I've grown into him!' And if we are honest, we often find ourselves saying and doing things in the same way that our parents did – especially the things that we didn't like about them. We have modelled far more than we bargained on. It is as if we have taken on a computer virus that only gets activated at a certain date – when we have reached our parents' age. I explained this to Andy, and told him that we could reimprint it in a way that was far more beneficial to him.

I asked him to imagine stepping inside his father (second position) in that memory, feeling what he was feeling at that time, and asking the question 'What is the positive intention behind this behaviour?' Andy's dad was punishing young Andy to stop him behaving badly towards his sister. His intention was to get Andy to behave in a more positive way, yet *how* he was attempting to get the message across was only making things worse. I asked him what was needed to get the message across in a better way. The reply was 'calmness'.

I asked Andy to search his memory for a time when he had experienced that kind of calmness for himself. Initially no answers were forthcoming. Then he remembered being on holiday abroad, on an almost deserted beach, with the sun high in a blue sky as he sat there contentedly for what seemed liked hours. We anchored this state, and as I prepared to beam it back to his father, Andy baulked, saying that his father did not deserve to feel that good! I explained that we were not really giving this to his father – only to Andy's *inner representation* of him. If he really thought about it, because the memory of his father was generated by his own neurology he was in fact only transferring resources from one part of his brain to another. In a funny kind of way he was actually giving the resource of calmness to himself.

On hearing this explanation he was more comfortable about beaming calmness back in time to the representation of his father. We felt that it would be best to back up the memory so that the calmness could be installed in his father *before* the altercation with young Andy – he would have been better prepared. I asked him to imagine stepping into his father and feeling what it was like to have that calmness circulating in his body *ahead* of time. He reported that it was a *really good feeling!*

I then asked him to consider young Andy. What was it that he really needed back then? The answer was 'to feel loved'. Again we searched his memory banks for an appropriate resource. However, Andy said that he had never really felt loved in this way – another dilemma! I asked him about his own son David, now aged 12 years. Had Andy given David that kind of love when he was aged six? With an affirmative answer we revivified a memory of Andy loving David in exactly that way, and anchored it. I then asked him to beam that resource back along his timeline to young Andy and to notice the look on his face when he received it. When in turn he imagined stepping into young Andy as he was 'filled up with love' he broke down and cried for several minutes – a powerfully moving experience for him.

Following this, the rest of the process went smoothly. We viewed what would have happened in that memory from the outside, in a dissociated fashion, if both his father and young Andy had had those resources available at the time. This radically changed the memory for the better. I suggested that he should step into young Andy at the beginning of that event and come up through time, in an associated fashion, all the way back to now, allowing the events between then and now to reorganise themselves in a more appropriate way. We continued to future pace the changes into the days, weeks and months ahead.

Over the next few months Andy reported feeling far more at ease with himself, and more accepting of the day-to-day vicissitudes of life, with less emotional turmoil. He found that he was more clear-headed, able to think straight at potentially difficult moments and, as he put it, 'much easier to live with'. He exemplified the kind of major integration and increased sense of personal congruence that can occur with an effective reimprinting process.

Reimprinting: the process

Many people believe that past negative experiences, whether they are remembered fully consciously or not, can drive current problem situations. It makes sense to pace that belief, find the imprinting experience and alter it sufficiently so that it no longer activates negative emotions. In fact, this process can actually turn the imprinting event into a positive resource that further fuels developmental change for the individual.

The NLP approach believes that, in some sense or other, all current problems have a major element of learning attached to them. Although genetic inheritance may predispose an individual to develop certain conditions, the experiences that we live through and learn from determine whether or not the condition actually develops. Of course, this is the old 'nature versus nurture' debate, for which there is no one 'right' answer. However, because we do not know how much of a part each plays in the process, it is often more useful (and productive) to assume that large elements have been learned. This prior attitude allows interventions such as reimprinting with timelines the possibility of facilitating major change – even in chronic conditions.

It is usually very instructive to imagine that all illnesses and diseases have a learned component, not only those that are considered to be psychosomatic or psychological. I encourage you to experiment with the following outline of reimprinting (based on Dilts' approach) in a whole variety of medical conditions.

Exercise 16:   The reimprinting process

1   *Identify a troubling problem or context* where the same symptom occurs time and time again. This could be an emotional state or even a physical symptom. Establish how this particular patient experiences their timeline – past, present and future. Float back along the timeline to *a recent experience* of the problem. Associate into it and *anchor the accompanying state* on a knuckle.

2   *Trigger the anchor* and, asking your patient to focus on the feelings, tell them to '*float all the way back in time*, until you come to the very first event ... the very first time you experienced all of this'. Many imprinting events have taken place under the age of 10 years, so keep going back until you get the very earliest event. The actual imprinting event may be a memory that at first appears to be irrelevant to the current problem.

3   When you have located the imprint, ask the patient to *review it from a dissociated perspective*. You can take them back to the here and now and have them 'look at it way back then in the past from the safety of the present moment'. Identify what happened in that memory, together with any other significant people involved.

4   *Step inside (second position) each of the characters involved.* Determine their positive intention in this situation, and *identify the particular resources which they needed back then* that would have changed this to a positive imprint.

5   Search your patient's personal history for times when they had those resources, even if only for a short period. *Revivify, amplify and anchor the resources.*

6   *Beam the resources back* to each individual, one by one. Notice from the outside (dissociated) how this changes the original experience. Then step inside that person (associated) and experience the resource from second position. Do this with each of the characters involved, finishing with the 'younger self'.

7   When you are satisfied that *the experience has been transformed into a positive imprint*, associate the patient into their younger self. Firing all of the anchors simultaneously, let them *grow up inside their timeline to the present day*, allowing the changes to ripple out as they do so. Seed the fruits of this new positive imprint *into the future*.

The reimprinting process using timelines is a very powerful tool for rapid change. 'Growing the person up' inside their timeline with the new resources allows generalisation of the changes into many different contexts simultaneously. It can often cause a profound reorganisation of a person's past, which then serves as a stable platform from which they can build an entirely new future – free from the previous limitation.

It is also an easily adaptable process which you can tailor to your patient's requirements. You can literally re-resource any previous negative memory that holds them back in some way and establish truly generative change. Robert Dilts and his colleagues have used it to tackle many clinical issues (both physical and psychological), with good results. Of course, although these reports are currently anecdotal, they do give a pointer towards future research.

There are several things that you can do to ensure that you can make the process go more smoothly and effectively.

1   Get the feeling state that is associated with the problem symptom and anchor it cleanly. The more precisely you can target that specific state, the easier it is to track back in time.

2   Problems that have been with a patient for some time, perhaps even involving several contexts, usually have an imprint below 10 years of age. If the patient's earliest conscious memory of the problem state is in their late teens or twenties, this is not usually the one to reimprint unless it is the most traumatic event. Often the imprint will bear no obvious relation to current events, yet it shares the same negative feeling.

3   Once you have reached the imprint, calibrate carefully to make sure you dissociate the patient from it so that they can review it and learn just what they need. You can use submodalities (smaller, black and white, distancing, etc.) to prevent them associating back into it. It can be very useful to establish a meta-position as a place of observation off the timeline altogether.

4   If there are significant others involved, ascertaining their positive intentions in the event, irrespective of their behaviours, is vital both for reframing and for adding resources. If your patient baulks at the idea of giving resources to the other person, because 'they don't deserve them', then remind them that they are not doing this in 'real life'. It is their *own* perceptual projection that you are re-resourcing – and *this* is clearly part of their *own* neurology. You are taking one set of resources and connecting them to another part of *their* brain, allowing *them* to function quite differently in the future.

5   If your patient does not appear to have the resources – in terms of personal experiences – needed for reimprinting the memory, you can find them elsewhere. You can go out into the future and imagine what it would be like to have such a resource. You could imagine someone (a mentor) who had

the resource and second position them to obtain it. You could even use any of the other anchoring techniques to build the resource from scratch.

6   After you have added resources to each significant other, including the person's younger self, run the event through as a dissociated movie to ensure that it turns out the way you want it. You can keep adding resources to each person until it looks right and you are satisfied with it. Only then can your patient step into their younger self and take this reimprinted state with them all the way back to now.

7   Imprints may not necessarily be single emotionally traumatic events. Sometimes it is the sheer repetition of the same message over a period of time that cumulatively builds into a problem complex.

Timeline interventions can be used in many different ways to change past limiting memories and release patients from previously conditioned responses. Floating above a timeline is quite easy for someone who is good at visual processing. However, for the more kinaesthetic members of the population, Dilts developed a walking timelines model which, although it utilises all of the above steps, does so externally rather than internally. The following case will demonstrate its usage.

Lucy's low self-esteem

Lucy was 31 years of age when we did this particular intervention. I had already treated her successfully to help her kick her smoking habit, and a few months later she opened up about issues of low self-esteem. Most of her life she had felt very 'needy', never matching up to expectations. Other people always appeared better than her in some way, and she felt very small in comparison. In her late teens and early twenties she had gone from one relationship to another, hoping that sexual fulfilment would ease her turmoil. Now in her second marriage, with two young children to look after, she seemed to be frenetically doing things all the time to prove that she was a good mother. She just wanted to 'feel normal and be just like everybody else'.

I decided to use a kinaesthetic *walking timelines* intervention with her. I asked her to imagine that she could project her timeline out on to the floor in front of her so that the past lay to her left, the future lay to her right and the present was just a step in front. We established a meta-position parallel to and just behind the present for dissociated observation of any events that we needed to discuss. I asked her to step into the present moment, facing the future, and to get in touch with the feelings that she associated with low self-esteem.

She put her hand on her solar plexus where the feelings resided, and focusing on this I stepped her slowly backwards along her timeline. I suggested that as she went back in time the feelings would intensify, and when they peaked this would probably represent the earliest event, whether she knew this consciously or not. She reached a spot on the line when her face quivered and went pale. Several silent tears fell. I asked her to step back *before* that event had occurred, and then to come off her timeline all the way back up to the meta-position, where we could review what had happened in safety.

From the meta-position she looked back in time and saw a six-year-old Lucy in tears, holding a rag doll, one of its arms on the floor. Her mother was chastising her for being a 'stupid little girl again'. She was ranting on about how she always made mistakes, never got anything right and was doomed to be a failure for the rest of her life. Now we do not know whether this event really occurred or not. And even if it did not, I take the view that this was an unconscious re-presentation which summarised the cumulative effect of a recurrent childhood message. Real or not, changing the representation can have profound effects.

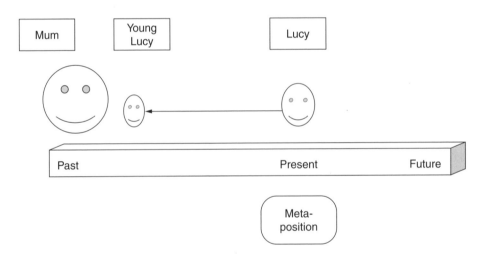

Figure 15.1:   Timeline intervention.

Interestingly, seeing it again from a dissociated perspective in the meta-position, Lucy could already begin to appreciate that the running commentary made by her mother was more about herself than about Lucy – changes were already beginning. She walked back and stepped inside her mother (second position). Through her eyes she sensed a great deal of pent-up frustration and general dissatisfaction with her 'lot' in life. Her positive intention was really to motivate Lucy to do better with her own life. Unfortunately, however, the words that she used gave a 'move away from motivation', with little direction as to what to move towards.

Lucy decided that the resource which her mother needed back then was a sense of acceptance of what was, together with hope for the future. Unfortunately, she did not appear ever to have had this resource for herself! I asked her if she had a friend – someone she knew, perhaps a mentor or role model – who displayed these kinds of qualities. Her friend Jill sprang immediately to mind. Lucy remembered a time in the recent past when Jill had been involved in a car accident. Although her car had been so badly damaged it had to be written off, Jill had accepted this setback and immediately started making plans for the future. Lucy imagined stepping into Jill (second position), and accessed the feelings of acceptance and hope for the future, beaming them back to her mother on the timeline.

We watched a rerun of the memory from an outside dissociated perspective as Lucy's mother behaved quite differently with the new resource. She was more loving and gentle, and used kinder words. Then I asked Lucy to replay the memory again, this time stepping fully into the associated perspective of her mother, seeing through *her* eyes the different effect on young Lucy. Next she stepped inside young Lucy and experienced it all associated at first hand. This time she felt bathed in powerful, supportive, loving feelings, and I asked her to walk slowly up her timeline taking all of these feelings with her so that the changes could seed throughout her personal history. Arriving at the present moment looking quite radiant, she continued walking into the kind of future that she wanted to create for herself instead.

Personally I have found *walking timeline* interventions to be very powerful inducers of change – perhaps reflecting my own kinaesthetic bias! The act of moving, together with accessing different postures and gestures, seems to allow a deeper level of integration to occur. I encourage you to experiment and experience it for yourself. Certainly in Lucy's case, low self-esteem disappeared as an issue in her life, to be replaced with a more congruent approach representing an inner locus of control. What she had looked for in vain on the outside she had now found inside herself.

How reimprinting works: connecting theory and practice

Although the process of reimprinting may initially seem quite complex, it is based solidly on both the learning theory and the practical interventions that we have already encountered. Many of our current problems and difficulties are based on *state-dependent memories* which are triggered by external contextual or internal perceptual cues – anchors, in other words. By obtaining a representation of a recent incident and anchoring the state that is engendered, we can track it back in time via a trans-derivational search to the earliest imprint.

Imprints are like *attractor basins*. The elements involved (pictures, sounds, feelings, other people, etc.) form a tightly bound molecular structure, the emergent property of which is the recurring display of a particular symptom complex – both physical and psychological. Added to this, of course, is a set of cognitive beliefs *about* both what has happened and what is likely to happen in the future as a result. Successful resolution can be thought of as occurring on many levels simultaneously.

At a fairly gross level, we can think of this as a *conditioning and counter-conditioning process*. Each of the elements – present experience, past imprint, significant others involved and resources – represents a state that can be accessed and anchored. In this sense, reimprinting is then simply a question of sequencing and collapsing anchors together to free up and change the state-bound information, allowing resolution to occur.

There is also a huge amount of *cognitive restructuring* going on at both a conscious and a non-conscious level. At the level of representation, the re-resourced imprint will show major changes in visual, auditory and kinaesthetic submodalities. Motor patterns involving posture, gesture and respiration cycles display significant shifts. Limiting beliefs are a major casualty of the process. Although the cognitive elements of the belief can be addressed directly during the process itself, most people experience the spontaneous emergence of new, adaptive, more empowering beliefs with an increasing internal locus of control.

Taking the reimprinted state into different future contexts allows a significant degree of *skills training*. The opportunity occurs – both consciously and uncon-sciously – to run through various imagined future scenarios with a changed behavioural product, noticing and updating responses both for self and for significant others. There is both the creation of a new set of expectations, and a belief in one's own *self-efficacy* for successful achievement.

Not to be underplayed is the *modelling* of the doctor or therapist by the patient, which occurs mainly at an unconscious level. This can be very significant in and of its own right. It can range from the provision of an anchor of safety and security (simply by having an already competent individual guide the patient capably through what might be a heavily charged personal encounter) all the way through to the non-conscious transfer of the prevailing beliefs and attitudes that the doctor or therapist has about whether or not the patient can successfully navigate the attractor landscape. Although I shall say more about these so-called *demand characteristics* later (*see* Chapter 18), it is important for the skilled helper to maintain a positive attitude for patient success.

Concluding

Timelines are not real – they are simply a construct of our minds which helps us to navigate the various sets of circumstances that we personally encounter. Yet if you really think about it, every symptom with which a patient presents – both physical and psychological – had a beginning in time. And before that time the problem simply did not exist. According to science, at a quantum physics level the notion of cause and effect makes no literal sense. Yet on a human level we define everything that has ever happened to us as having had a preceding cause.

Because we construct our view of reality in this way, it opens up the possibility that major change can occur quickly – if we know how. Taking resources 'back in time' changes the principal construct (reimprinting) on which the cause and effect are based. By the logic that holds that model of the world together, the ensuing domino effect promulgates the change throughout time. It simply cannot do otherwise. Philosophically speaking, there is only 'now' (the present moment) – we cannot literally alter past events. Yet our *representation* of the past is eminently malleable, and the changes that occur are palpable. What if you were to view patients' presenting problems in this way? Is this something that you could do more easily now?

Yet some people, when they are contemplating doing something new – perhaps thinking about putting into practice an idea like reimprinting – may suddenly find themselves in an old familiar state. You may call it mild anxiety, anticipation or even feeling overwhelmed, or perhaps you have another name for this sensation. It may start as a niggling feeling somewhere around your solar plexus which, as the time approaches, increases in intensity such that you find yourself questioning your ability, your aptitude, and even your belief that you can succeed in the task. Heaven forbid if it reaches the level of panic!

However, because it is an old familiar state, one that you may have encountered many times in the past, you might already find yourself connecting with certain images and sounds that arise. Sometimes these are of one event, sometimes of more than one, and occasionally they may be mixed together, accelerating the intensity of the underlying feeling. Often you can find that you momentarily lose contact with the present moment, drifting inside, somewhat lost in thought. And suddenly you are back there and then – exactly where it all started.

What if, for a moment or two, you allowed part of yourself to actually be in that experience, and at the same time the perhaps rather odd feeling of pretending that you could simultaneously observe from a distance? Is it only you there or is someone else involved? What might you learn? What would need to have happened differently back then? If you could name consciously what was required, what would it be? And what if you could only name it unconsciously instead?

You see, the interesting thing is that many people find the mere asking of the question allows the answer to percolate through – changing not only that experience, but also every other connection through time to the here and now, *very quickly*! What is more, from this perspective the future opens up very differently, doesn't it? So, as you continue to mull over all of this, which particular patients and which types of problems do you envisage helping now?

CHAPTER 16

Integrating parts

Introduction

Have you ever had the experience of being in two minds about something, when part of you wanted to do *this* and part of you wanted to do *that*? Perhaps you wanted that mouth-watering chocolate cake, yet you knew it would not be good for your diet, your figure or your health. Maybe you wanted to spend time on your own, but felt obligated to attend to family needs. Possibly one of your patients may have described how he could go without alcohol for some time but would then suddenly find himself 'inexplicably' on a drinking binge. Do you remember what it feels like in your body when you are at odds with yourself, torn between two different directions? Just what is going on here?

This kind of internal conflict is usually called an *incongruity*. We are *simultaneously incongruent* when both parts of the conflict are expressed at the same time – as in the chocolate-cake example. We are *sequentially incongruent* when both parts are expressed one after the other – as in the binge-drinking example. Although we do not really have 'internal parts', it is a very useful metaphor for describing internal conflicts. The tendency is for more serious medical problems, such as addictions, alcohol abuse and bulimia, to be represented by dissociated aspects of ourselves which 'take over and run the show' despite our best intentions. These are at one end of the spectrum of sequential incongruity, while milder addictions such as smoking are at the other.

So just how do we deal with this kind of conflict in order to facilitate a resolution? If you have ever acted as a mediator between two people (or between two groups of people), you will know that successful mediation is a bit like six-step reframing. First you have to find out what each side wants – their outcome – together with the benefits as they see it from their perspective. Then you chunk up on their respective positive intentions until you reach a level on which both can agree. Keeping this agreement in mind, you chunk down only as quickly as the details can be resolved from within the frame of this larger perspective. Then, of course, you organise various agreed steps for future action.

In this chapter, we shall look at how you can integrate conflicting parts using the standard *visual squash* process (it sounds painful – but it isn't!). We shall then consider a useful variation of the format, generated by Robert Dilts, which utilises *walking timelines*. I have used both interchangeably, with successful results. Of course, you will be able to adapt the principles of this method for any type of negotiation between two or more parties.

Kirsty's kids

Kirsty had two children aged 10 and six. Her husband, a fisherman, was only at home for a few days every two weeks. Increasingly she had found herself becoming angry and irritable with the children at the drop of a hat. She would shout and bawl at them with the slightest provocation, and afterwards she would feel very guilty about it. This recurring cycle was getting her down – she felt that she was a bad mother. It was as if she had no control over the angry outbursts, and they frightened her. She wanted to be 'a good mum', yet she was worried that she might actually hit the kids. Although she recognised that she was depressed, she was not keen to get 'addicted' to tablets – they were not the solution.

I explained to her that it seemed to me she had two 'parts' in conflict with each other. One part was very angry with the kids, and the other part wanted to be a good mother. Both parts wanted something for her that was for her ultimate overall gain. However, at the moment they did not yet know how to work in harmony as one. I suggested that we should use the parts integration process to see whether we could facilitate a worthwhile resolution. I framed it as if she were to be an observer in an argument between two parties, and she would help to mediate. I told her that although it might initially sound a little 'crazy', this process had helped many people come to a peaceful resolution. She agreed to give it a try.

I turned both hands over, palms up, about a foot apart and a foot above her knees. Then I said 'Kirsty, metaphorically speaking, I'd like you to imagine that each part can choose a hand to come out and stand upon ... so to speak. And as you think about that now, which hand belongs to which part?' She indicated that the left hand was for the 'angry' part and the right hand for the 'good mother' part. I continued 'Let's take each part one at a time, knowing that both parts will have an equal chance to have their full say ... (she nods) ... so starting with the angry part ... even if you can't *really see it clearly standing there* ... I'd like you to *imagine what it looks like* ... what it sounds and feels like ... how much it weighs ... how it breathes ... moves ... its gestures and postures ...'

She described it to me as follows. 'She looks really dark, forbidding and angry. She's dressed in black, has a harsh witch-like voice and feels very heavy.

I'm afraid I might drop her!' Building up a full visual, auditory and kinaesthetic representation in this way gives life and animation to a projected inner part. We did the same for the 'good mother' part. This was lighter, gentler sounding, was dressed in brighter colours, and was smiling and happy.

We started with the good mother part on her right hand, addressing it directly. We needed to find that part's outcome and keep chunking up until we had reached an intention that was highly valued in a positive sense. 'Now, Kirsty, looking at the part that wants you to be a good mother I'd like you to ask *her* ... what's important about being a good mother, in that way ... if she fully got that outcome, what would that do for her that is even more important?' I suggested that she might simply get a reply directly from the part itself, or that she might hear it as an inner voice of intuition which might or might not make complete sense. Her reply was 'The feeling of taking good care of others'.

We chunked up the levels in a similar way, asking the same question recursively of each answer:

- *'Knowing that I've done a good job.'*
- *'A sense that I'm doing something worthwhile.'*
- *'I'm really OK after all!'*

This last outcome, her highest intention, was accompanied by a major physiological shift – a deep sigh, facial flushing and a spreading smile of satisfaction. I asked her to thank the part for its co-operation so far, and to ask it to excuse us while we turned our attention to the part on her left hand.

I asked Kirsty to look directly at the angry part and ask 'When you're angry in that way, what is it that you want ... what is your outcome in that situation?' Her reply was 'She wants the kids to shut up, pay attention and do as they're told'.

I continued, 'And if she gets the kids to shut up, pay attention and do what they're told ... what does that do for her that's even more important? How does that really benefit her?' We asked that question of each answer, and obtained the following:

- *'Peace and quiet.'*
- *'A chance to think straight.'*
- *'A sense of relief.'*
- *'Feeling more relaxed.'*
- *'Confidence that I can cope.'*
- *'I can do anything!'*

With the last answer in the chain she again flushed, smiled and let out a long deep sigh – another major physiological shift. I said 'So that's interesting, isn't it? This part that had been angry ... what she really wants for you all along is to *have confidence ... confidence* that you can cope and then ... *you can do anything!* How does it feel to know that what initially started as a negative feeling ended up with her wanting something very positive for you?' She smiled a little bemusedly at first in response.

We moved on to the next step. I said 'Have you noticed, Kirsty, that when you really think about it ... the feeling that ... *you're really OK after all* ... and ... *you can do anything* ... are very closely related ... in fact so similar that you really can't have one without the other ... (she nods). I'd like you to ask each part to turn towards the other, and for them both to *contemplate* ... that *deep down inside* ... they really do both *want the same things* ... (she nods slowly and thoughtfully).' The acknowledgement that two parts which have started off almost diametrically opposed are actually united in their positive intention is a very powerful therapeutic experience.

'Kirsty, as each part looks at the other ... let them begin to think of a particular strength, resource or capability that the other has ... which, if they had access to it ... would really enhance their functioning.' One way to help the integration that is beginning to occur to proceed even more effectively is to identify resources and transfer them one to the other. The original angry part's strength was the 'ability to make tough decisions'. The good mother part's resource was a 'sensitivity to others' reactions'. Kirsty imagined each resource flowing from one to the other so that they could share each other's capabilities.

Now it was time to actually integrate the two parts as one. Remember that all this time Kirsty's hands had been hovering in mid-air, a foot above her knees. They had already begun to start some slow jerky movements towards each other – evidence that her unconscious processes were already starting to integrate. I facilitated this by saying 'That's right ... those two parts really do want to join as one ... and you can watch ... with an increasing sense of curiosity and wonderment ... as your hands ... almost of their own volition ... get closer and closer ... both parts merging together ... as one whole identity ...' She shuddered as her hands embraced, and her eyes closed.

With the fusion complete, I wanted to ensure that the new changes were available to her in future contexts with her children. 'Now Kirsty ... just allow those hands to rise up to your chest ... and as they do so ... *imagine* this new aspect of yourself ... the product of this *joining* ... *integrating deeply inside you* ... so that as you look to your future, now, you can imagine what it's going to be like *dealing with your kids differently* ... with the ability to *decide with sensitivity* ... and the confidence to feel that ... *doing the things you want* ... *can really feel OK* ...'

This completed the process known in NLP as the *visual squash*. When done well it can often have a profound effect, with an increased sense of congruence and a freeing up of energies that allow the patient to move in a different direction. Although there were no cataclysmic changes for Kirsty, she became much more tolerant of her children's behaviour, and they in turn 'spontaneously' seemed to behave better. Her angry outbursts faded and she found that she actually had more time on her hands. She had a good look at where she was in life, decided to get a part-time job that fitted with school hours, lost weight and generally became a lot happier in herself.

Jeri's eating disorder

In her late twenties, Jeri admitted that for several years she had gorged herself with food in the late evenings, regularly making herself sick in the bathroom – in disgust – in order to maintain her weight at a reasonable level. She came to see me at a time when her gorging was 'completely out of control'. She felt as if she had 'gone through a trapdoor' and found herself surrounded by food debris, with the half-eaten contents of her entire fridge spread across the kitchen table. This suggested to me that when the gorging was triggered she entered into a profoundly altered dissociated state which took her over without her conscious awareness. Returning to her 'self' in the midst of the debris was acutely painful, bringing on the remorse that led to the 'cleansing' act of vomiting.

In NLP terms, Jeri was displaying a sequential incongruity, when two markedly separated 'parts', each with their own belief systems and values, vied for control. Although I planned to use the *visual squash* as before, there was one step that I needed to add prior to starting the process. According to NLP trainers John Overdurf and Julie Silverthorn, it was important to convert the sequential incongruity into a simultaneous one so that we could gain full access to each part in the here and now. Failure to do this would make it less likely that we could achieve the eventual degree of integration which we required.

First of all I asked Jeri to get in touch with the part of her that wanted her to eat normally, and which felt such pain and regret after each binge. Since this was a state to which she had ready access on a day-to-day basis – indeed it was the main state that she lived out of 90% of the time – it was quite easy to step her into a full visual, auditory and kinaesthetic representation and anchor it on a knuckle of her right hand.

To get to the more dissociated bingeing state, I induced a light to medium trance state and floated her back in time to just before the last binge. As she stepped into what she had described as her 'inner zombie', right at the trigger point, I deepened the state, focusing on the feelings of gorging, and anchored that to her left hand. Then I brought her back to the here and now, fully aware in present time. We conversed a little about the experience to reorient her, and then I pressed both anchors at the same time. She really went into a *very* altered state as her breathing rate increased and her face alternately flushed and went pale. She felt quite dizzy and nauseated as she was pulled back and forth between each state – she literally swayed from side to side. I kept the anchors pressed for about three minutes to ensure that the two states had mingled together.

Now that we had converted a sequential incongruity into a simultaneous one, the rest of the process was exactly the same as the standard *visual squash*. The basis of the conflict was 'self vs. other'. It seemed that on the one hand, bingeing was one of the few things Jeri did that was wholly for herself – one of the few ways in which she could feel entirely filled up and completely satisfied. On the other hand, the disgusted part that made her vomit in remorse was more concerned about what other people would think about the breaking of society's rules by being 'selfish'. However, following and respecting the 'rules' led to respect from others, and finally to self-respect and satisfaction – both parts had the same overall positive intention!

The recognition that these two warring factions actually wanted identical outcomes was a profound learning experience for Jeri. Thereafter the joining together and integration proceeded very smoothly, as the main bulk of the reframing had been accomplished and little further negotiation was required. As is often the case when two very separate aspects of a person come together, Jeri had both a new-found sense of inner congruence and 'bags of energy'. Three years on, she no longer binges, has completed a college course and runs her own beauty salon.

Visual squash: the process

This is the NLP process to use whenever someone is in 'two minds' about something, displaying simultaneous or sequential incongruence. The giveaway is often the word 'or' – said or implied. When you can either do *this* **or** do *that*, you create what linguists call an 'exclusive or' – a boundary condition separating two functional aspects of self. The *visual squash* collapses these boundaries, allowing the free flow and exchange of information within neural networks. It is a very versatile tool, and you can conceptualise virtually *every* presenting issue in medical practice in this way. You can think about it as a far more sophisticated version of the earlier collapsing anchors paradigm.

The steps necessary for the successful use of this format are described below.

Exercise 17:   The visual squash

1   *Identify a context* in which a particular conflict occurs. *Identify the parts* involved and separate them out spatially – one on the right-hand side and one on the left. It may help to give each part a name.
2   *Build a full visual, auditory and kinaesthetic representation* of the parts on each hand. Imagine them as two distinct sub-personalities with their own voices, use of language and idioms, dress sense, postures and gestures, emotions, etc., even down to how heavy or light they feel.
3   *Establish the positive intention* of each part by chunking up. Save the part that has the most negative kinaesthetics until second. Ask 'What does this part want ...? And if it got that, fully and completely, what would it get that was even more important?' Keep chunking up each answer until you get a high-level positive intention. This is often accompanied by a major physiological shift.
4   Draw attention to the fact that *both positive intentions are very similar*, if not identical. At this stage you may find that the *hands spontaneously start to come together*. Establish that both parts need each other in order to get their outcomes fulfilled. Let each part find a particular strength, resource or capability that the other has, and to which it would also like access. *Exchange the resources*, one to the other.
5   *Integrate the parts together*. Using subtle language, suggest that the hands are coming together and both parts are beginning to integrate. Let them merge into one, blending the visual images, sounds and feelings together to *form a single image complete with all of the joint resources*.
6   *Future pacing*. Bring the new image 'inside' in a way that feels most appropriate. Imagine going out into the future to a time when the old conflict would have occurred ... *and notice what is different now*. Take the time to fully experience this new way of being before coming back to the here and now.

A good way to practise using this tool is to think about an outcome that you do not yet have and a problem that might be a barrier to achieving it. Perhaps you want to develop a particular skill but do not feel that you have the time to devote to it. Conceptualise these as two conflicting 'parts', and perform the steps as described above. Better still, get a colleague to help you out with it, and do the same for him or her.

Many people who come to medical consultations want to 'get better'. You can develop a full visual, auditory and kinaesthetic representation of what that outcome would be like and place it on one hand. On the other hand you can then develop a representation of the patient's presenting pathology as the part of them that is currently preventing that outcome from taking place. Then simply negotiate! As you improve, you will be able to do this conversationally and more covertly, using *your* hands to demonstrate *their* parts. At the very least you will help them to think in a completely different way about their issue, and simultaneously to develop a much deeper sense of rapport with their conscious *and* unconscious minds.

There are certain things that you can do which will make the process go more smoothly and effectively.

1   Lean over and lift each hand up into the air so that it is hovering about a foot above the patient's knee. If you do this with an ambiguous touch, moving their hand and arm minutely to get into the 'right' position, you will create catalepsy in the limb. This is the condition of 'waxy flexibility' that occurs during hypnotic trance induction. It has a powerful amplifying effect on the whole process.

2   It is best to use representations of parts that look like the patient, rather than abstract shapes and colours. Occasionally the parts may look older or younger than their current age, or even like a relative (father, mother, etc.). However, always ensure that when you do the eventual parts integration that this results in a representation of their own self-image, preferably at their current age.

3   Always leave the part with the most negative kinaesthetic to the second 'chunking up'. This part usually starts off two or three levels lower than the other part. There is often a major physiological shift when its intention flips to a positive outcome – especially with the concurrent recognition that, almost unbelievably, both parts which were initially polar opposites actually want the same thing!

4   It is important to frame the subsequent negotiation as both parts only getting what they really want if they work together. Always be respectful of each part in the same way that you would treat another person. If they are still squabbling, it means you need either to chunk up higher to obtain agreement, or to remind them that failure to agree means neither will get what they want! You may have to be quite creative at this point.

5   Sometimes, however, it is best for the parts to 'stay apart', metaphorically speaking. You may need to negotiate a working agreement whereby they let each other have the time they need in sequence. For example, an 'insomniac part' and a 'sleepy part' may agree that neither interferes with the other at inappropriate times.

6   When a profound integration has occurred, you might want to take advantage of this by future pacing the sense of personal congruence engendered into many different contexts (at work, home, play, hobbies, etc.).

As you get more skilled at this intervention, you will find yourself adding in many different nuances from the various processes that we have already covered so far. For example, you may want to take the integrated part on a timeline journey into the past to clear up and realign previous issues connected to the original presenting problem. Cleaning up the past and aligning this to their new future gives a tremendous sense of internal harmony and congruence. This is also the time to use the swish pattern, utilising their new self-image as a cross-contextual resource.

Integrating on a timeline

NLP pioneer Robert Dilts used the steps of the *visual squash* to develop a *walking timelines* pattern for integration of conflicting parts. It is a very useful alternative to the process that you have just learned. I have found it more effective with those who are less visual and more kinaesthetic in their processing. Below is a demonstration of the process involving Emily and her enuresis.

Emily's enuresis

Emily, aged 14 years, had been enuretic for many years. Initially dry and out of nappies by the age of two, she had relapsed increasingly, and by five years of age was regularly wetting through the night. In the subsequent years she had been investigated for genito-urinary problems and found to be 'normal'. She had had treatment with tricyclic antidepressants (amitriptyline), behavioural interventions with a buzzer and bell, and was now on long-term treatment with nasal desmopressin. She had had intermittent but no long-term success with any of these treatments, and was now quite desperate – sleepovers and boy-friends loomed large as major issues.

I initially started off with the *visual squash*, but it was clear that we were getting nowhere fast! I asked Emily to stand up and imagine an external timeline in front of her, with her past to the left and her future to the right. We stepped backwards off the present moment into an observing meta-position. We knew that out in the future she wanted to be completely normal, yet her past problems were a heavy weight dragging her down!

I stepped her on to the present moment in her timeline, and looking to the future I asked her to walk out to a time when she imagined she was completely 'cured', with everything the way that she wanted it to be. She walked forward a few paces and stopped. With her eyes closed, I built up an intense state of what she would look like, sound like and feel like when she had what she wanted. I went into detail about how she would walk, talk, breathe and move, her increasing confidence levels, and just what she would be doing differently as a result of feeling that good. When I was certain she was in a powerfully positive state, I anchored it on her right shoulder. We stepped back to meta-position and looked at that 'future Emily' from the outside – she really liked what she saw.

Then, standing on the present moment, I asked her to face the future 'her' and know that up until now something had been holding her back, stopping her from getting what she wanted. Focusing on that feeling of heaviness and sadness, I gently took her backwards on her timeline into the past. I told her that she would know by the intensifying of that feeling that we had reached the time in her life when this problem had started. Her physiology changed completely. Her shoulders hunched, her face went pale and she thought she might cry. I asked her to step back *before all of that had happened* and then come off her timeline back to meta-position.

The various positions are shown in Figure 16.1.

At meta-position we surveyed the timeline and the parts at either end. The 'future Emily' had a sense of freedom and the vision to see what it was she wanted and the many choices that she had for herself. Turning to look back into the past, she had the sense that she had been a young, small three- or four-year-old being scolded about an accident. This 'younger Emily' wanted to feel safe, secure and protected. At first she did not appear to have any strengths or resources. I suggested that in fact this younger part must have a great deal of strength and fortitude, given that she had prevented change from occurring for so long. Perhaps it was time for both parts to combine their respective capabilities so that they could both get what they really needed.

Standing in the 'future Emily', I fired off the anchor and she turned to look at her younger counterpart. She experienced an overwhelming feeling of wanting to go back and look after her, protect her and care for her. Focusing on her resource of seeing clearly what she wanted, she walked back along the timeline and stepped into the 'younger Emily'. As the two spatial anchors began to collapse together, I asked her to focus on the younger part's inner strength and fortitude. As she did this, she turned and walked up the timeline again to the 'future Emily', so that a full exchange of resources between the two parts could take place.

Emily stepped back off the timeline into meta-position once again. Now that the resources had been exchanged, the two parts were ready to come together. I asked her to mentally guide them by the hand so that they approached and met each other in the present. Here they blended into one, and we were ready for the final part of the process. I asked Emily to step forward on to the timeline and into the newly integrated part, as if she were trying it on for size like some

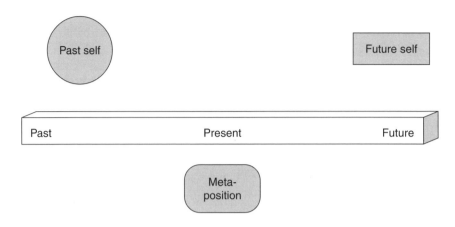

Figure 16.1:   Timeline integration.

new clothes that had been made especially for her – a perfect fit. Then she walked a few paces into her future, taking the sense of integration into the different contexts of her life.

Afterwards Emily was very surprised at how quickly her enuresis faded into the background, never to recur. That intervention took place seven years ago, and recently when I did her postnatal check after the birth of her baby girl, she reminded me of the event as I was gently enquiring about her genito-urinary function. One of the by-products of doing a successful in-depth NLP intervention in general practice is the development of an even deeper level of rapport and trust as time goes on – one of the benefits of practising medicine in the same place for many years.

How the visual squash works: connecting theory to practice

We can think about each of the 'parts' in this process as two different *state-dependent* entities. Each has its own neuronal networks which fire independently, with a neurological boundary condition keeping them separate. It is as if they are two *attractor basins,* kept stable by their own cognitive structures, with different beliefs and strategies pertaining whenever one part is 'in charge'. Broadly speaking, integration can be seen as an entrainment process – a relaxing and disappearance of the boundary condition allowing admixing of the networks to form a larger, more stable complex. This significantly alters the ensuing *attractor landscape.*

From a cognitive point of view there is a major restructuring of the limiting beliefs that have kept the problem intact. In a sense we have to reconfigure and restructure two sets of opposing beliefs. It is not that one is 'right' and the other is 'wrong', with the best prevailing. The *cognitive restructuring* actually encompasses both sets of beliefs, joining them together by finding the overarching belief (positive intention) that connects them. It is this cognitive binding that provides the basis for a stable realigning of strategies and behaviours that is akin to *skills training.* This is enhanced by the future pacing, which gives repetitive imaginal rehearsal of the new strategies in context – once again invoking the *self-efficacy* of future positive expectation.

In a more detailed sense, the restructuring and skills training occur at several levels simultaneously. We are literally creating a new self-image – not only in the visual modality but also within auditory and kinaesthetic modalities. The sequence of internal strategies (VAK) undergoes marked change, too. The external (and internal) triggers that were cues for the old behaviours now trigger a different sequence of modalities and submodalities, leading to new thoughts and behaviours in the previous context. Changes also occur at the motor level. With profound integration you may find that posture and movement undergo major shifts. Sometimes associated physical and biomechanical problems may disappear – yet more evidence that the mind–body connection not only exists but also should really be seen as a single functioning unit.

At a conditioning level, the two parts are actually powerful visual anchors for the contained states and strategies. The firing of each anchor is very similar to the activation of a *conditioned response,* albeit including internal cognitions as well as behaviours as triggers. Integration is the process of collapsing anchors together, akin to a *counter-conditioning* effect. However, it is vital to ensure that both adequate differentiation and cognitive restructuring occur *before* attempting to integrate the two parts. Failure to do so may lead to episodic confusion, resulting in the expression of simultaneous incongruence rather than resolution.

Concluding

Having read thus far, perhaps you are in two minds yourself about what to do next. Maybe part of you would really like to go ahead and put all of this into action straight away. You may even be conjuring up a detailed vision of what it would be like if you were already successfully utilising this in practice. Possibly you have identified several patients who would fit the bill. And of course, you are right to think that, like many other people, you can learn to utilise this approach to the benefit of both your patients and yourself. When you effectively apply this kind of process you derive an immense feeling of satisfaction with the results. It is the kind of feeling that may remind you of exactly why you came into medicine in the first place – and you will have your own particular way of describing that!

Yet you may feel strangely at odds with yourself – that niggling feeling inside that lets you know there may be an objection which prevents you from moving forward. Will you or won't you? On the one hand you'd like to ... yet on the other ...

Something may be feeling left behind. That niggling voice of uncertainty that tells you about all the pitfalls – lack of time, no training, and what if you made a mistake and it didn't go right? Of course, everyone needs a safety net when they are learning and doing something new for the first time. Building a stable sense of security in this way leads to the freedom to learn from every result you get – and the very important feedback of knowing whether that is taking you towards or away from your planned outcome.

So when you really think about it in this way, it becomes quite clear that anything less than the total security and freedom which lead to the kind of immense satisfaction that reminds you of just why you are in this job won't get you the results that both you and your patients deserve! Think about that now ... deeply.

As you reflect on it for a few moments, you may get a sense of the dust settling, the internal noise quietening down and the emergence of a future vision – perhaps a little hazy to start with – of a 'you' who is comfortable about using some or all of the steps in the *visual squash* ... singly or in combination ... with a wide variety of patients and clinical circumstances ... and perhaps even in areas, contexts and conditions that you had not previously contemplated ... paying attention to the feedback that is there all around ... incorporating everything as you are left to head in the right direction ... and just how good that really feels!

Possibility

CHAPTER 17

Clinical concerns

Introduction

In this chapter we shall look at specific medical problems – depression, anxiety, habit disorders, pain control and cancer – from an NLP perspective. Rather than focusing on a particular technique or format, I shall give a broad range of approaches based on applying everything that you have learned in this book so far. Although this will not be an exhaustive examination of these conditions (that would take a book apiece), you will get the opportunity to develop a raft of potential interventions for each clinical issue.

Up until now, NLP has generally eschewed diagnostic labels and categories. It treats everyone as a unique individual and is more concerned with *how* this particular person's thinking and behaviour contribute to their current problem. Diagnostic labels, it is argued, merely describe a cluster of symptoms – they do not tell you what to *do* differently. However, the *structure* of the subjective experience gives many clues for possible interventions.

Diagnostic labels are a double-edged sword. On the one hand, it can be extremely anxiety relieving for a patient with several different symptoms, who is worried about the potential causes, to know that they have a condition which has a name, that other people have had it and that treatments are available. On the other hand, the labels, once attached, are difficult to remove. They can rapidly become an identity-level statement – 'I am a ... (fill in the blank)' – that pervades and organises the foreseeable future and insidiously keeps them stuck.

Personally I think diagnostic labels are helpful. Well, I would, wouldn't I? I'm a doctor! Yet it is important to bear in mind that these labels are nominal-isations. They are process words dressed up as static nouns. It is necessary to de-nominalise the labels from time to time, and to turn the potential stuck state back into a process from which movement can occur. The meta-model can help enormously here (*see* Appendix 3). This de-nominalising gets us back to the inner workings of mind and body that can be addressed by NLP techniques.

In the rest of this chapter we shall examine the approaches and various techniques that you can use with each of the clinical conditions that have been selected.

Depression

Depression is a condition that we see daily in clinical practice in a variety of different guises. One or two people out of every five who are seen in general practice consultations are suffering from this disorder. The rapid worldwide rise in this diagnosis in the last decade or so is surely a potent indicator that it is attempting to cope with the increasingly frenetic pace of life in an instantaneous information age – rather than 'genetics' – which is the major cause. Both cognitive–behavioural therapy (CBT) and NLP approach depression as a skills-based deficit. They argue that the lack of specific thinking skills in particular makes people more prone to the problem. Teaching a cognitive package of relevant skills will both resolve the current issue and prevent future occurrences.

The good news about intervening at the level of thinking skills rather than simply relying on medication is that the relapse rates are significantly different. With medication alone, 50% of cases may relapse within two years. With CBT-type approaches this figure may be reduced to 20 to 25%. Utilising a teaching skills perspective like this can give lifelong immunity from a common problem.

Scene setting

There are particular kinds of thinking styles that make patients more prone to depression. Knowing what these are can give us many choice points for interventions.

Depression is a past-oriented problem. Patients ruminate over previous hurts, grievances and problems, often rehashing old events over and over again. This takes them out of the present moment and prevents them from thinking about the future. Both the present and the future, if they are seen at all, are coloured by this past perspective casting its dark shadow. One of the first steps, then, is to help them create a future that they want to move into.

People who are depressed are often motivated to identify problems to avoid. The difficulty with this kind of thinking is that if you only consider what you do not want to have, you are unlikely to move towards solutions. Focusing on problems tends to magnify them and make them seem unsolvable. Then they seem so insurmountable that 'it's not worth the effort of trying'. What patients need instead is an outcome orientation – something to move towards.

Depression involves global thinking. *Everything* is chunked up. Small problems become disasters. Issues get so big and overwhelming that change seems impossible. If people who are depressed fail at a particular task (behaviour), they chunk up so that 'I am a failure' (identity). It is important to use the meta-model to chunk down into the specifics of which one small aspect of the issue can be dealt with here and now.

When it comes to association and dissociation, depressed people have a tendency to associate with negatively charged past memories and to dissociate from happy occasions. Traumatic memories are easily relived, often with full bodily emotions involved, too. Good memories tend to be mostly out of sight – unreachable. The pervading negative state is unhealthy – depressing the immune system even more, and thereby increasing the likelihood of other illnesses, too. State-changing techniques are therefore paramount for effective treatment.

Depressed thinking often has an external locus of control – the person is the victim of uncontrollable outside factors. They are tossed and turned by the winds of fate. At times everyone and everything can appear to be against them. They minimise their own ability to take action, believing that they do not have the skills necessary to make a difference. Treatment involves strengthening their inner locus of control, and giving a sense of increasing personal mastery.

People who are rules dominated (should, have to, ought to, must, etc.) are more prone to depression. When you examine their 'rules' with the meta-model, you usually find that the rules really belong to someone else (parents, authority figures, church, society at large, etc.). They may try to live up to other people's expectations and get stuck in the rut of routine. They need help in formulating expectations for themselves that they want to live up to – and a procedure for generating these options.

Lastly, they may remain 'inside' their heads, talking to themselves in a never-ending stream of words that generate even more negative feelings in a recursive loop. They may say things about themselves in the kind of derogatory tone that they would never use with another human being. This usually goes on below the level of conscious awareness – all they notice is that they feel bad most of the time. It is important to break this strategy and replace it with more effective self-talk. This is a fundamental task in both CBT and NLP.

The sum total of all of this leads to the pervasive, deadly triad of feeling hopeless, helpless and worthless. Hopeless, because the depressed person cannot envision a future that is sufficiently different from the past to encourage them to move towards it. Helpless, because although other people may be able to create the kind of choices that lead to getting well again, the depressed person believes that they do not have the necessary skills – they are not capable. Worthless, because even if all of the above were possible for them, they believe that they simply do not deserve it – self-esteem is at rock bottom.

Next we shall consider the kinds of NLP interventions that you already know how to use.

Intervening

From a treatment perspective, one of the most important things you can do at the outset is to build a climate of positive expectation that the future can be different – this is vital. As an overall strategy within which to embed the various techniques, building a new future and seeding resources into every significant context is paramount. Patients with depression are already preoccupied with the past, and to continue to share and explore the details of that past is to court disaster. This is not to say that revisiting the past to deal with some critical incident is not necessary. However, if you do so, you must attend strictly to the *process* of the intervention, not the storyline content.

In the very first encounter you must use the *well-formed outcome* questions to delineate what they want instead. I keep on asking 'How do you want *your* future to be different?' until the patient has a detailed answer. Settling for 'happy' keeps your thinking at the same global chunk size as theirs – not a recipe for success. The *miracle question* is an excellent tool for conversationally chunking down on the specific details in a variety of contexts. Because of its versatility, it can be used to great effect in a short consultation. Even in this scenario, patients are good at keeping up their move away from strategy, telling you what they do not want in the future. It is really important that you keep obtaining counter-examples until they tell you what they want in positive terms. Begin any subsequent sessions with the questions 'What's gone well since your last consultation? What have you been doing differently?' Focus on the changes, no matter how small they may be.

Building *resources* is a vital part of getting well again for depressed patients. Thinking about dealing differently with future situations will uncover some potential impasses where particular skills are needed. It is always interesting how patients have many of the resources that they need locked up in other areas of life. With a little *reframing* if necessary, you can unearth some useful states. Then, using the powerful anchoring processes such as the *circle of excellence*, you can intensely revivify them and place them where they are needed. Pay attention to the VAK triggers in the future context, and time your anchors so that the new state is triggered instead.

I find it very useful to give patients a list of practical resource states which they can identify in their own time and practise accessing and anchoring themselves. This gives them an increased sense of control and mastery – they are doing something different that feels good. One strategy you can utilise before doing any other intervention is to elicit and use a stacked anchor for multiple states (five or 10 or more), including problem-solving skills. Once these have integrated together it will give a very different perspective on the patient's ability to deal with their difficulties.

However, they may need to be taught to associate and dissociate more effectively first. Some patients cannot seem to access good feeling states because negative feelings get in the way. If you elicit the *submodality* structure of these experiences – especially visual ones – then you can teach them how to reduce the intensity by distancing the image, making it black and white, and turning down the volume of any sounds. Then pace them by asking about 'those memories that should feel good but you can't seem to hold on to them'. They are often wispy and ephemeral at first, yet can be made bigger, brighter, more colourful, closer, etc. prior to stepping inside the image and trying it on for size. This strategy works just as well even if they pretend to do it without 'really' seeing the image.

The same kind of strategy can work with the *auditory submodalities* of critical internal voices. The volume can be adjusted downward and moved to a different location. Hearing the same harsh words being repeated in the tonality of a favourite cartoon character (Donald Duck, Sylvester the cat, Mickey Mouse, etc.) can take much of the sting out of them. Although this is not a major intervention in its own right, it can generate a useful state change – laughter!

Even though I suggested a future focus, there may be critical past incidents that need to be addressed. If these are traumatic in nature, the *phobia/trauma cure* is the best choice. If it is used on a few memories it will probably generalise into the rest of the past events. If there are significant other people involved in the past events, then *reimprinting* is the intervention of choice – provided that there are no overwhelmingly negative kinaesthetics. I have found this intervention particularly useful for self-esteem issues.

CBT models focus on identifying and writing down in a diary troubling automatic negative thoughts, together with the positive things that the patient could think about instead. This is a very useful externalising dissociative strategy. I have used the following version to combine NLP techniques as a homework task.

I ask the patient to write about any past event that is a problem for them in third-person language (he, she, it, they, etc.). They can write their own name, but not 'I'. They write as they simultaneously picture a black-and-white distanced video of the event in their past. With the event completed, they write down what they have learned from it and how they want things to be different in the future. As they do so, they picture a colourful movie of performing the new behaviours – still from a dissociated perspective. When they are satisfied with their new script, they try it on for size. This installs a very useful strategy. Each part of this strategy can be given to them as a piece of homework, one step at a time.

In depressed younger women in particular, I have often found a parts conflict based around self and other. Commonly work and family responsibilities and commitments may clash. Sometimes being a mother with several young children leaves little time for self. The *parts integration* model can work well here. Occasionally other relationships are involved, and the *meta-mirror* is usually a good choice. Another well-validated system for successfully treating depression, namely *interpersonal therapy*, is based on examining and updating critical relationships. The meta-mirror fits hand in glove with these precepts.

It is important to distinguish depression that is associated with prolonged bereavement reactions. The *grief resolution process* is very useful here. This can be combined with the phobia cure for particularly traumatic or gruesome experiences. Remember that 'loss' is not necessarily about the death of a loved one. Depression can also arise from loss of a job or a highly valued object.

Altering the depressed person's physiology is an important element. The psychomotor retardation that occurs in depression can take time to lift. However, aerobic exercise of one kind or another is a very quick state changer, and has proven beneficial effects in alleviating depression. Choose an activity that suits the individual. I have had patients do anything from brisk walking to disco dancing, as well as jogging, cycling, martial arts, etc.

Anxiety

Anxiety presents in medical practice in myriad ways, and may account for up to 30% of all consultations. Women tend to be affected twice as frequently as men. Any impending unpredictable life event, from sitting a driving test to having an operation, or from getting married to going through a divorce, can precipitate it. The increasing stresses of jobs that involve dealing with difficult people and situations, giving public presentations, etc., can make many individuals fearful and apprehensive. Quite commonly anxiety is a comorbid condition combined with depression and obsessive-compulsive disorder. In its more severe forms it may be triggered by phobias or post-traumatic stress, or it may even arise seemingly *de novo* as a panic attack. Other conditions such as excess alcohol consumption, drug abuse and eating disorders may develop as an attempt to cope with the underlying symptoms of anxiety.

Both CBT and NLP approach anxiety from the perspective of correcting the disturbed thinking and imagery that trigger and magnify the somatic responses of sympathetic nervous system overactivity (tachycardia, hyperventilation, paraesthesia, tension headache, gastrointestinal disturbance, etc). Behavioural approaches tackle the avoidant behaviour directly, preventing its occurrence.

Depending on the precipitating condition and comorbidity, interventional success rates range from 50 to 90%.

Scene setting

Whereas depression is a past-oriented problem, anxiety tends to be future oriented. The past and the present are literally forgotten as the patient focuses on unwanted potential future outcomes that they want to move away from. These unwanted outcomes are often pictured in vivid detail and loom large – so large that thinking other more realistic thoughts becomes impossible. In a way, patients with anxiety detach themselves from their past resourceful experiences in other areas of life and are unable to bring them to bear on this current context.

Moving away from negatively evaluated outcomes in this way causes much of the avoidant behaviour that typifies anxiety disorders. Every time a particular anxiety-provoking event is avoided, it not only installs further future avoidance but also classically conditions the negative feelings to occur sooner and more powerfully next time. These feelings, which are sometimes overwhelming in intensity, may generalise to other previously unrelated situations so that before long 'everything' may make the patient anxious. It is likely that conditions such as agoraphobia may develop in this way.

Anxiety sufferers are good associaters. Not only do they make big, bright, colourful pictures of potentially catastrophic events, but also they step inside them and experience the event as if it is happening now. If you imagined doing this now with one of your greatest fears, what would that feel like? You will quickly appreciate how many of the somatic responses (e.g. increased heart rate, dry mouth, trembling) are generated. The ability to dissociate effectively is a key skill that is worth learning.

Triggers for anxiety are usually synaesthesias. The more usual kind is a V/K synaesthesia where making a huge internal picture (e.g. of a spider, mouse, etc.) cues the unwanted response. For example, in A/K synaesthesias, imagining the sound of derisive voices following the humiliation of a failed task is enough to generate a fearful response. K/K synaesthesias involve imagining a feeling (e.g. being touched sexually in a particular way), having an aversive response, and becoming anxious about the consequences. Internal self-talk (AD) can also be used in a ruminant style to go over and over both the impending event and its consequences in a way that increases the anxious feelings. Often the internal voice is speaking faster and faster, at a higher and higher pitch, both driving and being reflexively driven by the somatic responses. This can easily bring on a panic attack.

As in depression, anxiety sufferers often have an external locus of control – events happen *to* them. They are usually unaware that although their feelings are unwanted, they are to a large degree creating them by their internal pictures, sounds and voices, which are often generated largely out of conscious awareness. They may identify a particular environment or context as the cause of their problem, not the thoughts and feelings that they have about that context. Successful treatment involves reattributing a sense of inner control.

Whether a person has generalised anxiety or a more specific disorder such as a phobia, the self-generated attempted solutions usually revolve around controlling the situation by avoiding it. Many patients can severely constrain their lifestyles in an attempt never to face their fears. The goal of NLP and CBT is to effect significant changes in thinking, feeling and behaviour, to enable them to be comfortable in doing what they previously thought was impossible.

Intervening

There are numerous ways of using NLP in the treatment of anxiety disorders. As usual, the first step is to set a *well-formed outcome*. Just how specifically does this patient want to be different in that context? What exactly will they be doing instead? In mild anxiety that is unicontextual, a detailed outcome elicited via the *miracle question* may be all that is required. Once they can see themselves successfully coping in the situation with specific behavioural responses that they can own for themselves, then the problem may already be resolved. However, a more detailed intervention incorporating one or more techniques is usually required.

Given that anxiety often prevents the accessing of valuable historical resources, a useful manoeuvre is to elicit these ahead of time and amplify them by anchoring techniques such as *kinaesthetic anchors* and the *circle of excellence*. Various resources can be stacked together and, through imaginal rehearsal, linked to the specific context. It is important to identify the earliest external trigger in the situation – usually something seen or heard – and to use this to cue the anchored state. Of course, the anchors can also be fired off in real time when encountering the problem context. This is best for non-phobic situations, and is less useful for generalised free-floating anxiety.

Collapsing anchors kinaesthetically is a variant of the above for use in specific, contextualised examples of anxiety, such as performance anxiety. In this scenario the negative feelings are accessed and anchored on the knuckle of one hand. Several resources are stacked on the knuckle of the other hand, ensuring that the positive kinaesthetics outweigh the negative ones prior to collapsing both together. I have used this successfully for patients with examination nerves, imminent driving tests and dental anxiety – and even with some minor phobias.

Chaining anchors is a way of installing a new strategy which takes a patient from feeling fearful and stuck through states such as frustration, impatience, curiosity, desire and 'going for it'. Although it is used for anxiety in specific situations, it can also be useful for free-floating anxiety, as it chains a common set of underlying feelings together to an outcome state which is valuable in many different contexts. It is important to use a 'moving away from' state such as impatience or frustration as the first link. This sets up the momentum for the rest of the chain. Rather than chaining directly to relaxation – a physiologically less energetic state – it is often more helpful to use higher-energy positive states to draw them through to the end point.

We can also install new strategies using *submodalities*. The anxiety-provoking pictures are often looming large and close, and are usually associated. Stepping out of the picture (dissociating) and draining all of the colour to a black-and-white still-frame photograph in the distance can markedly reduce the negative feelings. The new information that is gleaned from this perspective helps to formulate decisions about what to do next. This different outcome can be mentally rehearsed until it feels just right. Then it can be brought closer and made larger and brighter before the patient finally steps inside and 'owns' it. Rehearsing this new strategy in different anxiety-provoking contexts can allow the changes to generalise more rapidly. In simple cases the *swish* pattern can be quickly effective.

We can also use the *auditory submodalities* to provoke change. Often anxiety is maintained by the constant ruminating self-talk that occurs in the background of awareness. Localising the voice and identifying the words, tempo and tonality that are driving the anxious feelings is the first step. You can then alter the submodalities of location and tonality to effect change. Saying the same words in cartoon-character voices often provokes much laughter – a potent stimulus for counter-conditioning the negative feelings.

One important resource is that of the *counter-example process* – when is the patient not anxious? Finding a specific context when they should have been anxious and were not, or another situation where they never feel anxious at all, is very useful. You can elicit the structure of this experience both in terms of its submodalities and also by anchoring the states that the patient was experiencing instead. These can then be used as the new template on which the previously anxiety-provoking context can be superimposed.

The *phobia cure* can be used in patients with anxiety, but you must be careful about when to do this. It does *not* work for anticipatory anxiety *about* a forthcoming event. It is best reserved for severe instances of panic and phobic responses which have happened in the past. You must identify a specific past event that triggers today's symptoms. This method is most useful for single-issue phobias for which the patient can clearly recall a precipitating event. The arousal symptoms that are generated by PTSD flashbacks can often be readily ameliorated.

Anxiety and its symptoms can also be reframed. However, in my experience simply relabelling anxious feelings as 'excitement' about future choices rarely works. Much better in this regard is *six-step reframing*. Here the anxious feelings are initially redefined as a 'part of you' that wants something very important, such as safety, security and protection. Up until now this part has only had a very narrow set of choices, which have led to the production of various physiological symptoms. This step-by-step process allows the unconscious identification of new behaviours that fulfil the original positive intention, together with agreement for future utilisation. The *visual squash* method is a more refined way of doing this, by integrating the part that wants your future to be different and the part that is preventing this from happening.

Timeline interventions can be used in a variety of different ways, either in visual imagination or by walking on externalised timelines. For specific, unicontextual anxiety-provoking events, going out into the future *beyond* the successful completion of the event and looking back on it may be all that is required. Taking adult resources back along the timeline to a much younger 'you', prior to growing up with them in place, may realign past events in a positive way. The process of *reimprinting* can help to deal with traumatic past events where significant other people were involved in anxiety-provoking situations – the child may have introjected the adult's reactions. In these cases re-resourcing the other people who were involved may change the negative imprint and clear the anxiety from the timeline.

From a purely behavioural viewpoint, the symptoms of anxiety can be seen as those of over-arousal and preparation for action. Therefore actually engaging in action, such as mild to moderate aerobic exercise, dancing to favourite music, gardening, etc., can provide a useful diversion and distraction that lessen the symptoms. Paradoxical strategies, such as 'prescribing the symptom' (encouraging the patient to produce anxious behaviours on demand), can give conscious control to what were apparently unconscious phenomena. Although superficially this may seem nonsensical, at a deeper process level it is an excellent strategy for change.

Habit disorders

A habit disorder is a recurrent, repetitive behaviour over which a patient appears to have no long-term control. Smoking, alcohol abuse, overeating and drug addictions of one kind or another are all common problems in general medical practice. Many people can abstain from engaging in the behaviour for a short period of time. However, as the urge to engage increases, it seems to reach a point where the past and the future recede into the distance and having the 'fix' *now* becomes the dominant thought – one that is usually given into with relief all round!

Addictions and habit disorders are *present*-oriented problems. As the 'now' moment looms large, the future negative consequences of the current action are well beyond rational, contemplative consideration. By the same token, past problems caused by continued engagement in the habit are forgotten. Along with this is the apparent walling off of access to past resources that might have helped them to deal with the problem in the here and now. The main aims of CBT and NLP interventions in habit and addictive disorders are to correct the disordered thinking patterns that accompany the urge to indulge in the habit, to gain a wider perspective that includes marshalling past resources and forestalling future consequences, and to reassociate the trigger cues to result in different behaviours.

Scene setting

There are many ways in which habits and addictive behaviours can be acquired and maintained. It is useful to consider them from the perspective of the various models of learning, namely classical and operant conditioning, modelling and cognitive factors. This will give some insights into potential points of intervention.

Classical conditioning suggests that behaviours are acquired through associative learning. Taking a few deep puffs of a cigarette invokes diaphragmatic breathing, which in turn induces the relaxation response mediated by the parasympathetic nervous system. This naturally occurring physiological process becomes paired with the act of having a cigarette, and before long the conditioned response fires off automatically.

The conditioning cue can become paired with both external and internal factors. External factors may include the sight of a particular cigarette brand name, being with a certain group of friends, or seeing someone else smoke. Internal cues are usually mood derived – such as feeling tense or anxious – as well as being associated with particular mental imagery. This is of particular significance in eating disorders, where mood changes may trigger binge eating. Things can become even more complicated when the withdrawal symptoms that arise from abstinence can themselves become the triggering cue for the next binge (or cigarette). The addictive behaviour provides relief from its own withdrawal symptoms!

Operant conditioning requires that a particular behaviour is reinforced by the consequences of that behaviour. Positive reinforcement in smoking may come externally from social acceptance by a peer group, or internally from a sense of increased confidence or even the ability – once relaxed – to think through the solutions to problems more easily. And what about the post-sexual intercourse cigarette? The main negative reinforcer for many habits is the removal of withdrawal symptoms and states, such as anxiety and tension, that are caused by indulging in the behaviour.

Many addictive behaviours may be learned by *modelling* significant others – Bandura's social learning theory. The classic, of course, is smoking that is modelled on one's parents or peer group. The social influence of various media stars on children and adolescents can instil the belief that 'thin equals beautiful', with damaging consequences with regard to eating disorders in females. Of course, the risk taking associated with designer and lifestyle drugs can also be a potent attractor.

Cognitive factors include the mental imagery and self-talk that lead to addictive behaviours. Self-image in particular may be important in the case of smoking and use of drugs such as cocaine. A poor self-image may be bolstered by risk-taking behaviours. Others with poor cognitive-based coping and problem-solving skills may find solace in drugs such as alcohol. In the early stages, addictive behaviours may provide relief from difficult situations. In the later stages, the addictive behaviour itself exacerbates the original problem in a vicious circle.

From all of the above you will see that there are many sites of potential intervention.

Intervening

As usual, the place to start is with a *well-formed outcome* – sometimes easier said than done for habits and addictions. Most people want to simply 'stop using', and the more addictive the habit the less likely it is that they can come up with alternative outcomes. It may be hard to picture life after stopping. It is important to tease out the current benefits of the habit and chunk them up to the values that drive the behaviour. From there other choices may become apparent. In habitual smokers you must build up images of what they would look like if their lungs were healthier, how they could do routine tasks without getting breathless, and how they would smell and even taste different!

Building up and bringing *resources* from other contexts to the present moment is vital. In particular, ask about times when the patient was determined to do something and did it, times when they thought they might fail yet they succeeded, times when they said 'enough is enough' in other contexts and followed through with action, and any other resources that you deem to be useful, depending on individual circumstances. Anchoring formats such as the *circle of excellence* can build these up robustly so that they are ready for application to the internal and external triggers.

Aversion therapies have been popular in the past, but have obtained mixed results. Aversion anchors can be built in a number of ways. You can get your patient to think of something that personally disgusts them and magnify it markedly before anchoring it. For one patient, seeing himself in a coffin with his young children crying and asking why he had smoked himself to death was a very powerful aversive experience. For others, vomitus, faeces and even things that frighten them can be used. The aversion anchor should be attached to the trigger that cues the addictive behaviour or habit. Even more importantly – and in contrast to the more usual aversion therapies – once it has been triggered the aversion anchor should be *chained* to very positive resources that lead the patient towards achieving their well-formed outcome.

Submodality patterns such as the *swish* may have their uses as part of a total package of intervention. The dissociated outcome picture must be highly attractive, almost compelling in intensity, so that it draws the patient magnetically towards it. I have used this pattern with some success in smokers, although it is very important to get all of the triggering cues for each smoking context. Personally I find the other anchoring formats more effective. However, submodality changes can be very useful in the information-gathering phase to conversationally interrupt habitual patterns and loosen recurring strategies prior to other interventions.

The *six-step reframe* is a very useful strategy, especially with smokers and individuals with other habits that do not have an overwhelming addictive compulsion fuelling their behaviour. Identifying the positive intention behind the habit allows the substitution of other behaviours that meet the same overall goal. This method can also be used in patients with eating disorders of mild to moderate intensity, including bulimia, although I have found it less useful in anorexia. In binge overeating with or without bulimia, using the six-step reframe in conjunction with hypnotic trance seems to increase the potential for positive results, especially if the behavioural outcomes are kept at a non-conscious level, thus preventing 'sabotage'.

More severe forms of addiction and also habits that fail to respond to the above interventions usually suggest a sequential incongruence – two parts in conflict, with each surfacing at different times. A *parts integration process*, such as the *visual squash* done on or off the timeline, is almost certainly required. The 'addictive part' is usually quite dissociated from the rest of the patient's neurology, and 'takes over' after a mini-trance interlude. Patients often describe this as 'like going through a trapdoor'. It is usually important to have 'both parts together in the same room', so to speak. Doing a collapsing anchors process first will ensure that the subsequent visual squash goes more smoothly.

Timeline interventions – both visual and kinaesthetic – have a large part to play in more complex or resistant habits and addictions. *Reimprinting* processes can be useful for changing both the representation of and the prevailing beliefs surrounding the first time the patient ever engaged in the habit. Re-resourcing the 'younger self' allows a domino effect to spread throughout the rest of the past, present and future. Sometimes it is necessary to go back to the point of decision to engage in the habit, which may have happened well before the actual physical smoking of a cigarette, etc. Patients may have modelled significant other people (family members, friends, television 'heroes', etc.), deciding well in advance – usually at the unconscious level – to follow in their footsteps.

A habit or addiction can also be seen as a codependent relationship with an object (cigarette, etc.) or drug (nicotine, etc.), and even lifestyle (risk taking). This can be investigated and teased out even more by means of the *meta-mirror*. Many smokers project qualities such as self-confidence, manliness and control on to a cigarette. Having them identify with the cigarette by imagining stepping inside it – yes, a weird experience! – can help them to reclaim their projections and utilise them in a more positive, healthy way.

We cannot leave habits and addictions without talking about *recovery strategies*. In the real world the potential for relapse is high. Often the first slip-up leads to a wholesale relapse and complete reinstitution of the problem. This is a product of 'all-or-nothing' thinking – having one cigarette means that I'm a smoker again, one chocolate biscuit and I'm bingeing again. It is very useful to assume that a patient may be tempted and succumb in the future, and to plan for this possible eventuality. High-risk situations and the cues that trigger reusing can be identified beforehand. You can then rehearse various alternative coping skills and strategies and install them on the future timeline.

You can also take the patient out on their future timeline and get them to imagine slipping up and 'using' again. Having done this they can code it as a minor slip or lapse rather than a relapse, and see themselves subsequently getting immediately back 'on the programme', abstinent again. Occasionally I actually install a planned lapse: 'See yourself following a healthy eating plan for six days, have a day of 'pigging out', then another six days of healthy eating, etc.'. This seemingly paradoxical intervention may actually decrease the risk of relapse occurring by openly embracing and accepting its possibility. Of course, if you are dealing with a polarity responder (someone who does the *opposite* of what people say) you can tell them that they will most definitely 'use' again!

No matter which of the above processes you use, the fundamental approach to treating a habit or addiction is first to identify the specific context in which it occurs, and then to find the earliest triggering cue (internal or external) on which to attach a different state and resulting behaviour. If you keep this firmly in mind, you will increase your patient's chances of successfully overcoming their habit.

Pain control

Early models of pain focused on the physical factors that generate the sensation of pain, such as the chemical and nerve impulse changes which occur in localised tissue trauma. They suggested that psychological changes occurred as a result of pain, and not as a causal factor. According to this model, pain could be either organic or psychogenic – all in the body or all in the mind. However, wartime experiences with widely differing requirements for analgesia for similar types of injuries suggested that there is some degree of psychological mediation.

The gate control theory introduced the concept of pain as a perception, in much the same way that vision and audition are constructed representations rather than a faithful and unchanged reproduction of what is seen and heard. This theory suggested an interaction between physical, emotional and behavioural factors which could increase or decrease pain perception according to current mood, level of activity and medication. This led to the discovery that cognitive strategies and degree of self-efficacy (locus of control) were of prime importance in managing and reducing chronic pain. CBT and NLP interventions focus on changing the thoughts, beliefs, attitudes and behaviours that maintain unhelpful pain perceptions.

Scene setting

All of the major learning processes can be involved to one degree or another in pain perception. *Classical conditioning* allows any painful stimulus to be paired with an internal or external cue. If a child has a painful procedure performed in the health centre, they may link the discomfort to the doctor or nurse, the room in which the procedure occurred and their thoughts of going back there again. This can be easily generalised to all medical and nursing staff in other locations, such as hospitals. In chronic pain the typical postures, gestures and movements that accompany the painful feelings can become conditioned triggers which maintain the discomfort.

Operant conditioning also plays a part in pain perception. Pain generates certain behaviours, such as wincing, particular vocal expressions, postural changes (e.g. limping) and increased rest activity. This type of pain behaviour may be positively reinforced by the soothing sympathy and attention of loved ones, time off work, and even financial incentives such as benefit and insurance payments. This is sometimes called the secondary gain of the sick role. Pain can be negatively reinforced by intermittent painkillers that are given on demand, as the relief gained may reinforce more pill taking. This is more likely to occur in chronic than in acute pain. A potential solution that can be used to break this reinforcement is to give painkillers at fixed intervals and then gradually reduce the dosage.

A patient's emotional state influences how they perceive pain. Chronic unrelieved pain typically causes anxiety, which in itself further increases pain. States such as depression also magnify pain, which in a self-reinforcing loop makes the depression worse. The availability of a mechanism that gives patients access to positive states, such as relaxation, pleasure, etc., is a fundamental component in managing chronic pain.

The *cognitive* aspects of pain – our thoughts and beliefs about and attitudes to our experience – can have a major effect on how we cope with it. If you are a soldier wounded in wartime, your injury may allow you to escape from a dangerous situation. The meaning that you attribute to pain in these circumstances may actually reduce your perception of it markedly.

However, if you feel that you have no control over chronic pain, and have future expectations of it continuing unabated, this can exacerbate your discomfort in the present moment. Your previous experiences with episodes of pain, the level of discomfort and how you coped at the time, also act as a template through which today's discomfort is measured. Your internal imagery of past, present and future experiences – pictures, sounds, words and feelings – can both magnify pain out of all proportion *and* help to reduce it to a manageable level.

Different cultures have different beliefs about the meaning of pain and how to express it. Some reward stoicism, while others expect a display of almost hysterical proportions. What we believe about pain and how we cope with it can depend on what we were taught, mainly unconsciously, by the significant people in our lives as we were growing up. Personal and family belief systems provide a strong filter – often out of conscious awareness – for our perceptions of pain. Unearthing and modifying these belief systems appropriately can cause significant changes.

Both CBT and NLP offer approaches and specific techniques that focus specifically on adjusting, changing and amending perceptions of pain. This can vary from teaching a patient how to change their state to one of relaxation, to working directly on pain imagery itself, changing unhelpful beliefs and coaching the patient in various coping skills, such as distraction and differential attention. Alongside appropriate medication, these psychological strategies have proven efficacy in pain reduction.

Intervening

It is often very useful to begin with a detailed description of the pain itself, which may at first appear counter-intuitive. However, going into the details in this way involves both association and dissociation, as the patient initially feels the discomfort and then reports on it as an observer. By mapping out the finer points of the kinaesthetic submodalities (*see* Appendix 2 for details) the patient recognises that pain is actually composed of many distinct sensations, some of which are more amenable to change than others. In effect a large and amorphous generalisation ('I'm in pain') is subdivided into many discrete compartments. Very often this detailed observation can produce substantial pain reduction in itself.

Having identified the kinaesthetic submodalities, you can encourage the patient to experiment with them. Shrinking down the size and extent of the 'pain map' or paradoxically even increasing it to encompass the whole body can change the experience significantly for the better. Even if the discomfort initially increases, this can be taken as a signal that the patient has established a degree of self-control, the trick then being to find the changes that lead in the direction of lessening discomfort.

You can map across the kinaesthetic submodalities to visual and auditory representations. 'If your pain had a colour or sound, what would that be like?' You can then experiment with changing the visual and auditory submodalities and notice what effect this has. You can do this gradually and in small increments – for example, by slight changes in hue or sound volume, or even small shifts in location. Another useful question to ask is 'What colour (shape and size) or sound (volume and rhythm) would your pain have once it was gone?' From this information you can design a *swish pattern* to lead gently from one state to the other.

Certain contextual cues in both the external and internal world can trigger discomfort. Once you have identified these (e.g. places, times, people, sounds, words, external visual cues, internal imagery, etc.), you can attach different states to the trigger. You can *build and amplify resources* such as relaxation, pleasure, comfort, joy, etc., anchoring them to a knuckle. Then, in imaginary rehearsal, your patient can attach them to the various cues that are present in the original pain situation. You can use versions of *collapsing and chaining anchors* together to lead their experience in a different direction. Even if these interventions do not fully resolve the discomfort, they can result in useful pattern interrupts. The ability to lose oneself in a pleasurable past memory can be an effective distraction strategy.

It may be important to address the secondary gain and other benefits that pain may bring. Using the *six-step reframing* process you can identify the underlying positive intention of the discomfort. Once ascertained, this can be used as a basis for identifying other behaviours that bring the benefits of the intention in a different way. This is often useful in chronic recurring conditions such as migraine headaches. One question I often ask is: 'If your pain had a voice and could speak to you, what message would it give you?' It is often quite surprising what this can reveal that is directly helpful in alleviating or reframing the discomfort in some way.

Conceptualising the discomfort as a conflict between two parts can enable a useful *parts integration process* with potential resolution. In this scenario, one part is labelled as 'having discomfort' and the other as 'seeking relief'. Chunking up on the positive intentions of each part can lead to a common larger frame, even if this is expressed at the very high level of 'continuing survival'. You can chunk down again only as quickly as you maintain agreement while integrating or sequencing the competencies and skills that both parts exhibit. It can be challenging to think of the 'skill' that exists within chronic pain. However, this can be reframed as the skill by which the part is tenaciously able to persist in maintaining a particular state over a period of time – a skill which could be put to good use in other contexts in future.

Integration processes can be done on or off the timeline. The advantage of using spatial anchoring on a walking timeline is that it allows further exploration of the differing physiology, posture and gestures of each state. Given that chronic pain may be maintained by postural and physiological anchors, changing these by integrating the two states can lead to improvement. This is one way in which graded exercise to improve general fitness and posture may help to relieve pain.

Some patients store their memories of traumatic accidents as associated memories. Every time they think of the trauma they relive the event with the micromusclular movements, breathing patterns and physiology of the original accident. This often occurs outwith conscious awareness. Reprocessing the event with the *phobia/trauma cure* can not only relieve the negative emotions via dissociation but also, according to some NLP practitioners, it can allow the discomfort from chronic injuries to resolve. This is an area in which a most interesting research project could be set up.

Timeline processes (both imaginal and walking varieties) can be used in many different ways. Building up multiple resources and sending them back along the timeline to the 'younger you', at the time of or just before any event that precipitated the chronic pain, can allow a positive *reimprinting* of the mental perception that is still held. If any other significant people were involved in an original imprinting event, they can be re-resourced, too. Given that today's discomfort is impacted by previous pain episodes and future expectations of pain, it is possible to use timelines to dissociate from the past and future so that present discomfort is the only aspect to be dealt with. Dissociating from the whole timeline (past, present and future) can act as a pattern interrupt or distracter for short periods of time. It is a potent meditative state.

You can also create an imaginal future, beyond the time when the discomfort has gone. The patient can float out along the future timeline and build a fantasy of how they would behave differently – what they would see, hear, do and feel instead. Many people may initially object to doing this because they don't believe in the possibility of their pain going away. In fact, whether they believe it or not initially is immaterial. You can simply get them to build pictures that they *don't* believe are likely to happen, and then step into them and explore the scenario from the inside. This approach suspends both belief and disbelief and gets around the patient's inner critical faculty, which often prevents useful experimentation. Many of these types of strategies can be effectively enhanced and augmented by hypnosis.

As is usual in CBT and NLP interventions, backing up enough to get the earliest triggering cues of pain and discomfort is central to the process of effectively attaching different states and resources. Because pain is a perception, much can be done by creative experimentation with the various cognitions and internal imagery that are already present. Even a small change may lead to considerable relief. Patients may find that irrespective of what causes their pain, these interventions can foster an increasing degree of self-efficacy, resourcefulness and competency.

Cancer

Around 80% of cancers are avoidable. As a species we engage in many behaviours, such as smoking and dietary and alcohol excess, which are associated with the development of various types of cancer. There are also many claims that certain types of personality may be prone to cancer, and that lifestyle factors such as poor coping skills for dealing with stress, as well as adverse life events and even depression, may be either causative or promote its development. However, the research is not conclusive.

We have all met patients who have defied the odds and lived far longer than even the statistics have predicted. Was it solely the physical treatments that led to their longevity, or were other psychological factors involved? It is extremely difficult to tease all of this apart, but perhaps patients' beliefs, values, attitudes and behaviours may have a part to play not only in individual susceptibility to different cancers, but also in rates of disease progression, survival times and even 'cure'.

Notwithstanding the above, the very diagnosis of cancer can provoke marked emotional responses, such as anxiety, grief and depression, together with relationship difficulties and social isolation. Patients often search for meaning, attempting to understand both the causative and prognostic factors of their condition. Along with this may be an endeavour to gain a sense of mastery over current symptoms with both conventional medicines and alternatives such as meditation, guided imagery and 'positive' thinking. It is in this area in particular that CBT and NLP can aid symptom control.

Scene setting

The whole topic of pain control is a large part of symptom management in cancer care. Giving a patient the ability to have a degree of personal control over potentially distressing symptoms is very important. The previous section on chronic pain identified multiple points for successful intervention in adjuvant therapy.

Chemotherapy is widely used for many types of cancer, and is associated with the twin problems of nausea and vomiting (20–30% of cases), together with anticipatory anxiety (60% of cases) about the next treatment pulse. These problems are classically conditioned responses. As such they may respond to counter-conditioning techniques involving relaxation, visual imagery and other desensitisation techniques.

Some symptoms may be operantly conditioned. Pain behaviours and chronic coughing and regurgitation may be positively reinforced by the attention of carers (nurses, doctors, family, etc.). This can happen in hospitals, hospices and at home. Once recognised, it is possible to treat such symptoms and behaviours with extinction regimes and differential reinforcement of alternative behaviours.

There is currently much interest in various cognitive and imagery strategies that deal specifically with the cancer itself. In the 1970s, the Simontons pioneered the use of visual imagery whereby patients envisaged cancer cells being eaten up by the body's defences. This was also done by metaphoric means – for example, white knights on chargers scavenging for and killing aberrant cells. A gentler metaphor involved grazing sheep rooting out 'weeds'. Although it is difficult to be certain of the effect on longevity, this approach certainly gave patients an increased sense of personal control.

Specific cognitive strategies may also be used to build and bolster self-esteem and improve self-worth. Exactly the same interventions that were used in the sections on anxiety and depression can be utilised successfully here. Social skills training and group activities that foster relationship building can prevent isolation and improve the ability to become closer to loved ones. Group meetings can also expose patients to modelling of the successful strategies that others have used in specific circumstances.

CBT and NLP approaches therefore have a potentially large part to play in symptom control in cancer. Their role in actually reducing tumour size, preventing disease progression and increasing longevity is currently highly speculative, but is likely to be increasingly part of research in the next decade.

Intervening

NLP techniques such as *collapsing and chaining* anchors can be very useful interventions in the conditioned nausea and vomiting of chemotherapy. Stacking several positive anchors together and integrating them with the nauseous feelings can provide a one-session 'cure' of the problem. Anticipatory anxiety can become the first link in a chain of anchors going from frustration through impatience and curiosity to desire and 'going for it'. However, you can simply build resources and attach them to the anxiety triggers in the particular context. Giving patients the ability to generate and fire off their own positive anchors can lead to their having an increasing sense of self-control.

Submodality patterns such as the swish can also be used in anticipatory anxiety. You must build a clear, compelling picture of the 'you' who is confident, self-assured, able to handle things easily, etc. Find your patient's own value-based words for the ways they would want to be instead, and *swish* this with the triggering cues from the anxiety-provoking situation. Simple submodality changes such as dissociation can be used for patients who are undergoing uncomfortable medical procedures and interventions.

It is not surprising that some people, especially children, develop phobias of medical procedures, especially injections. Others have a fear of enclosed spaces such as scanners, getting panicky, claustrophobic feelings at the mere mention of the word. The *phobia cure process* can eliminate these responses fairly quickly in most individuals. It is generally most effective for specific memories of a prior precipitating event, although sometimes this may be outwith conscious awareness. The process is not useful for anticipatory anxiety.

Many people have fears about their cancer and its encroaching effects on their body. Most try to wall off these concerns, compartmentalising them in order to cope. This in itself may be a very useful skill. However, I have found that exploring thoughts about the tumour, even to the extent of having a 'dialogue' with it, can be very helpful, and for some may lead to a peaceful acceptance that allows them to live whatever life they have left more comfortably. The *six-step reframing process* can be very useful here. The key reframe is often around the cancer's uncovered 'positive' intention of death. When death can be reframed as a release from all worries and concerns and a step into peacefulness, the coexistence of cancer in one's body can be transcended.

The six-step reframe includes the elicitation of an involuntary signal system for 'yes' and 'no'. As well as aiding in finding the positive intention, it can also be used in other ways. In some circles, cancer can be seen metaphorically as the physiological expression of a lifetime of recurrent maladaptive behavioural patterns, or perhaps even as a response to some previous severe psychological trauma. The signalling system can be used to unearth these particular contexts, and the information so gained can be utilised when choosing updated new responses in place of the old ones. It is also possible to use the signals to assess the patient's congruency both in the expressed desire for future survival and in taking the necessary behavioural steps to increase the likelihood of this occurring.

The *meta-mirror* is another way to have a helpful interchange with the tumour, or indeed any other presenting symptom. The process deals with relationship issues and can generate new ways of dealing with difficult symptoms. More often, however, I have used it to help to heal estranged relationships with significant other people in the patient's life. The other person does not need to be physically part of the process, as it is done with the patient's own internal representation. I have never ceased to be amazed at the anecdotal occurrences thereafter, which include 'spontaneous' visits and phone calls 'out of the blue' from estranged relatives and loved ones – often with a healing of the rift and a renewal of the relationship. Not always, though!

The *grief resolution* process can be a very useful tool – and not only for bereaved relatives after the death of a loved one. Although cancer may ultimately involve loss of life, there may be many other smaller losses along the way. Some people can no longer work or take part in previously important pursuits. This kind of living loss – at the level of identity – can cause marked depression. Some types of cancer surgery may involve loss of a body part, such as a breast or limb, or other types of function. The resulting altered body image may be a permanent daily reminder of what *was*, engendering ongoing grief. All of these types of loss can be taken through the grief resolution process with imagery appropriate to the precipitating factor.

Some patients, recognising that they may not have much time left, struggle to deal with the inner and outer conflicts of so-called 'unfinished business'. This may relate to worries and concerns about finances, future provision for loved ones, and past guilts and regrets which may span a lifetime. It is often said that at death one's entire life flashes before one's eyes. Usually, however, I have found that this occurs ante mortem, often slowly, with the video pausing too long over past hurts. One useful goal for many cancer patients is to enjoy the present moment without undue interruptions from either the uncomfortable past or potential future anxieties. To this end, *parts integration processes* – with or without *timeline interventions* – can very usefully resolve these difficulties, leaving a sense of peaceful integration and the ability to focus on what is important here and now. There is also some conjecture that this integrated, parasympathetic-type state may in itself provide an impetus to healing at both mental and physical levels.

Timeline interventions can also be used to build compelling futures. Although the evidence remains anecdotal, I am sure that many doctors have encountered patients who seemed to have a dire prognosis, yet were able to live long enough to achieve a significant outcome, such as the birth of a grandchild or a memorable journey to some far-off place. People do need something to live for – and to make life worth living. The *well-formed outcome process* can initiate thoughts about what patients really do want to do and achieve. By utilising various other resources (determination, commitment, perseverance, fun, pleasure, etc.) you can help them to build a future timeline of events which both attracts and impels them to action. This results in a life truly worth living – no matter what the length!

Patients with cancer are more susceptible to anxiety and depression, and may also have chronic habits and addictions which they want to resolve. You can utilise all of the specific interventions described in the previous sections to help them to achieve their goals, giving a sense of mastery over their current situation. The only limits to using the principles of CBT and NLP for patient care are those of your own imagination and your ability to improvise creatively.

Concluding

I hope that I have covered these five areas – depression, anxiety, habits and addictions, chronic pain and cancer – in sufficient depth in this chapter to give you more than a flavour of what you could do to intervene appropriately in each circumstance. In truth, each area could easily have had a chapter or even a book to itself. However, I would encourage you to use and adapt the various tools that you have already assimilated in the second part of this book to fit whatever the unique patient in front of you at the present moment requires.

Although there may be a bewildering array of clinical presentations, you will find yourself being more easily able to *step back*, uncover the principle behind the symptom and disease process, and *select* the best intervention accordingly. Remember that you can use the *feedback* from any intervention you try out to guide you with regard to what to do next. You will find it increasingly easy to utilise the appropriate intervention in the best possible way for your patient.

CHAPTER 18

NLP, Freud and friends

Introduction

Throughout *Changing with NLP* we have focused mainly on a cognitive–behavioural explanation for much of how NLP works. This is a reasonable strategy given the undoubted research-validated efficacy of the CBT model. More outcome-based research has been done in this discipline over the last 30 years than any other form of intervention. Yet NLP, a plagiariser of the excellence of many disciplines, has also drawn key concepts from other fields of therapy. It is well worth elucidating just how NLP interprets and utilises material from these domains. This will, I believe, lay the groundwork for mutual understanding of each approach and perhaps even for future collaboration. However, first I shall give a brief history of the development of various therapies.

Some form of 'talking therapy' has been around for hundreds of years. However, the first specific enquiries into the psychological aspects of clinical problems arose with the interest in hypnosis that spanned the eighteenth and nineteenth centuries. Investigations by figures such as the German physician Franz Anton Mesmer, the French psychiatrist Hippolyte Bernheim and the neurologist Pierre Janet laid the foundations for interest in unconscious mental processing and functioning that stimulated Freud's entry into the field.

Dispensing with his early usage of hypnosis, Freud went on to develop psychoanalysis with its emphasis on repressed memories, imaginative fantasies, free association, transference and counter-transference. Melanie Klein extended this further in the development of 'object relations' with the notion of projective identification, which we shall explore further shortly. Psychoanalytical approaches were the mainstay of therapy until the 1950s, which saw the advent of behavioural and then cognitive therapy. They are still practised worldwide.

Cognitive–behavioural therapy arose in reaction to the so-called 'depth psychologies'. In summary, their practitioners believed that an 'archaeological' approach to the past was not required. Although most of the techniques tend to deal with the 'here and now', there has been some *rapprochement* with depth psychology in the development of integrative approaches. A close cousin to CBT is *interpersonal therapy* (IPT). We shall see how this contributes to effective treatment later in the chapter.

Creative therapies that make use of art, music and movement are intended to result in both a greater understanding and a resolution of psychological problems. Rather than relying on verbal wordplay, they engage many non-verbal emotive, symbolic and functional processes to facilitate change. We shall investigate Jacob Moreno's psychodrama in due course.

The advent of systems theory has led to the ability to look for the circular causality that typifies problem maintenance. Instead of seeking '*the* cause' of a problem, systems approaches explore the current pattern of engagement, eliciting multiple perspectives and acknowledging the positive intentions behind behaviours. 'Solutions' may arise as emergent properties of such exploration. This approach has been used in *family therapy* and, more recently, in narrative-based primary care.

Lastly, but by no means least, there are a range of factors common to all therapies that may lead to their success independently of the specific techniques that are utilised. Factors such as establishing a therapeutic alliance with the patient are of vital importance. These so-called *demand characteristics*, which are subliminally present within all contexts of therapy, merit further elucidation and utilisation.

In the rest of this chapter we shall focus on some of the key concepts and insights from an NLP perspective.

Freud and friends

In general, Freud's view of the unconscious mind was that it was the seat of emotional inner conflict, rooted in the past, often in suppressed or repressed memories with sexual undertones. It seemed to be a cauldron of drives and desires which, although mostly out of awareness, sought the light of day by expression in pathological thoughts and behaviours. Therapy was the act of tracing these superficial expressions, little by little, back into the murky past whence they came, shining the light of insight and liberating the released energies for useful work instead.

NLP acknowledges that the unconscious mind harbours the various patterns that lead to pathological behaviours. Yet at the same time, rather than viewing the unconscious mind as 'all bad' and the conscious mind as 'all good', NLP also recognises that the unconscious is the seat of every single resource and skill that we possess. The conscious mind may be the director of the show, but it requires the co-operation of the unconscious to perform meaningful tasks. The trick, of course, is to get the resources to the right place so that change can easily occur.

Freudian psychology is an archaeological approach – you dig and dig into the past in order to reach the 'buried treasure'. As we discussed in Chapter 15, NLP focuses on *process* rather than on content. It is not so much the story itself that counts, but rather *the way* in which those particular memories are structured which gives the clues for rapid change. However, in this section we shall concentrate on the usefulness of three psychoanalytical concepts, namely transference, counter-transference and projection.

Transference, counter-transference and projection

These three concepts are central therapeutic themes in psychoanalysis and its derivative psychodynamic psychotherapy. For non-psychiatrists, the very words themselves conjure up vague 'intellectual' processes. First we shall examine each concept and then we shall consider how it relates to NLP approaches.

Transference denotes the unwitting carryover of past experience into the present-moment encounter. Classically the feelings, attitudes and ways of responding to significant others in childhood (parents, teachers, authority figures, etc.) are unconsciously transferred to the significant figures in the current situation. Much of our rich inner imaginative life, of which we are generally unaware, forms a template for today's interaction. We unconsciously replay unresolved past traumas, conflicts and inner dialogues with similar recurring consequences (e.g. several consecutive relationships that end in the same way).

Counter-transference refers to exactly the same processes that occur in the therapist and are transferred towards the patient. These are all the thoughts and feelings that are stirred up in the therapist as the patient relates their current symptomology. They represent an important, albeit unconscious communication between patient and therapist. Freud stipulated that all therapists should undergo analysis to enable them to become consciously aware of their own unconscious bias – counter-transference – in therapeutic situations.

Projection was identified by Melanie Klein as a useful extension to the understanding of transference/counter-transference. Essentially this is an unconscious activity whereby 'split-off' parts of a patient – of which they are completely unaware – are 'embedded' in and become identified with the therapist. For example, the patient may unconsciously 'disown' her anger, which is projected on to the therapist. The patient then believes that the therapist is angry with her and, perhaps surprisingly, the therapist often actually does feel angry! This can happen with any disowned emotion.

It is probably true to say that this kind of projective identification is a normal occurrence in everyday life, and it seems to be one of the ways in which pre-verbal children in particular experience and begin to make sense of the world. We have probably all experienced it during consultations, especially with a 'heartsink' patient. The psychoanalytical therapist's main task is to be aware of and contain these projections so that gradually, over a period of time, the patient can reown them in a way that allows their full reintegration back into their personality.

The NLP approach

It may be surprising to some that the NLP approach can fit comfortably hand in glove with all of the above! Because we act out of our internal maps of the world, with patterns that repeat, we can profitably view the psychoanalytical transactions through this lens. Transference and counter-transference are like triggered anchors which replay out of conscious awareness. As an experiment, think of someone you met to whom you had a fairly instantaneous negative reaction. If you anchor these negative feelings and do a trans-derivational search, you will uncover the template from which the reaction occurs. Lost in the mists of time may be the memory of a person who had the same postures, gestures, manner-isms, looks or voice tone as the current 'suspect'. One of these has acted as the unconscious cue for your present response.

The NLP model (*see* Chapter 3) suggests that as much as 90% of all com-munication occurs non-verbally. Most of this is also non-conscious. When you are in rapport with another person, matching and mirroring their physiology and voice characteristics, you will find that you also experience similar emotions. In fact, a standard exercise on many NLP courses is to have one person silently relive a memory from the past while the other silently matches and mirrors as many parameters as possible. During the debriefing, many are amazed at the similar sequence of emotions that they both experienced. Some people also 'intuitively' picture similar events.

NLP explains projective identification as a natural consequence of rapport in a therapeutic situation. Obviously the question arises as to *who* is generating the feelings and *who* therefore 'owns' them. It can be terribly unsettling at first when negative feelings (e.g. anxiety, depression, anger, sadness, etc.) appear to arise unbidden in the therapist during a consultation, especially when the feel-ings seem to be at variance or even conflicting with what is happening 'on the surface'. However, they can be seen as a major clue not only to what is going on in the patient's inner world or map, but also as a pointer about what to do next. The key is to be able to identify the feelings and differentiate *what* belongs to *whom*.

I developed the following exercise after training with US trainers Tom Vizzini and Kim McFarland. It is very important to be able to identify – and even name – the various states that may arise in a therapeutic consultation. By deliberately stepping into the various states listed below, you can pay careful attention to their kinaesthetic submodalities. This will allow you to decipher their 'signature' when they arise unbidden. When doing this exercise, please make sure that you finish off with one or two very pleasant states!

Exercise 18:   Mapping signature states

Here is a list of states that you can elicit in yourself one by one. Add others as you wish. You can do them in any order you like, but do be sure to finish on some pleasant ones.

Anger, calmness, anxiety, excitement, sadness, playfulness, loss/bereavement, mischievousness, panic, happiness, depression, pleasure, frustration, joy, ecstasy ...

1   Choose a state and remember a time when you previously experienced it. See the pictures and hear the sounds again as you step inside it. If you don't have a particular memory, simply imagine what it feels like to be that way.

2   Turn your attention to your internal kinaesthetics of the state. Notice where it starts on your body (chest, solar plexus, lower abdomen, head, etc.). Where does it spread to next? Is it of high or low intensity? Is it continuous, discontinuous or pulsating? Does it move quickly or slowly? Is it heavy or light? Does it cover a small or large area? Is it hot or cold? Does it have a direction of spin?

3   Increase and then decrease the intensity of the state and notice what happens to the kinaesthetics. In particular, note again in more detail exactly where it starts and where it decreases down to again. How do the other kinaesthetics change when the intensity changes?

4   Now imagine that this particular state has a colour associated with it. Which colour fits best? If it had a particular sound associated with it, what would it sound like? How do the colour and sound change as the intensity changes?

5   Once you have mapped this state out on to your body so that you can recognise it whenever it arises, break state and go neutral for a few moments prior to moving on to the next one.

Finish off with a good feeling state and luxuriate in it!

Once you have mapped out the various states in this way, you can practise further as follows. Engage someone in casual conversation and establish a rapport with them. Ask them about a particular experience which they have had. Notice which state is triggered in you and check with them to see whether your experience concurs. Notice other people who are already in conversation. Choose one and imagine 'stepping into them' as if you had replaced them. Which state is triggered now?

You can also practise this during ordinary consultations. Whenever you are in rapport with a patient and you experience one of these other feelings coming up, you can say 'I don't know what's true for you at present, yet I have a feeling of ... (name the state) ... Does that make any sense to you on some level?' You can then of course check out their verbal *and* non-verbal response. Calibrating in this way prevents you from merely mind-reading.

Of course, occasionally the negative feelings and emotions that arise in the doctor/therapist during a therapeutic encounter belong to him or her, not the patient. You can view this as a signal that you have an as yet unresolved issue which you can deal with using any of the appropriate techniques described in this book.

Differences

One important way in which NLP differs from psychoanalysis is in the matter of conscious insight. Over a period of time, the analytical therapist will give a formulation of the transference/counter-transference and projective identification so that the patient has a major degree of insight into the causative factors. This insight is held to be therapeutic in its own right, bringing about changes in the way in which the patient views and acts in important relationships.

NLP, on the other hand, presupposes that major change can occur without conscious insight and that, in contrast to psychoanalysis, conscious insight may sometimes actually prevent useful change from occurring. The NLP therapist is more interested in the form and process of the patient's situation than in the content. Rather than going into the story in a detailed way, they look for the structure of the recurring problematic patterns of engagement. Changing the structure can lead to rapid change in symptomatology. Moreover, the effects are not confined to the symptoms alone – increased integration of personality and congruence also occur.

Psychodrama

Psychodrama was developed by the psychiatrist Jacob Moreno from his initial observations of children at play. He noticed that they easily stepped into and out of different roles during imaginative games, and he postulated that this activity – akin to modelling – was responsible for much of their emotional and cognitive development, as well as their ability to learn how to solve problems. He reasoned that adults could use similar processes to re-enact emotional conflicts in a way that led to resolution.

Psychodrama usually occurs in a group setting where various members are assigned roles in a current problem situation of one member. The setting can be made even more theatrical by the addition of a stage, lighting and other props, although this is not strictly necessary. However, it does encourage the 'players' to step even more fully into role, further emotionally dramatising the re-enactment.

Usually one group member is chosen who gives an account of the recent emotional conflict and chooses which of the other members will play each role. The 'director' (therapist) choreographs the action, setting up the 'theatre' in a similar configuration to the current problem. Action is the order of the day, with the protagonists being encouraged to display their emotion rather than just talk about it. When impasses are reached, the director will encourage role reversals in which the client of the day becomes the person on the opposite side of the conflict.

At times, the re-enactment of the current problem will reactivate past memories of similar issues, perhaps even in childhood. The scene then rapidly changes and the characters assume the parts of the significant players in this earlier event. The member whose problem is the focus of the group's attention is encouraged to experiment with stepping into the other roles as well as his or her own part. In this way past events can be relived from many different perspectives.

Insight and change can arise from many different sources. The other players in the drama are encouraged to act intuitively, and these intuitions may be the source of much useful material. The principal player, in role-playing parents or other characters, has an opportunity to 'see the other side of the coin'. He or she can also be encouraged to experiment and confront the other individuals in ways that he or she could not have done as a child. This can allow a dramatic 'reworking' of the original material and a subsequent improvement in current relationships.

The NLP approach

Interestingly, one of NLP's most widely used tools, namely the meta-model, was modelled in part from family therapist Virginia Satir. She was famous for 'parts parties' whereby acting out the various roles that encompassed a patient's problem could lead to a reconfiguration and even resolution. The other model for the meta-model, Fritz Perls, used the Gestalt 'two-chairs' technique to resolve conflict. The patient 'hallucinated' the person with whom they had a conflict sitting in the opposite chair, and was encouraged to actively and emotionally debate with this 'person' and then swap chairs and argue the case from the other side. This was the forerunner of the visual squash technique.

Moreno's psychodrama approach has much in common with the NLP techniques of meta-mirror and reimprinting. He encourages the patient to relive a current conflict from the perspectives of first, second and third perceptual positions – in particular focusing on the emotional feelings involved, often dramatising them to excess in order to ensure their full representation. The information gathered from each position can give much useful insight and personal change, as we saw in Chapter 14. Of course, the positioning of the patient during the re-enactment role acts as a spatial anchor for the elicited state. These anchors may be spontaneously 'collapsed' with others as the drama unfolds.

Moreno's patients may spontaneously regress to much younger memories with a similar emotional content. This is akin to a trans-derivational search that occurs when using timeline interventions. Here the negative state is anchored and tracked back into the past to an imprinting experience. Again the patient is encouraged to explore each role (perceptual position) with particular emphasis on the emotions that are aroused. Experimenting with new behaviours in the old situation reimprints the memory in a more useful way. In NLP terms, new resources are added, which changes the memory's configuration and structure, allowing the future expression of different behaviours. The patient now has a new strategy of interaction in place.

Although I have concentrated here on psychodrama, the other creative psychotherapies, such as art, music, dance and movement and play therapies, can all be interpreted in the light of NLP. This is not to promote one therapy – namely NLP – over another. The insights gained from this kind of analysis can be profitably used to enhance each approach. In particular I believe that NLP could benefit from incorporating much more movement into its techniques. Although many of the processes can be done visually, movement engages far more of the mind and emotions. Given that many problem states have a characteristic posture and physiology, this engagement could lead to more integrative change.

Systemic and family therapeutic approaches

According to systems theory, the current situation is kept in dynamic equilibrium by a series of cybernetic feedback loops between individuals that give a degree of homeostasis – keeping things mostly as they are. Instead of a linear process in which A causes B, systems theory proposes 'circular causality' in which A and B are both cause and effect at the same time.

For example, in a relationship, if one partner is aggressive and the other is submissive, the repetitive behaviours are kept going by the predictable and recurring effects that each set of behaviours has on the other. The same ending happens over and over again. For things to be different, something within the system must change. If A changes behaviour, then B will automatically change as well – and vice versa! In a sense it does not matter who the patient is, because changing another part of the system may in fact resolve the symptom.

In this way family therapists and those involved in the newer approach of narrative-based medicine focus more on the patterns of relationships than on diagnosing and treating the 'one cause' of all the problems. They recognise that a symptom arises as an emergent property of the system that the 'patient' is currently within. They seek to obtain the views and experiences of everyone involved in the situation – whether there are just two people or several. This often occurs in a family meeting where, using *circular questioning*, the underlying assumptions each person has about the situation can be explored. These assumptions, which until now have generally been unvoiced, provide much valuable information and in particular open up a dialogue about conflicting viewpoints and perspectives.

A key concept for the involved therapist/doctor is that of *neutrality and curiosity*. He is equally interested in all points of view, and does not presuppose the importance of one over another. He is curious about what people think might happen in different scenarios. Questions such as 'What would happen if nothing changed?' and 'What would you like to have happen instead?' can be most illuminating. Of course, all other members of the system get to hear the verbal (and non-verbal) responses, which can open up other areas of dialogue.

Another concern is to fully hear the stories of those involved. A family *genogram* – which is like a family tree – records three generations of the key life events, including births and deaths. Out of this can come a joint 'family story' or narrative about the current situation. Solutions may well arise by helping the family to retell the story in a more helpful and useful way.

It is important at all times to maintain a *positive connotation* – that is, to see a positive motivation underlying even the most debilitating and damaging of behaviours. Often the presenting symptom can be explained as the best or only option that the 'patient' has of reaching a valuable goal which is in the family's overall interests – even if they are not yet consciously aware of that possible positive interpretation. This kind of reframing is an important part of strategic therapy with groups. Of course, making a family decision about the next step can be therapeutic in its own right.

The systems approach used in family therapy has been shown to be of benefit in adolescent eating disorders, psychosomatic issues and various behaviour problems, together with depression. For an excellent overview of the use of systems methodologies in general medical practice, the reader is referred to *Narrative-Based Primary Care* by John Launer (*see* Bibliography).

An NLP interpretation

NLP has a great deal in common with systems theory approaches to therapy. We tend to look at problems as arising out of a recurring pattern, the structure of which can be changed in a variety of ways. In particular, Robert Dilts has developed what he calls *Systemic NLP* – although to be fair to others in the field, whenever you alter the structure or process of a presenting issue you are altering the system of which it is a part. Sometimes the systemic effects are too small to be noticed (first-order change), and sometimes they are large and ripple out into other contexts (second-order change).

The *neutrality and curiosity* exhibited by the family therapist are an integral approach of the NLP practitioner. They are a reflection of the NLP presuppositions that *everyone has their own unique model of the world* and *the meaning of your communication is the response that it gets.* Respectful listening to a person's perspective without judging their internal map as right or wrong creates a 'field-space' for appropriate updating and change.

Positive connotation is synonymous with the NLP concept of an underlying positive intention behind each behaviour, no matter how bizarre it may seem. The subsequent reframing to allow the manifestation of that positive intent with new behaviours, thus allowing systemic change, is identical. Much of the circular questioning that is used is contained in the meta-model challenge 'What would happen if ...?' The concept of the situation remaining the same or changing in some way can be explored without commitment at this stage to do anything new. In NLP terms, 'the map is being expanded'.

In the narrative-based approach, the primary focus is to help the patient/family tell their story in a better way – recognising that some stories are better than others. NLP also recognises that some maps are more useful than others. However, rather than being somewhat restricted to the verbal retelling in the narrative approach, NLP brings all of its other tools to bear. Using representational systems and visual, auditory and kinaesthetic submodalities together with movement, we can expand the retelling of the story dramatically, adding further scope and dimension to the words themselves.

NLP really comes into its own when using the concept of the *genogram*. From an NLP perspective, we all carry around in our minds our internal representations of the significant other people and relationships in our lives. These representations contain far more information than we consciously know. This includes a summary of all our historical interactions with these individuals, together with our usual automatic behavioural patterns in their presence. They act as a template that governs our actions and reactions when we are interacting with these individuals in real life. However, they are mostly out of our everyday awareness.

Using techniques such as the meta-mirror and parts negotiation, we can externalise these projections and gain valuable new information from first-, second- and third-position perspectives. Changing, rearranging and updating our mental representations in this way can lead to profound changes in the way in which we relate to these significant other people when we meet them again. The updated representations can be seen as systems attractors around which new behaviours can arise as an emergent property. We can literally build a new attractor landscape in which to move through daily life. The beauty of this approach is that 'family therapy' can be undertaken with only one member of the family present!

Another advantage concerns the realm of deceased relatives. Obviously they are no longer here in real life! However, the patient's internal representation of a deceased relative still lives on inside their neurology – for good or ill. They can tap into this information and perhaps place them in a more appropriate position in their internal landscape (*see* Chapter 12).

Sometimes it is not the current situation which is causing the problem, but the 'family template' from childhood. This representation can be reconstructed with family members who were present at, say, the age of five years arranged around the patient in projected mental space. Occasionally the space which is occupied by someone with whom there is a relationship difficulty today is exactly the same space as that occupied by a person with whom there was a problem in childhood! Reimprinting (*see* Chapter 15) this earlier template with new resources can lead to changes in the current situation.

Psychologist and NLP trainer Lucas Derks has expanded this concept into the *social panorama model* (*see* Bibliography). He gives multiple examples of how to utilise and change internal representations in contexts that might normally be thought of as family therapy. In summary, NLP, systems and family therapy together with narrative-based approaches have a great deal in common, and have much to learn from one another.

Interpersonal therapy (IPT)

Interpersonal therapy, together with CBT, has proven efficacy in the treatment of depression and eating disorders. It is a model of therapy based on the premise that all problems occur in a social and interpersonal context which must be understood for improvement and even resolution to occur. The presenting problem is seen in the light of the patient's current relationships, and the insights engendered are then worked through to effect changes in future expectations. Links are made between the problem and the following four main areas of intervention.

1   *Grief reactions.* The main concern here is to facilitate a mourning process. This is not necessarily only for bereavement of close friends and relatives, but can also be for the loss that occurs when relationships end or when people move on to different jobs, or even the grief engendered by loss of dreams and ideals.

2   *Interpersonal role disputes.* Many problems can be seen within the framework of conflict or dispute with other people. Recurring relationship difficulties are often due to maladaptive communication patterns and strategies which may have been modelled on significant others in the patient's life. Identifying the specifics of the conflict and making a plan of action with regard to future choices is pivotal.

3   *Role transition problems.* Throughout our lives we are transitioning from one role to another (single, married, parent, grandparent, etc.). These are sequential transitions over time, yet there are also simultaneous roles occurring in the same time frame (parent, child, lover, friend, co-worker, boss, etc.). Transitioning into new roles in a positive manner improves self-esteem and self-efficacy.

4   *Interpersonal deficits.* Many patients may be socially isolated because of a lack of particular skills. Examining past relationships and the current relationship with the therapist can identify the skills that are needed to develop more effective future new relationships.

IPT tends to focus on the here and now, and in particular on how patients express emotions. Therapists identify the various recurrent patterns in thoughts, feelings, actions and relationships. Some who are more psychodynamically oriented will place more emphasis on the past. Generally there is an exploration of patients' main areas of avoidance or their engagement in the kinds of activities that preclude problem resolution. Throughout there is an emphasis on the therapeutic relationship as a key model for the future.

IPT has been used to good effect in depression of all types (including adolescent, postpartum and late-life onset), eating disorders (e.g. bulimia), somatisation of symptoms (e.g. irritable bowel syndrome) and deliberate self-harm.

The NLP perspective

NLP has much in common with and a great deal to add to the IPT approach. Processes such as the meta-mirror and reimprinting are central to this understanding. Much of the other NLP technology you have learned so far can be utilised to facilitate resolution of relationship issues.

Grief is a prime example. The grief resolution process (*see* Chapter 14) is a very versatile approach for a variety of situations of loss. It can be used successfully at the ending of any relationship, whether this is due to death or estrangement, and even if the relationship was with a treasured personal object or a previous job. Often in these scenarios it is important to deal with any concurrent anger that may prevent effective task engagement.

When it comes to resolving interpersonal role conflict, both the meta-mirror and parts integration processes provide a very useful working template. The skills involved in chunking up to find the positive intention underlying each part of the conflict are paramount as a first step towards a negotiated settlement. Maladaptive communication patterns may result from unconscious projections which can be reowned and integrated. This can be a major step in improving congruence and self-esteem.

Role transitions always involve change to some extent. How well we have managed this in the past is often a predictor of future success – although not always. NLP modelling processes that utilise the various perceptual positions can help the patient to acquire role expertise more rapidly. Effective role play in imagined future scenarios aids skills integration.

Interpersonal deficits may be caused by an inability to access state-dependent resources that are 'locked up' in other life contexts. NLP revivification and anchoring techniques can help to spread these resources generatively into all areas of life. However, with the best will in the world, some patients do not have these 'locked-up' skills and must rely on skills training. NLP has extensively modelled the kinds of skills that are required for managing relationships effectively, and these can be acquired in a step-by-step format through imaginal rehearsal and subsequent role play.

NLP and IPT can mutually benefit from each other's approach. IPT's strength in particular has been in identifying the four main areas in which therapeutic work can lead to improved outcomes. Within each of these categories the addition of specific NLP skills can further hone the process of intervention, leading to more precision and perhaps shorter overall treatment times.

Common factors across all therapies

Common factors across all therapies are those that are not just specific to one approach or technique. They are present whether you are performing psycho-analysis, cognitive–behavioural therapy, creative therapies or NLP. They are a powerful aspect of achievement of therapeutic outcomes, and are embedded within the very substance of the *context* of treatment. They are sometimes called the *demand characteristics* – a set of factors that are mainly out of aware-ness and which are present in every encounter and role therein. A broad group-ing of these commonalities includes the following:

1   a patient who has a positive expectation that treatment will help him or her
2   establishing a therapeutic relationship that is based on rapport and trust
3   a convincing therapeutic model that gives an explanation for the patient's problems and a method of addressing them
4   a 'technique' that requires the active participation of both the patient and the therapist/doctor.

Analysis of these common factors consistently shows that they contribute more to the therapeutic outcome than the specific type of therapy itself! It is therefore well worth finding out exactly how we can optimise these conditions.

Key components of the common factors include support, learning and action. Any kind of intervention provides scope for an empathetic encounter and the opportunity to address a troubling issue in a supportive way with an expert who can communicate a new and helpful perspective. A huge amount of learning can take place both consciously and unconsciously through advice, insight, integration of problematic experiences and cognitive restructuring. Factors that encourage the patient to take subsequent action in the real world, such as skills practice, cognitive mastery and the positive feedback established through experiencing success, are vital for optimistic expectations and self-efficacy.

The factor which is most frequently mentioned as being of primary importance in achieving outcomes is the degree of therapeutic alliance that the practitioner and patient realise together. This good working relationship encompasses the patient's ability to focus on the agreed task, the therapist's ability to empathise, and the level of commitment that both bring to the encounter. This allows the tolerance of ambiguity and conflict, which may be required to resolve certain difficulties. It is not surprising, then, that therapist training emphasises the de-velopment of interpersonal skills, such as empathic listening and development of a working alliance.

All therapeutic models have some degree of underlying theory about why and how this particular problem has occurred and what – if anything – can be done about it. The more this rationale makes sense to the patient, the more they 'buy into' the model, and the greater the chance of therapeutic success. In fact it is often very worthwhile to have an orienting session in which the therapist explains the basic tenets of the model and its application together with what the patient can expect as a result of following the therapy over time. This form of 'education in the therapy' can pay dividends by increasing the likelihood of achieving a successful outcome.

The congruent application of the subsequent technique by the therapist is also a factor in determining whether or not an outcome is achieved. A therapist who 'believes in' his or her model and what he or she is doing, together with a belief that the patient can succeed, is more likely to actualise that outcome. Incongruence, where the therapist doesn't fully 'believe in' their therapeutic model, can be picked up unconsciously by the patient. This may result in a less than optimal outcome for the patient.

Patients come for therapy with different degrees of readiness for change, and different expectations about whether they can be helped. This is not an all-or-nothing phenomenon – the degree of readiness and expectation of success may fluctuate over time. The *stages of change model* of Prochaska and DiClemente is a trans-theoretical model of the current stage of readiness of the patient. It is not specific to any one type of therapy, but is common to all approaches. The stages are as follows:

1 pre-contemplation – the issue is not consciously acknowledged by the patient
2 contemplation – acknowledgement of the possibility of change – in 'two minds!'
3 decision – the resolution of ambivalence and a commitment to change
4 action – actually taking the steps
5 maintenance – consolidating the change over time.

Regardless of the intervention you are going to use, you must ensure that your patient is at the right stage to implement it. It is well worthwhile asking yourself what needs to be done to move them from one step to the next. A mismatch caused by pressing for action without resolving the ambivalence of the contemplation stage will probably lead to failure and exasperation.

The common factors are very important, yet are often glossed over in the rush to get to the learning and application of technique. We shall now consider how NLP approaches can enhance the effectiveness of these factors even further.

The NLP approach

NLP is of great practical value in enhancing the non-specific factors that are common to all therapeutic encounters and modalities. In fact, we could say that

NLP was the first discipline that not only examined what worked and why it did so, but also answered the *how* question – dealing with structure and process. There are many applications both to the therapeutic encounter and to the context in which it takes place.

The setting up of an effective field of rapport is a *sine qua non* of an effective NLP intervention. Rather than referring to the large-scale nominalisations that are used to discuss this process, NLP has developed specific skill-sets for the rapid acquisition and utilisation of this important state that exists between practitioner and client. The details can be found in *Consulting with NLP*, but a brief overview is provided here.

The state of rapport is demonstrated in action at the level of physiology when both practitioner and patient match and mirror one another. They adopt similar body postures, gestures and movements so that they are in synchrony. Simply acting as if you are the client's bodily mirror will easily begin to elicit the state. Speaking at a similar rate, volume and intensity will also achieve this. Patients usually speak using a combination of the various representational systems (visual, auditory, kinaesthetic, etc.), often preferring one over another. Reflecting this back in your own speech will allow them to feel that you have followed their train of thought.

Because rapport is a state that exists between two people, it is possible to anchor it and use it over and over again. If you think about therapeutic encounters in which you did develop an excellent rapport, you can revivify them in your mind's eye and anchor the resulting state to a knuckle. You can trigger this anchor in any subsequent encounter. You can also establish rapport at the level of beliefs, values and identity. Respecting the fact that a patient's beliefs about their current situation are true for them, whether or not you agree with their content, is very affirming. This non-judgemental status is a harbinger of the deeper levels of trust that evolve in a therapeutic relationship.

The psychogeography of the layout of your room is an environmental message that can increase or decrease the level of rapport. Whether you sit on facing chairs, at an angle or side by side, or use a couch, etc. makes a significant difference. There can be quite a disparity in levels of rapport when comparing a cramped office with one in which there is space to walk around. Large piles of patients' records lying about and dirty coffee cups convey more than you might intend.

Patients also project images of their mental experiences into the space around them. Noticing where they glance when thinking in a particular way, and gesturing to that area in subsequent discussion lets them know unconsciously that you made a deep connection. Closely calibrating to your patient in this way can make it seem as if you are a mind-reader. This skill and the others described above are all taught within a fairly short period of time on basic-level NLP courses. They foster the development of a strong therapeutic alliance.

The effective therapist must have a therapeutic model and a set of techniques that he or she believes are valuable for successfully gaining outcomes. During training, NLP practitioners practise the techniques on one another as well as observing how others interact. They have first-, second- and third-position perspectives on every intervention and, having used them fruitfully in these circumstances, they have an increased level of congruence when using them in the clinical situation. They have personal experience of what works!

Explanations of what is happening to a patient in terms of a coherent model which they can understand increases that model's efficacy in eliciting change. NLP can provide simple – yet not simplistic – explanations of the current situation and what needs to be done in a way that fits the patient's model of the world. This increases compliance and commitment, deepens rapport and helps to actualise outcomes.

For each step of the *stages of change* model, NLP has a particular orientation that can help to move a patient swiftly through to action and maintenance. In pre-contemplation, issues of possible change can be suggested with close calibration to unconscious responses, without any pressure to do anything more than 'think about it'. Contemplation – the 'two minds' scenario – is really concerned with the resolution of ambivalence with regard to change. This can be aided both conversationally and by specific techniques, such as parts negotiation. Decision is the result of such resolution, and states such as determination, inner strength, confidence, etc. can be brought to bear to aid commitment. Action is the exhibiting of the particular change technique, and maintenance is the future pacing and rehearsal for re-entry to the real world.

The *stages of change* model is a very useful framework for engaging patients in conversational change processes. I shall explore how this can be further integrated with NLP approaches in a forthcoming book entitled *Persuasion in Practice*.

Common factors across all therapies are a hitherto neglected area of practice, mainly because the 'non-specific' issues involved have been conceptualised at too high a chunking level. Most people prefer to get straight to the active utilisation of the various techniques. De-nominalising and chunking down of these non-specific entities into detailed skill-sets, as is done in NLP, learning them step by step and applying them in the therapeutic encounter, can help us all to increase our effectiveness and achieve improved patient outcomes – regardless of therapeutic orientation.

Concluding

We have explored various currently active therapeutic approaches from an NLP perspective. Although the comparisons in each field are not completely exhaustive,

I am sure by now you can see that all of the contemplated models actually share much in common with NLP. Each of the therapeutic tasks is similar in each field, and what starts out as appearing totally unique and foreign can be readily approached and explained through the NLP lens. There are actually far more similarities than differences.

However dissimilar they may appear, each approach incorporates the same fundamentals for change. Each has to make sense of the patient's current symptomology. Each needs a mechanism of exploration and a methodology for incorporating an autonomously functioning aspect of self into an integrated whole again. Whatever their initial perspective, their overall objective is very similar.

Yet we have also seen that the commonalities which all approaches share may in fact account in large measure for their therapeutic efficacy. Although it is easy to get caught up in the 'right' approach or the 'right' technique, it is very important that, whatever we do, we pay close attention to the factors that build the therapeutic alliance. This is the edifice without which useful change is unlikely to occur. And it is one area in which NLP has a great deal to offer.

CHAPTER 19

The dark side of the force

Introduction

Having read this far, and having practised and incorporated the various techniques presented, you may have come to the conclusion that NLP is indeed a very powerful change technology. And without a doubt it is! Yet, like me, you may also have wondered whether such mechanisms are entirely safe and can do no harm. NLP as promoted in commercial and public forums is heavily advertised as a potent force for gaining control of your life and positively influencing others. But is there a negative side too?

More than a decade ago, Michael Yapko, internationally acclaimed psychologist and a leading Ericksonian therapist, wrote what for me was a very influential book, entitled *Hypnosis and the Treatment of Depressions*. The following quote has remained lodged in my memory:

> *Anything that has the potential to be therapeutic has an equal potential to be antitherapeutic;* a clinician unwittingly can establish, despite the most benevolent of intentions, associations that are harmful for the client.
>
> (Yapko, 1992: 37, italics as in the original)

It has certainly been my own personal experience over the years with NLP that there is potential for both great uses and great abuses. Of course, with any powerful tool there can be accidental mishaps despite the best intentions. And it is important to delineate areas of possible problems so that you can avoid similar pitfalls. Yet the tool can also be used deliberately to 'persuade' people to do things that may not be in their best interests. Now I hasten to add that it is an individual moral responsibility of those with potent tools to use them with integrity. Very occasionally, however, this does not happen – not through the fault of the tool, but through the fault of the user.

Myths abound, even in NLP! One such myth is to 'trust your unconscious mind – it always knows what's best for you'. Poppycock! If you have the unconscious mind of a therapeutic genius then perhaps that myth is at least partly true. However, most of us are not so equipped. If our unconscious minds were really that powerful, why did they let us have problems in the first place? Or why can't they solve the problems themselves? Conscious minds are required, too – for structuring and sequencing change patterns. A well-functioning human being has well-*integrated* conscious and unconscious functions.

In this chapter we shall take a closer look at these and other areas of potential harm. When we can recognise and name what is happening, we have an increased opportunity to do something different.

Clinical scenarios

In my early days of NLP skills acquisition I was keen to use my newly developed resources creatively in all kinds of therapeutic encounters. In most circumstances this is an excellent thing to do, as it generalises your skills into multiple areas very quickly and gives good feedback about what works, what does not yet work and the differences that can help you to improve. I was undoubtedly rather zealous and learned a great deal from the two following cases.

Finding Maggie's memory

Maggie was in her mid- to late forties and had developed a phobia about travelling outside Buckie (where she lived) in a car. Three years earlier she had been travelling to Aberdeen as a back-seat passenger in a car driven by an acquaintance of her husband. He was also present, together with an elderly woman whom she had not previously met. Half-way through the journey the driver had overtaken a car in front which had inexplicably veered out on to the highway and slewed into a vehicle coming in the opposite direction. They somersaulted twice and ended up in a field. Maggie, her husband and the driver all survived without serious injury. The elderly woman died.

Since that fateful day she had only been able to travel by car within a 15-mile radius of her home. Any further and she panicked and had to be brought home. She had developed a vehement dislike of the driver, whom she blamed for the incident. He had received a caution and a small fine through the courts, which she believed was not a harsh enough punishment. Whenever she met him in the street she would shout abuse at him! This by itself should have alerted me to complicating underlying factors. However, all I saw was an opportunity to practise the phobia cure.

Maggie was very agreeable and the process went remarkably smoothly. In a dissociated position she gained a lot of new information about what had happened. We ran the memory backwards several times, and I suggested that with each repetition it would be increasingly difficult to get it back. By now I was on a roll, and I finished off with the collapsing anchors process to neutralise her angry feelings about the driver. Pleased with the apparent success, I suggested that she should see me in a week or so for follow-up.

She didn't last the week. I was on call that Sunday, and at one o'clock in the morning I got an angry phone call from her husband telling me to 'get your fucking ass over here right now … she's gone completely loopy!' With a degree of trepidation, wondering even at this stage what the Medical Defence Union would say, I went over to the house to find her in a distressed fugue-type state. She was sweating, babbling and almost incoherent. She had cleared out all the contents of her drawers as she searched for something.

It turned out that what she was searching for was her memory of the accident. The phobia cure had worked too well, and she could not remember the incident at all – the harder she tried, the worse it got and the more agitated she became. She thought that she might have hidden it somewhere – but where? She had turned the house upside down looking for it. I realised at that moment that the accident three years previously had had a profound effect on Maggie's thinking and behaviour. In fact, her whole life had been organised around the subsequent phobia and her hatred of the driver. I had removed the one thing that gave meaning to her life. As her husband demanded that I admit her to a psychiatric hospital, my sinking feeling got worse.

I thought quickly about the options open to me – tranquillising medication, admission to hospital, or one last chance to see if I could repair the damage. Recognising that her current fugue state was akin to a trance, I laid her down on the couch. Using relaxing and deepening suggestions, I induced a much deeper level of trance. Her breathing slowed, her face became symmetrical and her arms became flaccid by her side. I breathed a sigh of relief.

Suddenly she started to shout, scream and contort her body around. I realised that she was having a hypnotic abreaction – she was back inside the accident, reliving it again from the inside out as if it were real! After a few moments, the reaction was over and she settled again, looking much more peaceful. I gave her many suggestions about integrating everything she had learned from the experience so that it could accompany her wherever she went in life – with a clear memory of the incident whenever she wished to review it.

When she reoriented she was much calmer, and thankfully her husband – who had witnessed it all – was happier with my suggestion that I should review her in the morning rather than hospitalise her. To be on the safe side I gave her some tranquillisers, and I then went home to a rather sleepless night myself!

Maggie was actually much better in the morning. She was delighted that she had her memory back – and so was I. She actually maintained an element of her phobic reaction for several years, although she was able to travel much further than previously. When the original driver of the car moved out of the area this seemed to be a signal to her that she could finally let go and move on.

When I looked back through her case records I found that she had seen a psychiatrist several times in her late teens. He had diagnosed a 'borderline personality disorder with hysterical overlay'. Although these kinds of diagnostic labels do not really give much of a clue as to the structure and process of the underlying thinking involved, the whole situation certainly prompted me to take a good look at a patient's previous medical and psychiatric history in future, prior to intervening!

Gina, George and a pair of scissors

Gina, who was now in her early thirties, had reputedly been a victim of multiple episodes of sexual abuse as a child. Although she was a capable mother in her own right, she was also at times deeply unhappy and had regressive experiences which occasionally overwhelmed her. At these times she would appear as if she were a frightened child, uncommunicative and often exasperating to those who tried to help her. I was asked to see her with a view to using NLP technology, and I jumped at the chance to see whether my toolkit could really make a difference.

People who have been abused in the past are often remarkably good trance subjects. They have developed the protective skill of being able to dissociate readily – a function which helped them to escape into their mind when the actual physical aspects of the abuse occurred. Gina undoubtedly had this skill. I decided that I would undertake the NLP interventions in a trance state, and she readily agreed to this.

Using the phobia/trauma cure in the trance state, we re-viewed several memories from a comfortable distance. I really had no idea of the actual content of the memory, other than that several people were involved and the events had a ritualistic element. I decided to add into the process a representation of courage and inner strength to give her more power and control over the incidents. I suggested that she could introduce 'George', a huge gorilla completely under her control, whom she could direct to do her bidding at will. Well, George entered each memory and ripped the perpetrators limb from limb, extracting revenge on her part! I finished off this section by integrating the younger part in the standard way.

Once more on a roll, I decided to use a process for severing any other links that continued to bind Gina to the abusers. In her mind's eye she imagined being attached to each one of them by a string – in much the same way as an umbilical cord. Using a 'magical' pair of scissors she cut all of the ties with a flourish, simultaneously watching the abusers getting smaller and receding into the distance. On rousing she looked radiant and felt as if a great burden had been lifted from her. I silently congratulated myself on a good job.

Late that evening, I was once more on call, and the phone rang at 11 o'clock. It sounded like a child's voice at the end of the phone, sobbing and crying. It turned out to be Gina, once more in a regressed child-like state. I asked what the problem was, and she replied 'It's George, he's after me with a pair of scissors ... and he says I've been a very naughty girl and need to be punished'. That sinking feeling rapidly returned again!

Hitting on a brainwave, I said 'I need to speak to George directly ... put him on the line'. Well, of course George declined to take the call! I told Gina that I was going to talk to her for a few moments and that she was likely to get very sleepy and drift into a deep trance while she was still carefully holding on to the phone and listening to every word I said. I gave her a countdown induction, and when she was in a trance I spoke directly to George. I asked him to safely dispose of the scissors, and then delineated a complete job description for him, stating that his one and only overriding intention should be to protect Gina fully at all times. I further suggested that he should completely reintegrate himself with Gina so that this protection could be fully expressed in ways that served her, context by context. He grunted in the affirmative! I led Gina out of the trance so that on 'awakening' she was completely back to her adult self.

Thankfully Gina had no more problems with George or the scissors, and I breathed a sigh of relief that this creative incident passed by without further event. I certainly learned more about the ecology of change work, and especially the importance of ensuring complete reintegration after the phobia cure and deep-trance work.

Other caveats

These two cases have been the only ones I have experienced over the last decade of practising NLP that had initial untoward outcomes which were later remedied. However, the point is clear – powerful technology can have powerful adverse effects.

Although I am quite happy to continue using NLP interventions in cases of anxiety and depression, I do now carefully check the patient's previous psychiatric history, looking for comorbid conditions. Personally I would not countenance working in depth with patients who have underlying psychosis and borderline personality disorders unless you either have specific training and expertise in this area or are working under the supervision of someone who fulfils those criteria.

This perhaps flies in the face of those in NLP who say that every condition has an underlying subjective structure, and simply changing that will 'cure' the patient – a somewhat simplistic view in my opinion from those who have little clinical experience 'in the trenches', and which on the whole does NLP no long-term good. However, there is encouraging work which shows that CBT interventions can be a useful adjunct to medication in treating these conditions.

There is always debate as to whether we should use NLP interventions in those who are on continuing medication (e.g. antidepressants). The theory goes that medication induces state-dependent learning, and that any NLP work which is undertaken when the patient is on medication will not carry over when they are better and the medication stops. This has not been my experience in general – there is often good carryover of therapeutic effect.

We can certainly argue about the efficacy of antidepressants which show a 50% recurrence rate of depression over two years, compared with CBT, which has a recurrence rate in the region of 20–25% – and even the question about whether antidepressants are any better than placebo. Yet trials combining CBT and antidepressants do show efficacy, and my view is that sometimes NLP combined with medication primes the patient for a better response rate. No comparable follow-up studies have ever been conducted with NLP alone, so the point is at best moot.

Unfortunately, anyone in the UK with any background whatsoever can train in NLP and begin to offer services to all and sundry from the high street. As long as this is confined to areas of performance enhancement and the treatment of habit disorders such as smoking cessation, little harm is likely to ensue. The Association of NLP (ANLP) has a psychotherapy division which is affiliated to the UK Council of Psychotherapists (UKCP). Membership requirements include annual assessment and ongoing supervision practices – a major step forward towards good clinical practice.

Propulsion systems

You will recall that a propulsion system occurs when a negative anchor is chained to a positive one in single or multiple steps. This gives a combination in sequence of 'move away from' and 'move towards' motivation. In general it can be useful in the treatment of some habit disorders, such as smoking cessation. However, there is little in the way of ecology in the system itself. Moreover, the negative anchor – the original problem stimulus – is left unchanged. It still needs to be accessed in order to give the initial 'push' to the system. It is probably all right to use this for minor issues, but you must be very wary of using it in patients with major issues.

Some schools of NLP use propulsion systems in a massive way to facilitate change. You may be asked to imagine just how bad life could get if your problem remained unchanged or even worsened. This is magnified out of all proportion and then associated as the negative anchor. Next you imagine just how good life could get once the problem was fully resolved. Massive amounts of pleasure are associated to this in turn. We now have a major propulsion system that is ready for action.

The problem with using propulsion in this way is that some people become stuck in the negative state and cannot get out of it. They become swamped by the unresourceful feelings and find that their problem may spiral out of control. Worse still, they may feel that there is nothing further they can do about it.

Instead of that worst-case scenario, they may be left with a polarity response. Sometimes they feel really good – sometimes they feel awful. This can have an effect similar to using the 'on–off' switch of a light. It is akin to having had two parts installed which communicate only poorly, if at all. This is not unlike the structure of manic depression.

If either of these alternatives arises, then you must do something to resolve the issue. First, it is important as a prelude to parts integration to ensure that you reduce the negative feelings associated to the 'move away from' part. You can do this by dissociating and then adding resources, much as in reimprinting. After all, the original positive intention of the negatively created aspect was to participate in a process to help to improve matters, so this aspect is still being honoured. The second step is to integrate and realign the parts, taking them into a new future. In his book *Transforming Your Self*, Steve Andreas suggests several ways to do this gently and ecologically.

Propulsion in sales

Propulsion systems are also used deliberately and covertly in sales as a technique to persuade the buyer to proceed with the transaction. During the discussions, any negative state or customer objection that is elicited is anchored spatially to one hand, and the positive states are anchored to the other. The salesperson can fire off the negative anchor when speaking of the consequences of not buying the product, and the positive anchor when discussing the benefits. I have seen this used with great precision and to good effect – in the sense that the customer bought the product.

The anchors can be used in other ways, too. Any talk that involves your competitors can be associated covertly to the negative anchor and the positive anchor can be used to attach good feelings to yourself. You can also elicit the client's decision-making strategy for a satisfying purchase and run your product through it. If you are very good you may also inoculate against buyer's remorse. This may seem a little far-fetched, but – believe me – it is entirely possible! Of course, many a good salesperson uses this as a natural part of their approach without being consciously aware that they are doing so. And many different types of sales training – both NLP and standard sales – teach what are essentially similar approaches.

Entrepreneurial sales approaches are a feature of many NLP training advertisements. The promise 'Change your life in a weekend' can be very alluring to many who are unhappy with their lot. Much of the advertising focuses on eliciting great states (of curiosity, wonder, excitement, etc.) and attaching them to your attendance at the seminar. Sometimes, however, it is all window-dressing, and the beautifully wrapped present turns out to be an empty cardboard box! Yet it is quite easy during the event to covertly install feelings of attraction, even compulsion to attend the next seminar in the series. Don't get me wrong – it is desirable to have the ability to access powerful feelings and states. However, do be careful about any financial decisions you make when you are in that kind of state!

It may be difficult to decide on the ethics of all this. On the one hand it may seem decidedly unfair, unethical or downright immoral! On the other, perhaps a salesperson is entitled to do what is required to make a living for himself and his family. There may be another way around this. If you first pre-qualify the buyer, you can ensure that your product fills a specific need that they have, and that this would be of value to them. If you get a congruent 'yes' at this point – conscious and unconscious calibration – then you have the green light to go for clinching the sale using all of the skills at your disposal. If not – then stop there. You can always send the buyer elsewhere.

In a sense, whether we are in sales or in therapy we are dealing with the same bottom-line – generating good feelings about the future. This may involve a greater or lesser degree of persuasion skills, depending on the individual concerned. I have certainly experienced its abusive side – and also seen it done with the integrity that allows both parties to get what they want. I shall leave you to decide on what is ethical and what is not, based on your own interpretation.

The myth of positive intention

One of the most widely quoted presuppositions of NLP over the years is that *'behind every behaviour lies a positive intention'*. It seems to me that much of the field of NLP has been built around it – so much so that the presupposition itself has become a reified truth. I have heard NLP practitioners and even trainers arguing vehemently that not only is this fundamental to all change work, but also it is an absolute requirement in the way that the unconscious mind preserves the contextual ecology in any intervention. At times this has been preached in such a fundamentalist way that we are in danger of mistaking the map for the territory.

Let me be clear from the outset that my belief – for what that is worth – is that the notion of positive intention is indeed a useful myth. Not the truth as such – simply a lie that we can utilise effectively. To find out why this is the case, we need to ask ourselves the question 'What is the purpose and function of this lie?' And before we answer it we need to step back and consider what the conscious and unconscious minds actually do.

One of the great attributes of the much maligned conscious mind is its tremendous ability to plan and organise. Without it we would still be living in caves with stone tools, surviving on instinct alone. Conscious minds are good at thinking about what we want to have happen in the future – and the kind of sequencing and ordering that is required to get us there. They help us to reflect on and make meaning out of our lives. What conscious minds are very poor at achieving is the actual *act* of getting there – the actual *doing* of the thing. Left to their own devices, they interfere with the very complex and poorly understood processes that co-ordinate our ability to do what we want. As an analogy, they would dig up the roots of a plant on a daily basis just to see how fast it was growing.

Unconscious minds, on the other hand, are very powerful beasts indeed. They co-ordinate, without interference, the multitude of physical and mental tasks that we undertake each day. If you are thirsty and decide to get a drink, you do not consciously move each muscle in an attempt to fill the glass. Having set the outcome, you trust your unconscious processes to get the job done without interference. Unconscious minds are the repositories of the kind of wisdom which, properly utilised, is concerned with ecology over the longer term – something that the conscious mind is too narrow in scope and function to accomplish adequately. The main drawback of the unconscious is its poor organisational abilities. When left to its own devices it will simply keep doing the same thing over and over again – ingrained habits and patterns.

So what does this have to do with positive intention? Well, the conscious and unconscious minds must learn how to work together in an integrated fashion. To do so, the conscious mind must set up the terms and conditions within which scope the unconscious mind can then function. Put bluntly, the conscious must organise the unconscious in some way – and then get out of the way! This is where the myth of positive intention is most useful. It operates as an organiser of change by creating a set of rules and conditions that act as a container for unconscious processes giving a direction for change. The positive intention is actually created by the procedure itself – mapping a linguistic category on to a set of neurological transforms. Positive intention *per se* does not exist at the neurological level.

Of course, we could equally well have the opposite presupposition – that behind every behaviour lies a negative intention. Some people live exclusively out of this model of the world, too! It will have a different direction for organising the unconscious mind, and equally powerful results. It is no more true or false than the preceding presupposition. The simple question is 'Which map do you choose to live your life from?'

Thus positive intention is simply a way to organise unconscious processes. Its critical function is to act as a *state changer*. A patient comes to see you with a particular problem. When that problem is seen through the lens of its positive intention, this causes a change in state. This new state offers a much wider perspective, where the problem behaviour is included in a much larger set of behaviours that can achieve a similar outcome. The *state change* is the catalyst here. So why not simply choose and apply any state at random to the negative situation?

It is, of course, quite possible to do this by applying any standard anchoring format. In theory, then, you could consciously choose a state which you think fits better, elicit and anchor it, and then collapse the anchors together. And the technology is sufficiently powerful for it to be possible that the change may last. Proponents of the positive intention model claim that over time, however, using the anchoring format in this way, the original problem will gradually surface again relatively unchanged. John Grinder states that any change which is consciously chosen without consulting the unconscious mind (*see* Chapters 5 and 13) has the odds stacked against long-term success. And I have to agree that this is often the case.

However, there is a way round this. Instead of just collapsing anchors with one or two elicited states, you can create a whole plethora of all the patient's best states and resources over time and integrate these together first as a 'super' state. This can then be added to the problem-state triggers, giving a whole new range of states and behaviours in response. In these circumstances, finding the positive intention becomes a moot point – the patient's unconscious is 'wired in' to all of its own problem-solving resources.

In New Code NLP (*see Whispering in the Wind* by Bostic St Clair and Grinder) there are a number of 'games' that fulfil this function. Various mind–body interactive games get the player into a high-performance flow state, completely in tune with all of their resources, and responding intuitively in the moment to novel experiences. When this state has been developed sufficiently, the player then steps into the previous problem context, where the triggers and contextual cues for the problem become 'rewired' to the flow state – completely changing the response. There is no reliance on the elicitation of historical states – the flow state is entirely here and now. As I see it, this flow state is a logical level above, and thus contains access to, the 'super' state. Again, positive intention becomes moot.

In summary, then, positive intention is simply a presuppositional tool for organising experience in a particular way. It is very useful, but it is not the 'truth'. There are other ways of organising resources for useful change that do not require the action of positive intention. The ability to continue to discriminate between the map and the territory is an important one.

Perception, projection and beliefs

One powerful approach which is utilised in some schools of NLP is the view that perception and projection are synonymous. That is, mind creates the world 'out there' as a projection of what is 'in here' – reality is entirely observer created. The intention of this presupposition is to suggest that we are the sole creators and masters of our own world – if we created it, then we can change it. Its purpose is to acknowledge and accept that we 'cause' whatever happens to us either as a conscious or an unconscious choice. It turns the individual from being a victim of the world to being a master of his own fate. Accepting this can lead to rapid and sometimes profound change.

However, applying this notion universally, so that you have complete responsibility for everything that happens in your world, can have unfortunate and deleterious effects. Presuppositions such as this can be a double-edged sword. For example, if your spouse is angry with you or depressed in him- or herself, then somehow you have 'caused' this to happen. If you have developed cancer or some other illness, then you have made an unconscious choice to have this disease – perhaps to learn a particular lesson in life. You could easily escalate this even more to perceive that the entire condition of the world today is projected by your mind, and thus you are responsible for wars and pestilence. A series of very depressing thoughts is generated which could end up becoming psychotic hallucinations and delusions!

Consider the more minor example of going for a job interview. By this token you are completely responsible for whether or not you get the job. A well-meaning NLP practitioner may anchor various powerful states in his client and tell him to hold in his mind the outcome picture of actually getting the job – despite the fact that there are several other applicants who are perhaps better qualified. He may be told 'Perception is projection. You create your own reality, and to the extent that you accept this you will easily be able to persuade the interviewers to give the job to you'. Of course, the client may fail to get the job for any number of valid reasons that are nothing to do with him personally, yet he will still feel like a failure. Insidiously he has also been victimised by the practitioner, who has encouraged a false appraisal of the various factors at work in employee selection.

I am a firm believer in the mind–body connection, and am aware of many anecdotal reports of cancer cures and remissions due to the use of visualisation techniques of one kind or another. There is no doubt that manipulation of internal representations can, by a whole variety of as yet incompletely explained neurohormonal and endocrine changes, cause major beneficial effects in serious illness. Yet I do not believe that it is ethical to say, in effect, that you have unconsciously chosen to create your cancer and are thus responsible for healing it. For the patient who is excited about mind–body interventions yet fails to manifest the sought-after changes, such failure may bring about intense guilt and self-blame. Worse still, I have heard grieving relatives being told that the deceased had an unconscious death wish and had chosen to die! This I believe is a completely unprincipled forcing of one person's model of the world on to another.

There is no doubt that, in one sense, people are responsible for the behaviours that may lead to cancer, such as choosing to smoke. Perhaps our part in the relationship with our spouse has contributed to their anger or depression. And we could probably all do a little more to promote the cause of world peace. Yet as I see it, this conflation of NLP with a particular philosophical approach – idealism – can insidiously cause an individual to become even more of a victim by virtue of self-blame: 'What has happened is my entire fault – I am completely responsible'. There is no discriminatory strategy at work here (as an aside, I suggest that you apply the entire meta-model to 'perception is projection' – you may get some interesting answers).

The opposite philosophical viewpoint is that of materialism – the mind is a mirror that faithfully reflects exactly what is 'out there'. Instead of being a projector, we are more like a camera that faithfully attempts to reproduce what it 'sees'. You cannot change it – only accept what 'is'. Given these two contrasting and opposite viewpoints, it is not surprising that a parts integration of sorts must take place.

We saw in Chapter 4 that data from the external world have to pass through a whole series of neurological transforms prior to our forming a representation of what is out there. The information is changed in a number of ways during this process – by deletion, distortion, and generalisation – so the mind is definitely *not* simply a mirror reflecting exactly what it sees. In the case of 'perception is projection', there is a simple experiment you can try. Choose a busy road, step out in front of a truck and see if you can stop it by changing the perception in your mind. Try something smaller first, like a bicycle – it hurts less!

Integrating these two perspectives gives *co-construction* – a much more helpful stance. In effect this view states that the world out there really *does* exist and we perceive it through a set of neurologically modified perceptions which gives us a mental and linguistic interpretation of what is actually there. It is this aspect that is entirely malleable. The changed interpretation once again interacts with the world in a recursive loop to co-construct something else – in a continuum.

In the case of a physical reality such as a mountain, you can change your interpretation of it, yet it remains the same physical entity. You can change your perceptions about another human being and, although they are still physically the same, your revised interpretation may cause them to behave differently. This is because you yourself will have changed the way in which you approach them – you are communicating differently, and they may well do likewise. You may have a creative idea about a new product which exists only in your mind – yet over time you bring it into existence. If you look around the room you are currently in, everything you see was at one time no more than a thought.

Approaching a job interview, an altercation with your spouse or a patient with cancer in this way allows you to let go of the effort of having to be responsible for everything. In essence you take charge of those things which you can personally do something about, and acknowledge that there are other variables about which you can do little. You can discriminate one from the other. However, you can take the feedback from each encounter as new information to help you to plan your next response. Your responsibility as such is in *how* you respond.

Co-construction is – in my view – a more balanced way to approach NLP interventions. It follows the old adage of controlling what is within your sphere of influence, and not wasting time or energy on what is outside that. Of course, knowing where the boundaries lie between the two helps a lot! For those of you who are more interested in the philosophical aspects of this section, I suggest that you read any work by Ken Wilber.

Beliefs

Before we leave this section altogether, I want to mention something about beliefs, which are also filters for perceiving the world. As a keen and enthusiastic investigator of all NLP matters, I have travelled far and wide attending one seminar or another. When some delegates find out that I am also a medical practitioner, there often ensues a lively debate where I am taken to task for the failure of the medical profession to fully incorporate NLP principles and practices – and also for the beliefs that the profession holds, especially about the causation and treatment of mental illness.

Strangely enough, these debates occasionally centre on conditions such as multiple personality disorder (MPD) – there is still great medical debate about whether or not this condition truly exists. Certainly from a lay perspective it is a condition that catches the eye. Usually once the practitioners have learned the visual squash method for integrating parts they can see no reason why MPD should not be cured by such a process – in about 20 minutes or so! When I attempt to explain how challenging it is to treat chronic enduring mental illness, and that there are no 'quick fixes', I am usually subjected to a barrage of views, generally stating similar things, the commonest of which is that 'of course it takes a long time if you believe it will!'

It seems that it is my belief which is preventing rapid resolution of the problem. If only I changed my belief, my patients would get better more swiftly. Since beliefs shape and alter our reality, there is no doubt that changing them can have profound effects. Yet I have serious misgivings about the idea that MPD will get better in 20 minutes whether I believe it is so or not! This kind of response is not uncommon in NLP circles, as there is a general failure to understand that delusions are also types of beliefs – it is important to separate one from the other. Convictions are also strong beliefs, and those who have worked with deluded individuals will know how difficult it is to shift them once they are embedded.

As usual, an invitation to practical experience can sometimes help to sort this out (not always, though). My usual counter these days is to ask 'Do you think you could survive being electrocuted in the electric chair?' If the answer is 'Yes', I happily offer to organise the demonstration and sell tickets for the event. If the answer is 'No', then I reply 'No problem ... we can simply use an NLP belief-change technique of your choice ... change the belief so that you believe you will survive ... then we'll do the demonstration ...' To date I have had no takers.

Another common area where beliefs are invoked is in the realm of behavioural change. This goes along the lines that a patient must believe that the intervention is going to work for it actually to do so. If the intervention fails, 'your beliefs prevented the change – they stopped you letting go of the problem'. This is of course a fail-safe for the practitioner – as the patient is fully responsible for making the change. If the change fails to materialise, then the patient 'caused' this to happen by faulty thinking. Some practitioners try to stack the odds for change by charging large sums of money for each session. This, they argue, increases commitment and belief in the outcome, thereby markedly increasing the likelihood of success. Sadly, if that were really true then all we would have to do would be to charge extortionate sums, perform any 'magic ritual' and change would occur – and undoubtedly this *can* occasionally happen. To their credit, some therapists do offer money-back guarantees!

There is no doubt that some patients can and will resist change. As Michael Yapko says, 'a depressed patient can defeat the therapist simply by doing nothing'. Yet for many change processes, beliefs are in a sense irrelevant. Many patients do not believe that the phobia cure will get rid of their problem. When they have had the process explained to them, some are even more sceptical. Yet change happens – and belief in the process is not necessarily required. Many techniques, such as anchoring, work directly on conditioned responses that are found in the subcortical processes of the limbic system. It is the result – a new and changed *experience* – which forms a new belief. In this case beliefs are changed *after* the fact. In effect, beliefs are an integral part of the state you are in at the time. Change the state and the belief changes, too – and vice versa. You can intervene on many different levels.

Rather than working on beliefs directly, you can change them indirectly by therapeutic tasking. This is when you give the patient a particular behavioural task to do, such as a homework assignment, the completion of which allows the belief to change naturally. Essentially you are prescribing a behavioural counter-example to their current situation, yet it must be 'dressed up' in such a way that the patient has no conscious clue about the covert outcome. There are many different ways of performing tasking. One that I like is the paradoxical intervention of 'symptom prescription'. Essentially you ask the patient to 'perform' their symptoms at a particular time and place. The act of consciously doing what was an unconscious process can be very powerful.

The aggressive battle-cry, 'That's just a belief ... you can change it' can be heard on almost any NLP training course. Yet some beliefs are more useful for change than others. Limiting beliefs about self and core identity issues are generally more fruitful targets. John Grinder has a different approach. He suggests that beliefs act as feedforward filters which can actually prevent you from having direct experience of the world – better to have no beliefs at all! He recommends that you develop the ability to congruently step into *any* belief system you choose – much as you would change your shirt. When you can do this in a variety of different contexts and conditions, it is functionally equivalent to having no beliefs at all. The benefit is that you are then more open to what is happening right now – with less judgement.

Models and change

The tremendous excitement, curiosity and experimentation that were around in the early formative days of NLP must have been very heady indeed. The early practitioners and investigators dived headlong into exploring new approaches and methodologies. They had a tendency to learn a particular technique, experiment with the effects that it had in a variety of situations and then, having noted their successes, lay it aside. This was so that they could push the edge of their map towards completely new and different approaches which could achieve similar or even better results.

Today things are a little different. Many aspects of NLP seem to have become reified truths over time (timelines, logical levels, meta-states, etc.). Several different schools of NLP offer their own championed methodologies, the covert statement being that this is the 'right' way to do NLP. In one sense it is useful to put together a training package that can allow new practitioners to rapidly acquire powerful therapeutic change methodologies and techniques and have a structure as an *aide-mémoire*. However, prepackaging in this way may cause many to fail to explore the other equally valid approaches – each of which has something valuable to offer.

It is not uncommon at conferences to hear practitioners of one persuasion or another arguing about the merits of a particular approach to utilising timelines. What most fail to realise is that each approach is simply one way to organise perceptions so that the conscious mind can be convinced that change has occurred. In fact, teaching clients about timelines and going into detail about how change occurs through their use is a form of psycho-education, so that they 'buy into' the model of change. By providing a conscious mind rationale for the technique you are about to apply, you can increase therapeutic rapport and fulfil many of the demand characteristics that we explored in Chapter 18.

In truth, it does not matter a whit which change technique you use – it is simply a model, not the real thing! For the same presenting issue you can employ a behavioural change mechanism that occurs in the here and now (extinction by *in vivo* exposure), float into the past and find the root-cause imprint, or float into the future to the time when the problem has been solved. Each of these approaches can work with exactly the same set of problems. In fact, all change happens in the here and now. What differs is the client's specific perception that you work on in order to make that change. All that these techniques do is to format the unconscious mind for more streamlined transformation.

In a sense, all of the techniques you have been exposed to in this book are lies – there, I admit it! For you to believe that they are NLP is to risk the reification of a specific tool so that it remains unchanged. These tools are simply a by-product of a way of thinking about change which incorporates excitement, exploration, intense curiosity and a desire to push back the frontiers of current knowledge and application. This is NLP! All the different schools of NLP have within them some 'golden nuggets', and we should celebrate these aspects of their excellence. I encourage you to learn about the different approaches, whether by reading, listening to tapes or attending courses. However, most of all you should learn how to do the modelling process for yourself. Then you will simply make up your own techniques as you go along, as well as incorporating the best that other role models have to offer.

Concluding

Any powerful technology for change has both an upside and a downside. There can be adverse effects caused by the techniques themselves, regardless of the good intentions of the practitioner who is using them – good intentions alone have never guaranteed underlying skill. It is vitally important to be aware of both your strengths and your limitations when engaging with patients, particularly those with chronic or severe mental health problems. These patients deserve particularly skilled attention, not some haphazard technique from someone who has attended a training course and read a book or two.

Thankfully, many NLP practitioners whom I have met have had a strong sense of personal integrity, and willingness to use the tools both for their own development and for respectfully assisting others in changing. However, there are a few who appear to use this powerful technology for their own personal gain. They have no qualms about covertly using potent persuasion tools to get their own way – at the expense of others. At least if you know a little about how NLP can be used unethically, you can be better prepared both to spot it and to do something about it.

In ending this chapter I would like to make a strong plea for using NLP with congruence and integrity. In particular, I believe that it is unhelpful for the practitioner to delve too deeply into content, or indeed to inflict their own personal content on the patient. Interventions should be carried out at a process level, with much respect for and calibration to unconscious processing. With these intentions in place, inadvertent mishaps are less likely to occur and our patients can be assured of a better matching of skills to their presenting issues.

CHAPTER 20

Further along the path ...

Introduction

This is the final chapter of *Changing with NLP*, and I trust that you have both enjoyed the read and developed your skills – whether you know this consciously yet or not. And not only that – I hope the topics included in this book have whetted your appetite to pursue your further exploration and development, whether by reading more from the Bibliography, listening to audiotapes of seminars or actually attending a training course.

This is a time not only to reflect on what you have learned thus far, but also to contemplate how the future – your future – might be different. Many things can happen when you begin to incorporate a body of knowledge such as NLP into your everyday life. Some may simply elect to have things remain more or less the same as before. Many will already have begun to contemplate just how to integrate this material fully within their consulting practice. Others may be thinking about just what new directions and pathways have opened up for them now – and how to take the next steps.

Yet before this it is important to mention one or two things about the body of knowledge that you have been learning and integrating into your daily behaviours. One major fallacy that often occurs is to reify this knowledge into something called 'The Truth'. The processes and techniques that you have been assimilating so far are only the crest of the current wave of development in the field. They are only the historical products of the best of today's thinking. If you accept them as the right way, the only way, the best way, then you will be doing yourself – and NLP – a major disservice. In 100 years' time people may look back and laugh at our rudimentary knowledge and understandings of today. The past is not necessarily a good predictor of the future!

The 'truth' is that we do not yet know what is possible or what the future holds in terms of further developments. If you cast your mind back over the last 25 to 50 years of development in your current field, you will notice that change does not occur at a steady, linear rate along a well-defined trajectory. More often than not there are fits and starts, interesting tangents and diversions with some cul-de-sacs and dead ends, together with the occasional unpredictable quantum leap that may revolutionise a field. Our current body of reified knowledge is tenuous to say the least – grasp it lightly, and not as a drowning man clutching at a straw.

There is always so much more to learn in every field of human enquiry. So how should we proceed? Personally I think that it is important to take the time to digest carefully all of the current offerings. The process of digestion has several phases. First you eat until you are replete – satisfied without being overstuffed. Then, of course, there needs to be a gap before you indulge further. And during this time period what is useful to our continuing growth and development is assimilated, while simultaneously there is a sorting out of that which needs to be eliminated. This sorting, sifting, assimilation and elimination occurs in a continuous cycle from our first breath to our last. It is an apposite metaphor for knowledge management.

So with that under our belts we shall now consider what developments are already taking place and which areas we can speculate on further.

What is in store for NLP?

Even as I write this book I am aware of other developments in the field which have exciting potential. Rather than attempting to include everything that is happening, I shall look briefly at two areas which are in some senses at opposite ends of the NLP spectrum. Steve Andreas has written about his developing model of self-concept and John Grinder has written about New Code NLP games for high-performance states of excellence. Andreas deals with the more lofty generalisations that we might call beliefs and attitudes about ourselves, whereas Grinder stays more at the level of sensory-based behavioural description. Both approaches are providing interesting results.

Steve Andreas has actually been working on a model of self-concept for the last decade, patiently piecing the parts together. His book, *Transforming Your Self* (*see* Bibliography) gives all the details of how to use it for best effect. Steve has taken concepts such as resilience, tenacity, thoughtfulness, honesty and (his favourite) kindness, and found out exactly how, using submodalities, various people build these generalisations about themselves. He provides a very thorough and detailed exploration of the basis of self-esteem, which is our evaluation of our self-concept – for good or ill.

As well as modelling how all of these parts fit together, he has formulated simple and ecological methods not only for changing and updating conflicting aspects of self-concept, but also for building from scratch previously non-existing elements. This approach is particularly useful for 'parts' conflicts of minor to major degree. The whole process is gently integrative, and in my view it super-sedes the more blunderbuss visual squash – the cusp of the next wave of develop-ment. I believe that it will be a useful tool for conceptualising, investigating and treating conditions such as depression, manic depression and even paranoia, which can all be formulated as disorders of self-concept.

Steve Andreas has also been exploring states such as certainty and uncertainty, self-reference, recursion and paradox (especially of the double-bind variety). He has clarified how each relates to the other and the way in which linguistic interventions can produce change. It is interesting how you can begin to create a therapeutic double bind whereby the patient gets better no matter which choice they make. Our understanding of the whole area of scope, category, levels of meaning and logical types is woolly at best, so reformulating these with suggestions for application merits further exploration. This will help to clarify further such concepts as meta-states and show more clearly which types of intervention do what.

John Grinder has further developed what he calls New Code NLP in *Whispering in the Wind* (*see* Bibliography). This is an aspect of NLP which looks to incorporate more effectively aspects of non-conscious functioning that have hitherto been ignored. One major aspect of this is *high-performance states*. These are flow states in which the performer is fully engaged in the here and now, adapting to and dealing with novel stimuli as they arise. A good example of this would be a champion athlete of any sport in full flight. So just what is happening here?

A high-performance state is one in which you have full access to any and all of your resources at a moment's notice. You are fully engrossed 'in the game', and in a sense you have 'forgotten' all about your self. Rather than thinking about what you are going to do and what resources you are going to deploy in a particular situation, you are totally in the moment, dealing spontaneously with what happens next. There is no self-consciousness – you are in the flow. Grinder has developed a series of New Code games which can generate this type of high-performance flow state within any individual in 10 to 15 minutes.

In a sense a high-performance state is the set of all states available to a person at any one time. At one level you can access and anchor a single state, such as confidence or determination. The next level above that is when you collapse several resource states together, so that no matter which one you start from, the rest are available simultaneously – a stacked anchor or super-state. The high-performance state exists at a logical level above, yet includes access to this super-state – as well as any other super-states that you have set up co-temporaneously. It is a content-free state in comparison with states that have been anchored in the usual way, because it does not depend on taking the content of the historical past state into the present moment.

Having identified a context for change and the triggering cues, Grinder asks the patient to 'play the game', calibrating to ensure that they are in a flow state. At a certain point (after 10 to 15 minutes) he abruptly steps them back into the problem context while they are in the high-performance state, with instructions just to notice what happens rather than try to 'do' something consciously. Thus there is a non-conscious choice of the most appropriate resource for that situation. Grinder has identified several different types of game which fulfil his criteria for high performance, and it appears to be a very generative model which is worth exploring with a variety of problem presentations.

So far NLP in the clinical domain has mainly confined itself to treating standard mental health problems (e.g. anxiety and depression) and psychosomatic conditions (e.g. irritable bowel syndrome, asthma, etc.). There are also anecdotal reports of treatments for what would be termed diseases and disorders, such as cancer. There is now room for clinical studies of the first two categories mentioned above by trained medical (or other) practitioners to seek to validate NLP methodologies and techniques by evidence-based research. Given that the mind and the body are part of one whole system of interaction, it would be fascinating to utilise NLP techniques alongside conventional medical therapy for chronic conditions such as neurological degenerative disease (e.g. Parkinson's disease, multiple sclerosis, etc.), ischaemic heart disease and chronic obstructive pulmonary disease, as well as the myriad cancers. Finding out how a patient represents their disease process internally (VAKOG) and then manipulating the submodalities would be most intriguing.

One way to think of illness is as a kernel of disease surrounded by the patient's attitudes, beliefs and future expectations about what that disease personally means to them, and its future prognosis. NLP can certainly deal very effectively with the illness cognitions, and changing these may possibly alter the underlying disease process. However, what if we conceptualised the disease itself being held in place by and even consisting of a series of anchored responses (both internal and external)? What if the disease itself actually caused a state-dependent phenomenon which maintained its existence?

Whether this is a 'true' representation of the situation or not is a moot point. However, if we acted 'as if' it were true and targeted our interventions to alter and change the underlying state, this might have potential for a therapeutic response. Oncologists are refining their approaches to chemotherapy to seek a 'magic bullet' that targets and can be delivered to cancer cells alone, leaving the other healthy cells intact. We know that different states of mind and body have different chemical signatures, both neurologically and physiologically. Perhaps, then, we can look for a similar 'magic bullet' of states which could perform a parallel function. You may well be able to think of other suitable areas of potential intervention.

Finally in this section, just a brief word about the explosion of neurological research that has occurred during the last decade. The advent of fMRI scanners has revolutionised our ability to see what is happening in the brain moment by moment in a whole host of disorders. These highly accurate scans – which will become even more accurate in the near future – are beginning to trace the subtle interplay between ordered and disordered thoughts, neuronal pathways and networks, together with the fluctuating brain chemistry in disease and health. The studies which have already been conducted can do much to help us to specify which interventions to use and when (e.g. conditioned fear and the amygdala). However, scanners may become sufficiently sophisticated for interventions such as NLP techniques to be followed and tracked in real time in order to determine their mechanisms and pathways of action. The future is definitely not what it used to be!

What will happen if ...?

Having just thought about the future from the perspective of NLP, we need to turn our attention to a future that is even more important ... your own. One of the problems that many people may face after reading a book like this is deciding what they are going to put into action first. We have covered a huge amount of material in *Changing with NLP*, and thinking about it all at once may leave you feeling rather overwhelmed. There is literally so much choice about what to focus on for the next few days, weeks or even months ahead.

Overwhelm is a strategy of chunking up on *all* of the things that you feel you have to do and seeing them *all* together at one time. It is a little like trying to see the whole forest at once, rather than focusing on each tree individually. Many authors leave you completely to your own devices in this regard, which can sometimes mean that although you enjoyed the read, and gained some new knowledge, concepts and attitudes, as yet you have failed to put any of it into practice. However, I would like you to have a different fate – one that gives you the maximum opportunity to gain new behaviours from your endeavours.

When you think about all the ground that we have covered so far, some aspects will spring directly to the front of your mind, while others will be tantalisingly at the edge of conscious awareness. Some of the approaches and techniques will seem intuitively correct, while others, like Pavlov, may be ringing a bell somewhere inside. I would like you to keep all of these thoughts in mind as you go ahead and complete the last exercise in this book. You may well be glad that you did ...

Exercise 19:   What will happen if ...?

1   As you examine your thoughts and look back through the various chapters of this book, choose three areas that stand out for you. Choose those that would make the most difference if you incorporated them into your future behaviours. You can note them down if you wish.

2   Take each area and get really specific about what it is that you are doing differently. As you picture yourself, notice how you walk, talk, move and gesture differently. Listen to the sound of your voice and the words as you say them. Adjust all the internal imagery until it feels just right.

3   Examine each area in turn. Notice how others are responding to you differently. Look at the expressions on their faces and their body language. Listen to their words and voice tones as they reply, and notice their different behaviours.

4   Now, as you settle back in the theatre of your mind's eye, allow these three areas to coalesce in a collage. You don't need to see them clearly ... just pretend that you do. Imagine that all of the skills are merging and integrating and, as they do ... step inside, try them on for size and luxuriate in the feelings.

5   Now let's go for a trip into the future on your timeline. Take all of the feelings, skills and resources and imagine that you are in next week ... in a specific context where you work ... and notice how things are different. Do the same for one month, three months, and then as far out in time as you'd like to go now.

6   And from that point in the future, look all the way back to now ... sensing how your skills have continued to develop over this time ... even in ways that you're not yet fully aware of. Allow yourself to come back to the here and now, only as quickly as you're integrating everything in your best interests ...

You can use this exercise or adapt it to a walking timeline approach to help sow the seeds of change in any future direction that you wish to take. It can have very powerful, aligning effects as it helps to increase your self-efficacy. It is well worth repeating again at some point in the near future with three different areas of your choosing.

First steps ... reprise

We have come a very long way in this particular journey since the opening few pages of *Changing with NLP*. Those very first patients who experienced my initial interventions after I had read *Frogs into Princes* have survived a decade to tell the tale. What has happened to them during that time?

The woman whose mother was terminally ill remains a non-smoker to this day (her mother was less fortunate and died shortly thereafter, though). What was it that caused her to stop smoking after a simple pattern interrupt of 'Just how surprised will you be when you stop smoking next week?' The answer lay partly in her reply: 'I *will* be surprised!' She used and emphasised the word *will* rather than *would*, which in itself seems a minor detail. Yet this emphasis on the definite future-tense *will* as opposed to the conditional-tense *would* is very important. The former makes the change far more likely to take place than the latter. How many times do we say 'I would if I could' – yet we don't!? The word *will*, when accompanied by a completely congruent physiology, increases the chances markedly.

The other factor was that I slipped this into the conversation as a non sequitur which abruptly interrupted her thought processes and induced a mini-trance state, which for all its brevity was quite deep. The fact that I knew this patient well and already had a good level of rapport that had been built up through many encounters was also of paramount importance in ensuring the result. As for my own state, I was in experimentation mode and had no vested interest in the outcome either way. I was just practising! Yet the result was a major indicator to me both that lasting change could occur in such a brief encounter – and of the power of language in a well-timed question. From that day on I also began to pay more attention to the works and words of Milton Erickson.

You will recall that Janine's dental phobia had been cured in one session. A few years later she reminded me of the fact as she proudly showed me her new false teeth – she had had a total dental clearance under general anaesthetic! The NLP fast phobia cure has undergone some revisions since those days to ensure that the changes are more easily locked in. The submodality shifts and movie reversal in fast time make it one of the more effective NLP techniques available. And I hear that some people are using an even faster process for simple phobias, with good results!

Janine also had a mastectomy for breast carcinoma eight years ago. She had been intrigued by the success of the fast phobia cure, and as well as her conventional medical treatment she used meditation and guided imagery to help her get well again after surgery. I cannot say for certain whether any of these adjuvant procedures made any difference to her recovery and continued survival.

However, Janine believes that they did. More importantly, though, they gave her a feeling of personal mastery, control and fighting spirit which she displays to this day.

Marilyn, you will recall, had suffered a double bereavement, yet my clumsy attempts with a collapsing anchors process had paid huge dividends, with a complete and sustained resolution of her symptoms. The Medical Defence Union did not need to be involved, and my main learning point was to use knuckles rather than knees for anchors! Of course, these days I use a version of the slightly more sophisticated grief resolution process of Steve and Connirae Andreas, which employs visual anchors instead. Again it is one of the most useful tools in the NLP toolbox.

Two years ago Marilyn was severely tested once more, and I had a first-hand opportunity to witness the generative learning that had taken place following our initial encounter. Unfortunately, another son who suffered from a chronic medical condition died suddenly. Marilyn displayed the normal and appropriate signs that I would have expected of anyone in acute grief. I arranged to see her for some follow-up visits over the next few months. However, within a few weeks it became apparent that things were different this time. When she spoke of her son it was of past remembered good times rather than sadness. And her memories were stored visually in a similar place to those of her other son and her father. She had spontaneously and automatically reorganised her perceptions – evidence of the kind of deep learning that is possible with NLP processes.

Concluding

The final section of any book is awash with a mixed set of feelings. There is the undoubted satisfaction of being able to look back and acknowledge the vast amount of ground we have covered so far in our journey together. There may even be particular highlights that spring to mind, particular areas and topics that you have enjoyed immensely – special favourites. For some there may also be a tinge of sadness, almost a feeling of loss that the last chapter of this adventure is nearly at a close. Yet for others there is a sense of completion and a turning towards writing your own future chapters – well, metaphorically at least!

I have gained an enormous amount from putting down on paper my thoughts about the mechanisms of learning and changing together with exploring the vast potential of the NLP approach. I hope that you have gained as much through your own commitment to reading this far. I have tried to be as thorough as I can, yet at the same time to sow the seeds for your own further investigations. So with these thoughts very much in mind, what is it exactly that you have gained for yourself?

For the counsellor, nurse and those in professions allied to medicine, what is it that you have learned which will help you to deal with the multitude of issues that are presented to you on a daily basis? In particular, I hope that the sections on grief resolution and dysfunctional codependent relationships have given you more ways to facilitate resolution in these situations. What do you believe now about rapid change? And what are your own next steps?

For the psychiatrist, I hope that you have been given enough information to help you to expand your choices in dealing with chronic and enduring mental illness. Which approaches in particular will you be adding to your repertoire? Would you benefit from further training? Or do you want a period of consolidation before you move forward again?

If you are a physician, surgeon or hospital doctor in another specialty, what exactly have you learned anew? How do you see yourself dealing differently with difficult diabetics or patients with chronic lung disease, high anaesthetic risk, chronic pain and cancer? The ability to deal with challenging issues in a new way will give you another string to your bow. What would happen, both for you and for your patients, if you were to continue to develop these skills?

As a general practitioner, you may already have identified a whole host of different areas to which you can apply your learning. You are the first point of contact in the chain of medical care, and you have an opportunity to deal with the entire spectrum of illness and disease presented at different stages of advancement – from early to late. How will you be dealing differently with the nicotine addicts, the grossly overweight, the worried well, the anxious, the depressed – and any others that come to mind? Which particular issues will you focus on first? Which of the techniques are you completely comfortable with and which need more practice? Of all the health professionals addressed so far, you may have the potential to make the biggest impact across the board.

So finally, for you the reader, as you *really* think about it, just how easy is it for people to change? Given the skills that you have now acquired, how easy is it for your patients – and you – to develop new thinking patterns, new behaviours and new responses to old situations, so that they and you really can *do something different* – both subjectively and objectively? The process of effective change can be disarmingly simple and rapid when you attend to the underlying principles. I wish you good fortune as you use the tools of *Changing with NLP* to go about making a considerable difference in lives – both theirs and yours.

Glossary of terms

Accessing cues The subtle behaviours of eye movements, postures and gestures indicating which representational system (VAKOG) a person is thinking with.

Anchoring Associative classical conditioning whereby an external trigger is linked to an internal response or state. This can be reaccessed overtly or covertly.

Association Seeing, hearing and feeling the world as if one is completely inside the experience, whether it be right here and now, or a remembered or imagined event.

Auditory The sensory modality of hearing, speaking, sounds and words.

Behaviours External observable actions; 'what' we do.

Beliefs The operational rules that connect values to behaviours. Beliefs form three main categories about (a) causation, (b) meaning and (c) boundaries in (1) the world around us, (2) our behaviour, (3) our capabilities and (4) our identity.

Break state An abrupt interruption of the current state, especially if it is negative or unresourceful.

Calibration The ability to read non-verbal responses and behavioural cues accurately, linking them to specific internal states.

Chunking The amount of information that is considered at any one time. Chunking up leads to more abstraction, chunking down leads to more details, and chunking laterally leads to analogy, simile or metaphor.

Congruence A state in which all parts of yourself are aligned and working together in harmony.

Content The who and what of a situation.

Context The where and when of a situation; the environment in which it takes place.

Criteria The standards by which something is evaluated; values.

Critical submodality The driver submodality which, when changed, automatically changes the rest.

Dissociation Experiencing an event as if you are outside yourself, observing.

Ecology The study of consequences; ensuring that outcomes and changes fit with the rest of the system.

Embedded commands Using a downward tonality to _mark out_ what you want someone to do.

Environment Where and when something takes place; the context.

Eye-accessing cues The specific eye positions for remembered and constructed pictures and sounds, feelings and self-talk.

Feedback The external response to your behaviour which gives you information about what to do next.

Future pace A rehearsal of future actions connecting present resources to specific behaviours.

Gustatory Relating to the sense of taste.

Incongruence The experience of being at odds with oneself, in inner conflict; wanting one thing yet doing another. Simultaneous incongruence occurs when both parts of the conflict are expressed together. Sequential incongruence occurs when one part is expressed at a later time.

Kinaesthetic Relating to body sensations, feelings and emotions.

Logical levels The various levels of experience divided into a hierarchy of environment, behaviours, beliefs and values, identity and beyond. Useful for organising thinking about problems, resources and interventions.

Matching and mirroring The behavioural elements of establishing rapport at the level of physiology and voice.

Meta-model A set of questions to specifically explore deletions, generalisations and distortions.

Metaphor The process of thinking about one thing in terms of another; a story that can be used to generate change.

Metaprogramme A fundamental out-of-awareness information filter that acts across many contexts and determines our general responses to experiences.

Modelling The 'how to' of finding out about and replicating another person's skills; finding the difference that makes the difference.

Model of the world A description of a person's internal map of experience.

Neuro-linguistic programming The study of the structure of subjective experience; the process of creating models of excellence.

Olfactory Relating to the sense of smell.

Outcome A goal which meets the criteria for a well-formed outcome.

Pacing and leading Building rapport by matching part(s) of another's experience prior to moving in a direction of mutual gain.

Parts A metaphorical way of talking about our needs, desires and behaviours in different situations. 'It's like part of me wants X and part of me wants Y.'

Perceptual positions Moving mentally between being in your own shoes (*first position*), the shoes of another (*second position*) and a fly on the wall (*third position*). Very useful for negotiating successfully.

Predicates The words that indicate which representational system is being used: visual, auditory, kinaesthetic, olfactory, gustatory or unspecified (digital).

Process The 'how' of a situation, as opposed to the content (the 'what').

Quotes Richard Bandler was quoted as saying 'You can give people information by saying what someone else said, thus removing your overt influence'.

Rapport The mutual dance of responsiveness as you align with another person.

Reframing Changing the meaning of an event by changing the frame that surrounds it. There are many ways to do this, including the 14 verbal reframing patterns.

Resource state Usually a positive past experience which can be brought to bear on the here and now to effect change.

Sensory acuity The ability to detect the more subtle nuances in what is seen, heard and felt.

Sensory-based description Describing what is happening or has happened in terms of what can be seen, heard and touched.

State The sum total of all mental and physical activities and feelings that are going on at one time.

Strategies A set of explicit thinking and behavioural steps for achieving a specified result.

Submodalities The basic building blocks of experience. The qualities of each of the five sensory modalities (VAKOG).

Synaesthesia See–feel and hear–feel circuits whereby accessing the first automatically accesses the second simultaneously. Phobias are a prime example.

Timelines The unconscious arrangement of past experiences and future expectations, usually seen as a line from left to right or from front to back.

Translation Rephrasing words from one representational system to another. For example, 'see what you mean' (V) and 'loud and clear' (A).

Values The answer to the question 'What is important to you?'. Important standards that we aspire to, such as honesty, integrity, making a difference, achievement, etc.

Visual Relating to the sense of sight.

Well-formed outcome criteria Goals that are stated in positives, initiated and maintained by the self, have sensory-based evidence for evaluating success, preserve current by-products, and have an ecological fit.

Bibliography and other resources

In this section I list the various texts that have been used as reference material for *Changing with NLP*. The psychology and neurology references are the specific books that have formed the cognitive backbone of learning and changing theory, against which the NLP techniques have been contrasted and compared. Also included is a general NLP reading list together with a list of other books that I personally have found useful in my own studies of the theory and practice of effective change.

Psychology and neurology references

- Carter R (1998) *Mapping the Mind*. Weidenfeld and Nicolson. Draws on the latest brain-imaging techniques to disclose human behaviour. Very well illustrated.
- Cash A (2002) *Psychology for Dummies*. Hungry Minds, Inc. A light-hearted and down-to-earth approach to the psychology of behaviour. An entertaining read.
- Damasio A (2000) *The Feeling of What Happens: body, emotion and the making of consciousness*. Vintage. A professor of neurology, Damasio is a leading world expert on the neurophysiology of emotions.
- France R and Robson M (1997) *Cognitive Behavioural Therapy in Primary Care*. Jessica Kingsley Publishers. A practical book on how to use cognitive–behavioural interventions effectively in day-to-day general practice.
- Gross R (1996) *Psychology: the science of mind and behaviour* (3e). Hodder and Stoughton. A complete textbook on the nature and scope of psychology geared to undergraduate level. A weighty reference work!
- LeDoux J (1996) *The Emotional Brain*. Touchstone. A book by the foremost researcher on the brain mechanisms of conditioned fear responses.
- Ogden J (2000) *Health Psychology* (2e). Open University Press. An accessible and comprehensive guide to all of the major topics in health psychology. Well referenced and easily readable.
- *Psychiatry*. The Medicine Publishing Company Ltd. A continuously updated textbook of psychiatry published chapter by chapter on a monthly basis.

Each chapter, with various editors, gives multi-author views on all aspects of psychiatry. The series advisors are George Szmuckler and André Tylee. An excellent resource.

- Ramachandran VS (1998) *Phantoms in the Brain*. Fourth Estate. A book written by a world-renowned neurologist who uses fascinating case histories to artfully illustrate the neuroanatomy of how we perceive the external world. It gives major insights into phantom limb pain and its treatment.
- Salkovskis PM (ed.) (1996) *Frontiers of Cognitive Therapy*. The Guilford Press. A compilation of current interventions across the spectrum of psychological disorders by many noted researchers and clinicians.
- Spiegler M and Guevremont D (1998) *Contemporary Behavior Therapy* (3e). Brooks/Cole Publishing Company. A superb resource with many behavioural interventions across a wide spectrum of disorders.

General NLP reading list

- Andreas S (2002) *Transforming Your Self*. Real People Press. Describes the process of building self-concept and self-esteem. Cutting-edge material at the forefront of NLP development.
- Andreas S and Andreas C (1990) *Heart of the Mind*. Real People Press. Each chapter details a client problem together with NLP tools for change. Many useful patterns are included.
- Andreas S and Andreas C (1987) *Change Your Mind – and Keep the Change*. Real People Press. An in-depth look at various submodality patterns, including timelines.
- Andreas S and Faulkner C (1996) *NLP: the new technology of achievement*. Nicholas Brealey Publishing. An American-based introduction to NLP with plenty of submodality exercises. Comprehensive coverage.
- Bandler R and Grinder J (1975 and 1976) *The Structure of Magic 1 and 2*. Science and Behaviour Books. An in-depth study of the meta-model.
- Bandler R and Grinder J (1979) *Frogs into Princes*. Real People Press. The first edited transcribed seminar. Contains many techniques, and is fun filled and irreverent!
- Bandler R and MacDonald W (1988) *An Insider's Guide to Submodalities*. Meta Publications. An intriguing look at various submodality patterns for change.
- Bostic St Clair C and Grinder J (2001) *Whispering in the Wind*. J & C Enterprises. Covers the epistemology of NLP and the development of New Code applications.
- Charvet SR (1995) *Words That Change Minds*. Kendall/Hunt. Excellent examples of the use of language to influence change processes. Published for business, yet applicable in every context.

- Derks L (2003) *Social Panoramas: changing the unconscious landscape with NLP and psychotherapy*. Crown House Publishing. Social psychologist Lucas Derks has used NLP to explore the structure of the way in which people think of other people. A very useful addition to family therapy practices.
- Dilts R (1990) *Changing Belief Systems With NLP*. Meta Publications. Covers several approaches to belief change, mainly using kinaesthetic timelines.
- Dilts R (1998) *Modelling with NLP*. Meta Publications. A description of the NLP modelling process and its application.
- Dilts R (1999) *Sleight of Mouth: the magic of conversational belief change*. Meta Publications. A cognitive and categorical approach to verbal reframing patterns, which is a mine of useful information.
- Dilts R, Hallbom T and Smith S (1990) *Beliefs: pathways to health and well-being*. Metamorphous Press. An in-depth look at various belief change mechanisms in health.
- Gordon D (1978) *Therapeutic Metaphors*. Meta Publications. Considers the generation and application of isomorphic metaphors for change.
- James T and Woodsmall W (1988) *Time-Line Therapy and the Basis of Personality*. Meta Publications. The authors' particular version of utilising visual timelines for change.
- McDermott I and O'Connor J (1996) *NLP and Health*. Thorsons. An excellent application of the basics of NLP applied to health and disease. Well worth reading.
- McDermott I and O'Connor J (1996) *Principles of NLP*. Thorsons. A good short introductory overview. Easy to read.
- McDermott I and Jago W (2001) *The NLP Coach*. Piatkus. Combines NLP with the field of coaching, providing many useful conversational approaches that are adaptable to everyday general practice.
- McDermott I and Jago W (2001) *Brief NLP Therapy*. Sage Publications. Key concepts and applications of NLP in numerous clinical situations. A good overview from a Rogerian perspective, plus two detailed dissected case histories.
- O'Connor J (2001) *NLP Workbook*. Thorsons. A practitioner-level training in workbook form, from one of the best NLP authors in the field. An excellent resource, well worth the investment.
- O'Connor J and Seymour J (1990/1994) *Introducing NLP*. Thorsons. A comprehensive introduction and clear overview.
- Walker L (2002) *Consulting with NLP: neuro-linguistic programming in the medical consultation*. Radcliffe Medical Press. The application of NLP formats to effective communication with patients in everyday general practice.

Books on Milton Erickson and allied approaches

- Battino R and South T (1999) *Ericksonian Approaches: a comprehensive manual.* Crown House Publishing. An in-depth guide to learning the fundamentals of Erickson's approach.
- Grinder J and Bandler R (1975 and 1977) *Patterns of Hypnotic Techniques of Milton Erickson, MD. Volumes 1 and 2.* Meta Publications. Describes how Erickson used language exquisitely to obtain therapeutic results.
- Haley J (1993) *Uncommon Therapy.* Norton. The various psychiatric techniques of Erickson applied across all ages and all problem areas
- Overdurf J and Silverthorn J (1994) *Training Trances.* Metamorphous Press. An integration of Ericksonian and classical strategies for change. A truly outstanding example of multi-level communication with individuals and groups.
- Rosen S (1982) *My Voice Will Go With You.* Norton. The teaching tales of Erickson. Many, many short stories about Erickson, his patients and his unique approach.
- Rossi E and Ryan M (1998) *Mind–Body Communication in Hypnosis.* Free Association Books. Milton Erickson's views on psychosomatic medicine and healing approaches.
- Yapko M (1992) *Hypnosis and the Treatment of Depressions.* Brunner/Mazel. An excellent introduction to the various cognitive and strategic aspects of treatment of depression in its various guises.
- Yapko M (2001) *Treating Depression with Hypnosis.* Brunner-Routledge. This is a follow-up and extension to Yapko's previous work, and it utilises cognitive–behavioural and strategic therapy approaches in conversational change.
- Zeig J (1980) *A Teaching Seminar with Milton Erickson.* Brunner/Mazel. Describes the man and his approach to therapy.

Other useful books

- Assagioli R (1965/1990) *Psychosynthesis.* Mandala. A manual of principles and techniques for psychological change and growth. In many ways a forerunner of NLP.
- Bridges W (1991) *Managing Transitions.* Nicholas Brealey Publishing. Discusses helping people to cope with organisational change. Includes many good adaptable individual strategies.
- Cialdini R (1993) *Influence: science and practice.* Harper Collins. A professor of social psychology, Cialdini expounds on the six fundamental rules of

influence. Backed up by an impressive array of research evidence, this is a best-seller!

- Csikszentmihalyi M (1997) *Living Well*. Weidenfeld and Nicolson. A discussion of the psychology of flow states in everyday life.
- De Shazer S (1994) *Words Were Originally Magic*. Norton. Solution-focused approach that incorporates the miracle question. Includes plenty of client transcripts.
- Farrelly F and Brandsma J (1974) *Provocative Therapy*. Meta Publications. Farrelly's approach to therapy and change is fun filled, humorous and paradoxical, yet it gets results. A good read.
- Gleick J (1987) *Chaos: making a new science*. Viking. A very readable introduction to complexity and chaos theory.
- Jackson P and McKergow M (2002) *The Solutions Focus*. Nicholas Brealey. Although it is ostensibly a business book, this has tremendous application for brief solution-focused therapy. Contains many helpful hints for medical practitioners.
- Kopp S (1972) *If You Meet The Buddha on the Road, Kill Him!* Science and Behaviour Books. An enjoyable read that cuts through the myths and legends of psychological treatment.
- Launer J (2002) *Narrative-Based Primary Care*. Radcliffe Medical Press. Describes the use of elements of family therapy and systems theory in daily medical practice. Has much in common with the NLP approach.
- Lawley J and Tomkins P (2000) *Metaphors in Mind*. The Developing Company Press. Describes the use of symbolic modelling to effect client transformation via 'clean language'. Interesting applications for medical practice.
- O'Connor J and McDermott I (1997) *The Art of Systems Thinking*. Thorsons. A practical introduction with everyday examples, including health applications.
- Pryor K (1999) *Don't Shoot The Dog!* (revised edition). Bantam Books. Describes the principles of operant conditioning in action, from training dogs to changing human behaviours. Provides many examples of positive reinforcement in an easy-to-read style. Immediately applicable.
- Rinpoche S (1992) *The Tibetan Book of Living and Dying*. Rider Books. Random House. A Buddhist text that is a mine of information for palliative care.
- Rossi E (1993) *The Psychobiology of Mind–Body Healing* (2e). Norton. Contains detailed explanations and evaluations of the bodily chemical changes that are caused by thinking processes.
- Rossi E (1996) *The Symptom Path to Enlightenment*. Gateway Publishing. The application of complexity and chaos theory to biological systems, with specific reference to psychological change mechanisms. Outstanding!
- Simonton C and Matthews Simonton S (1982) *Getting Well Again*. Bantam Books. Discusses medical professionals working with creative visualisation

in the field of oncology. One of the first intensive investigations of mental adjuncts to standard cancer therapies.
- Sinay S (1997) *Gestalt for Beginners*. Writers and Readers. The life and times of Fritz Perls, and the precepts of Gestalt therapy, upon which many aspects of NLP were built. All in cartoon form!
- Sweeney K and Griffiths F (2003) *Complexity and Health Care*. Radcliffe Medical Press. An introduction to complexity, chaos, self-organising systems and attractors in everyday medical practice.
- Watzlawick P (1978/1993) *The Language of Change*. Norton. A clear exposition of the elements of therapeutic communication.
- Watzlawick P (1983) *The Situation is Hopeless But Not Serious*. Norton. Describes how people make life miserable, and what they can do about it.
- Watzlawick P (1983) *Ultra-Solutions: how to fail most successfully*. Norton. 'The operation was successful but the patient died' sums up this book perfectly.
- Watzlawick P, Weakland J and Fisch R (1974) *Change: principles of problem formation and resolution*. Norton. One of the original Palo Alto group studying effective communication in therapy.
- Wilber K (2000) *Integral Psychology*. Shambhala. A fascinating integration of Western and Eastern psychology from its beginnings up to the present day.

Audiotapes

- James T. *The Master Practitioner Collection*. A set of 28 advanced training tapes, the next step up from Practitioner. Well edited and professionally produced by the originator of timeline therapy, a well-known US trainer.
- McDermott I. *Tools for Transformation*. A four-tape set, extracted from a Practitioner-level training course, that covers several useful skill-sets.
- McDermott I. *Freedom From the Past*. A two-tape set that contains demonstrations of the NLP phobia cure in trauma resolution.
- McDermott I and O'Connor J. *An Introduction to NLP*. A two-tape introduction that includes several easy yet powerful exercises.
- McDermott I and O'Connor J. *NLP Health and Well-Being*. A single tape that includes several health applications.
- Overdurf J and Silverthorn J. *NLP Practitioner Tape Series*. A set of 32 tapes of a live Practitioner-level training by two of the best American trainers in the field. Well edited, the material flows and is an outstanding resource in place of doing the training yourself. Contains plenty of material about using NLP for therapeutic change.

- Overdurf J and Silverthorn J. *NLP Master Practitioner Companion*. For use in preparing for their accelerated training, this includes sections on verbal reframing, metaprogrammes and values.
- Overdurf J and Silverthorn J. *Beyond Words*. A six-tape set from a live seminar, with plenty of demonstrations of the use of language patterns for change.

Internet resources

- www.itsnlp.com The website of Ian McDermott. Articles and training schedules for a variety of short and longer seminars.
- www.anlp.org The website of the Association of NLP (UK). Has a quarterly magazine, *Rapport*.
- www.nlpu.com Robert Dilts' website. Many excellent articles and extracts from the *Encyclopaedia of Systemic NLP*.
- www.anglo-american.co.uk The Anglo-American Book Company specialises in mail-order NLP books. An extensive catalogue.
- www.iash.org The International Association for the Study of Health. Linked to Dilts, Hallbom and Smith's Health Certification Trainings.
- www.nlp.org A large collection of articles and links to other sites. Includes reviews of training and books.
- www.nlpwhisperinginthewind.com Grinder and Bostic's website, with an excellent discussion forum on New Code NLP.
- www.steveandreas.com Many interesting articles from trainer, author and developer Steve Andreas.

Great states

Alive	Autonomous	Wide awake	Adaptable	Appreciated
Great beauty	Bright	Calm	Cheery	Compassionate
Committed	Challenging	Courageous	Creative	Curious
Determined	Decisive	Dignified	Dynamic	Delighted
Elegant	Excellence	Excited	Energetic	Enthusiastic
Focused	Free	Fulfilled	Friendly	Fascinated
Full of fun	Forgiveness	Flexible	Graceful	Grateful
Grandiose	Glamorous	Caring	Happy	Healthy
Honest	Harmony	Helping	Humour	Hopeful
Innovative	Inspired	Integrity	Interested	Keen
Playful	Joyful	Jovial	Justice	Learning easily
Loving	Luscious	Loyal	Laughing	Making a difference
Mastery	Optimistic	Organised	Ordered	Peaceful
Persevering	Passionate	Powerful	Revolutionary	Relaxed
Resourceful	Resilient	Safe	Secure	Stimulated
Service	Simplicity	Problem solving	Sharing	Successful
Truthful	Unique	Useful	Unstoppable	Vitality
Wisdom	Warmth	Zest	Centred	Grounded
Synergistic	Winner	Wonderful	Brilliant	Contented
Carefree	Confident	Cool	Collected	Fabulous

I have listed above a large but not exhaustive number of different positive states. You can choose the ones that attract you and vividly remember, with all of your senses, past memories with that particular feeling. Or you could just as easily imagine what it would be like if you had that state right now, and build it up, intensifying it so that it is strong and stable. Then, of course, you can attach it to any anchor of your choosing. Experiment, like a great chef, with mixing several of them together, and imagine what it would be like to experience that mixture in some future event. You can use the list to generate various options and alternatives for your patients. You can even photocopy it and give it to them so that they can practise for themselves. The choice is yours!

Submodality charts

You can use these submodality charts to explore the structure of any subjective experience. They are the brain's basic building blocks. You will find that changing them will change the coding of the experience itself *and* its meaning. Certain submodalities are drivers. Shifting them will cause others to shift, too, like a ripple effect. Sometimes one apparently small shift can cause major therapeutic change.

It is often useful to compare and contrast the submodality structure of different experiences. NLP calls this *contrastive analysis*. You can elicit the submodalities of the problem in its context and compare this with different contexts where the problem is absent. *Mapping across*, whereby the submodalities of the first experience are changed into those of the second, can have a profound effect. You can compare pairs such as boredom and curiosity, failure and success, grief and gratitude, problem and opportunity, doubt and belief, or confusion and certainty. Experience what happens when you change one into the other!

Submodality chart		
Visual	*Experience 1*	*Experience 2*
Black and white or colour		
Associated or dissociated		
Bright or dim		
Near or far		
Location in space		
Still-frame photograph or movie		
Bordered or panoramic (all around)		
Clear in focus, or fuzzy out of focus		
Life size, bigger or smaller		
Three- or two-dimensional		
Single or multiple images		

Auditory	Experience 1	Experience 2
Loud or soft		
Near or far		
Surround sound or point source		
Location in space		
High or low pitch		
Clear or muffled		
Normal speed, faster or slower		
Rhythmic or arrhythmic		
Moving or stationary		
Kinaesthetic	Experience 1	Experience 2
Location of feeling		
High or low intensity		
Hot or cold		
Continuous or discontinuous		
Still or moving		
Fast or slow		
Heavy or light		
Small or large area		
Direction of spin		

Have fun exploring the various submodality shifts. You can make any experience appear, sound and feel better than it was originally. Use these submodality shifts to make your outcomes more attractive, more motivating and more compelling.

The meta-model

Below is the complete meta-model, in detail, as it appears on standard NLP trainings. You will recall that *distortions* operate on *generalisations*, which in turn operate on *deletions* in a linguistic hierarchy. You will obtain far more impact and potential for change by challenging distortions first. However, you are *not* from the Spanish Inquisition! Remember to preface your questions with softeners (I'm wondering ... I'm curious ..., etc.) to gently extract the appropriate information.

The meta-model			
Distortions	*Example*	*Intervention*	*Effect*
Mind reading	*'You're angry with me'*	*'How do you know I'm angry?'*	Recovers the source of the information
Lost performative value judgements	*'It's difficult to get better from this'*	*'Who says?' 'According to whom?'*	Recovers the source of the belief
Cause and effect (X causes Y)	*'Not having a job makes me depressed'*	*'How does not having a job make you depressed?'*	Recovers the choice. Provides a basis for alternative choices
Complex equivalence (meaning)	*'Asthma means I have weak lungs'*	*'How does having asthma mean that your lungs are weak?'*	Further specifies how X = Y. Reframe by counter-example

Generalisations	Example	Intervention	Effect
Universal quantifier (all, every, never, etc.)	*'This illness will never get better'*	*'Never?'* *'What would happen if it did?'*	Elicits counter-examples
Modal operator of possibility (can, can't, will, won't)	*'I can't see myself getting over this'*	*'What stops you?'* *'What would happen if you did?'*	Recovers prior causes and future effects
Modal operator of necessity (must, have to, should)	*'I have to look after my elderly parents'*	*'What would happen if you didn't?'* *'Or ... ?'*	Recovers consequences

Deletions	Example	Intervention	Effect
Simple deletion	*'I feel uncomfortable'*	*'About what, specifically?'*	Recovers the detail
Comparative deletion (better, worse, less, etc.)	*'She's much better than me'*	*'Who is better?'* *'Better at what?'* *'Better in which way?'*	Recovers the specifics of the comparison
Unspecified verbs	*'He hurt me'*	*'How specifically did he hurt you?'*	Recovers the details of the act
Lack of referential index (fails to specify person)	*'People just don't like me'*	*'Who specifically doesn't like you?'*	Recovers the performer of the act
Nominalisation (process words turned into nouns)	*'Our relationship is not working out'*	*'How are you relating at present?'* *'How would you like to relate instead?'*	Turns the event back into a process, recovering deletions

One important use for challenging deletions is when you are helping someone to enter a resource state, or to recover more information about a pleasant experience. By going into detail in these circumstances you will help them to reaccess the state fully in the here and now, and you can then redirect this for future utilisation. However, getting all of the details about their recurring depression is only likely to make them feel worse!

Use meta-model challenges sparingly, lest you become a meta-monster!

Eye-accessing cues

It often seems that our eyes move randomly when we speak. Have you ever noticed, though, that if you ask someone a question and they have to 'go inside' to think about it, their eyes may move to a specific location – up, down, left or right? It seems that these types of eye movements help us to access our stored information and memories in a particular way. The originators of NLP noticed this and studied the connection between eye movements and representational system predicates. They asked themselves '*Do eyes move to a particular location when people are thinking in pictures, sounds, words and feelings?*' This gave birth to NLP *eye-accessing cues*.

Now what follows is not necessarily the 'truth', but merely a useful generalisation. Although it is not true for all people at all times, it can be a very helpful aid for determining *how* someone is thinking about a particular experience. When answering a question, when people look up they are usually visualising. *Up and to their left* is remembering a past image or memory. *Up and to their right* is constructing a picture, perhaps of a future possibility. *Straight ahead and defocused* is often visualising as if watching a video. *Across to their left* is remembering sounds from the past, and *across to their right* is constructing what something might sound like. *Down to their right* usually accesses feelings, and *down to their left* is internal dialogue. You can verify this for yourself by watching television interviews.

The eye patterns as seen in Figure A4.1 are the most common ones. Some left-handers and a few right-handers may have the cues reversed. This is simply normal for them. By seeing whether patients access down to their *right* when responding to questions about *feelings*, you can assume that the rest of the cues are as above. If they access down to their left instead, then the other cues are likely to be reversed as well.

So this looks rather complicated. What is its practical use? Well, first, eye-accessing cues give you a clue as to *how* someone may be thinking. If you ask a question to which the answer is '*I don't know*', accompanied by the patient looking up to their left, you can assume that they are making a picture of which they are not yet consciously aware. You can follow up with '*If you did know ...*

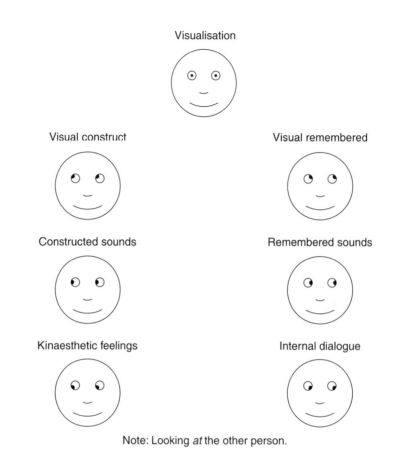

Figure A4.1:   Eye-accessing cues.

how would you picture that?' This subtly paces their ongoing experience and also deepens rapport.

Perhaps you have asked a question about what is making them feel so down, and they shake their head and look down to their left. You can follow up with *'Could it be something that you're saying to yourself?'*

Or perhaps, in response to a general question, they sigh and look down to their right. You could ask *'How do you feel about that?'* By pacing the patient's current experience in this way it can almost seem as if you are mind-reading. Most people will get the feeling that you really understand them at a deep level.

What I believe is even more important than the eye access itself is *where the eyes go to immediately after that.* Think of it in this way. The eye access is like finding the relevant file on a computer. It can be stored in a variety of areas in a variety of ways. However, once accessed it needs to be projected on screen to be read. In the same way, it is as if we project our memories, imaginations and experiences into the space around us.

As you now begin to notice more clearly where people look immediately after accessing, you will see what I mean. And what are the benefits of this? Well, by noticing where people store these things you can easily gesture to the area of projection and thus pace their ongoing experience when talking to them. It can also give you a handle on whether a problem is still a current issue or whether it has been resolved. The projected location will have changed!

Useful questions are the answer

Here is a list of questions that can prove useful at each stage of your intervention with patients. It is not an exhaustive list, and although I have laid out the questions under the headings of the *meta-pattern* format, you can – with a little modification – use them in several of the stages. They will give you ideas about the many varying ways in which you can elicit the information that you want.

Before you start an intervention, and at any stage throughout, there are certain questions that you can ask yourself, the answers to which can set you up to move in the most appropriate direction at that time. These set the frame for the ensuing encounter.

Frames

- What is the most useful question I can ask right now?
- What am I missing that is important?
- What is the most useful way to think about this?
- What am I assuming about this situation?
- What is the intention behind my question? What am I eliciting here?
- What is the unspoken question in the patient's body language?
- Am I in the right state for the job in hand?

Associate to problem

- What is it that you want to change?
- What do you want to work through today?
- Just exactly how do you 'do' that problem (X)? (elicits their strategy)
- What lets you know that it is time to ... (X) ...? (backs up to the beginning of the strategy)

- Where/when do you ... (X) ... .?
- How do you know that is a problem? (elicits reality strategy)
- What do you think keeps this behaviour going?
- What do you want to accomplish by engaging in this behaviour?
- When you are in the context, what do you see/hear just before you ... (X) ...?
- Where in your body do you feel that feeling?
- What are you saying to yourself as you feel that?
- What has stopped you from changing up until now?

Dissociate from problem

Asking any of the well-formed outcome questions will start this phase off.

- How do you want to be different?
- Where/when do you not have the problem ... (X) ...? (elicits counter-example)
- Tell me about times in your life when this is not an issue ...
- Can you teach me how to do that problem step by step? What would I have to picture in my mind's eye? What would I have to say to myself on the inside? (dissociates them as they teach you!)
- If you looked back on this from 100 years in the future, what would you think?
- If you were a fly on the wall watching *that you* ... what would you notice? (elicits third position)
- How would your best friend see the situation? (elicits second position)
- If your friend had this problem, what advice would you give to him or her?
- If, as a result of meeting here today, this were solved to your satisfaction, what would have changed?
- What are the benefits that the problem brings you? (chunks up to positive intention)
- What would change in your life if you got what you wanted?
- Who else might be affected or benefit?
- What is this person really teaching you? (for a relationship difficulty)

Access resources

- What would help to set you up differently next time?
- What would let you know that you are succeeding next time? How are you different then?

- How would you incorporate what you have learned so far?
- What are your attributes and strengths? What do people compliment you on?
- What things do you really enjoy doing ... (Y) ...? (you can find many resources here)
- What is it like when you are ... (Y) ...? (conversationally elicits resource state)
- When you are (Y) ... how do you know you are ... (Y) ...? (elicits reality strategy)
- If you were ... (Y) ... right now, how would I know just by looking at you?
- If you were ... (Y) ... right now, what would you be saying to yourself?
- Who do you know who can handle this easily? If you were to imagine actually being them, doing it that way ... how does that feel?
- Remember a time when you were ... (Y) ... As you *go be there now* ... what are you feeling/saying to yourself/picturing in your mind's eye?

Associate resources to problem state/future pace

- What is the first step you can take to change this situation in the way *you really want to ... don't you?*
- As you look at it through this perspective ... (Y) ... how have things changed?
- As you are feeling this resource (Y), try to feel that problem (X) you had ... do you notice what is different now ... ? (conversationally collapses anchors)
- So how do you really know it is different now? (elicits reality strategy of solution)
- How does it feel looking back on what used to be a problem ... ?
- As you look ahead, what else does this allow you to do ... ?
- What other things have you not yet noticed that are different as a result of this change? (presupposes other changes)
- What is the first thing your family/friends are going to notice as a result of today ... ?
- Will it be the second or third time you have done this automatically that lets you know consciously that things really are different?
- If it were six months from now and this change had seeded into every area of your life ... what is that like? And, looking back on today, how do you know that?

What to use when

Many people, when exposed to the various NLP techniques for the first time, may wonder just which one to use with this particular patient today. They ask 'How do you know which approach to use with whom?' There are no right answers to this question, although some techniques are better suited to some individuals than others. Of course, if you have used them all in practice on yourself then you will have a better, more intuitive idea of which one fits best. As usual, starting off in one direction and modifying what you do based on the feedback you receive is paramount.

NLP trainers Richard Bolstad and Margot Hamblett developed a useful model based on the Myers–Briggs inventory. Here we shall simplify it and use the concepts of *association, dissociation, general* and *specific* to form a continuum generating four quadrants. Patients generally come with the ability to do some things better than others – this may be why they have developed specific problems. Those who are good associaters will easily get into resource states via the various anchoring formats. However, they may find it difficult to dissociate, which is a key skill in the phobia cure. Good dissociaters, on the other hand, may find it easy to use visual timeline techniques, yet find it difficult to associate into experiences in the here and now.

The chunk size of attention – big picture or details – is instrumental in combining with association and dissociation in certain clinical conditions. Depression and mania both involve chunking up associated feelings (negative and positive, respectively), whereas psychosis can be thought of as chunking up and dissociating. Allergies are associations to a specific allergen (chunking down), whereas grief is dissociating from positive memories of a specific deceased person. Anxiety disorders generally involve associating to negative feelings while thinking about specific things that could go wrong. These definitions may appear a little simplistic, yet they can be very useful in deciding your first steps with patients.

General ·

Walking timelines Timeline parts integration Six-step reframing Meta-mirror Metaphors	Visual timelines Visual squash Dissociative hypnosis
Building resources Collapsing anchors Chaining anchors Counter-example process	Submodality patterns Swish Phobia cure Outcome setting Grief resolution

Associated   *Dissociated*

Specific

One way to approach this is to start off by using the techniques from the quadrants that seem to fit with the structure of the patient's presenting condition. In the case of anxiety or phobia sufferers, you may first want to associate them to specific positive states instead. Often you may need to teach them a skill from the opposite quadrant, such as how to dissociate effectively via the phobia cure. Those who are depressed need to associate into good feelings first. Then they can learn to chunk down on and dissociate from negative experiences. The structure of grief is to dissociate from past good memories of the deceased – the cure is to reassociate with those feelings. Addiction is an intense association to the drug or habit, with dissociation from past resources and future consequences, often as a sequential incongruity. Chunking up with a parts integration process is a very useful strategy.

Of course, none of the above clinical conditions or techniques fits exclusively into one quadrant only. They each have elements of association and dissociation – the meta-mirror, for example. However, if you can help your patients – and yourself – to develop the skills that lie within each quadrant, then you will have a formidable array of potential interventions for all kinds of problem issues.

Index